Whittle's
GAIT ANALYSIS

SIXTH EDITION

Whittle's
GAIT ANALYSIS

Edited by

Jim Richards, BEng, MSc, PhD
Faculty Director of Research and Innovation
Research Lead for the Allied Health Research Unit
Faculty of Allied Health and Well-being
University of Central Lancashire
Preston, UK

David Levine, PT, PhD, DPT, CCRP, FAPTA
Board-Certified Clinical Specialist in Orthopaedic Physical Therapy Emeritus
Professor and Walter M. Cline Chair of Excellence in Physical Therapy
Department of Physical Therapy
The University of Tennessee at Chattanooga
Chattanooga, Tennessee, USA

Michael W. Whittle, BSc, MSc, MB, BS, PhD
Formerly Walter M. Cline Jr Chair of Rehabilitation Technology
The University of Tennessee at Chattanooga
Chattanooga, Tennessee, USA
Director, H. Carey
Hanlin Motion Analysis Laboratory
The University of Tennessee at Chattanooga
Chattanooga, Tennessee, USA
Formerly Acting Director
Oxford Orthopaedic Engineering Centre
University of Oxford
Oxford, UK

ELSEVIER

Notices

Practitioners and researchers must always rely on their own experience and knowledge in evaluating and using any information, methods, compounds or experiments described herein. Because of rapid advances in the medical sciences, in particular, independent verification of diagnoses and drug dosages should be made. To the fullest extent of the law, no responsibility is assumed by Elsevier, authors, editors or contributors for any injury and/or damage to persons or property as a matter of products liability, negligence or otherwise, or from any use or operation of any methods, products, instructions, or ideas contained in the material herein.

ISBN: 978-0-7020-8497-3
Printed in Scotland
Last digit is the print number: 9 8 7 6 5 4 3 2 1

Content Strategist: Trinity Hutton
Content Project Manager: Arindam Banerjee
Design: Bridget Hoette
Marketing Manager: Belinda Tudin
Art Buyer: Narayanan Ramakrishnan

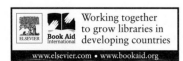

CONTENTS

The additional online resources can be found on our Evolve learning system.

For access please go to http://evolve.elsevier.com/Whittle/gait and follow the onscreen prompts. Contents include:
- Video clips
- Image collection from the book
- MCQs
- Appendix 1 – Conversions between measurement units
- Appendix 2 – Contributors to Whittle's Gait Analysis, Sixth Edition
- Glossary

PREFACE TO THE SIXTH EDITION

Gait analysis is the systematic study of human walking, using the eye and brain of experienced observers, augmented by instrumentation for measuring body movements, body mechanics and muscle activity. In individuals with conditions affecting their ability to walk, gait analysis may be used to make detailed assessments and plan optimal treatment.

The first five editions of this book have made a significant contribution to the use of gait analysis worldwide, supported by the fact that the current editors and contributors were all influenced by Professor Michael Whittle's earlier editions. We hope this latest edition, as with the previous editions, provides a text which does not require a high level of academic learning to be understood, yet gives a good grounding in the science and application of gait analysis. In this edition we have added the contributions of more subject matter and clinical experts in their respective areas of gait analysis.

Over the past decade, gait analysis has 'come of age' and many clinicians now use it routinely to provide the best possible care for many groups of patients. This is most notable in the management of cerebral palsy; however, gait analysis is also now being used more widely in the management of other neurological and musculoskeletal conditions. This textbook has been updated accordingly throughout, but particularly in Chapter 4, Methods of Gait Analysis; Chapter 5, Applications of Gait Analysis; Chapter 6, Gait Assessment in Neurological Disorders; and Chapter 7, Gait Analysis in Musculoskeletal Conditions, Prosthetics

and Orthotics. It also now contains a chapter focusing on two growing areas: gait analysis in running, and injury management (Chapter 8, Gait Analysis in Running and the Management of Common Injuries). Since the advantages of this approach have been well established, it is to be hoped that its usage will continue to spread so that many more will benefit from the treatment decisions which can be made when gait analysis is used.

Continual improvements in the ease and speed with which gait data can be collected and interpreted, coupled with decreases in the cost of the equipment and the skill level needed to use it, have led to significant strides in gait analysis since the fifth edition of this book. This edition aims to show the current uses of gait analysis and provide guidance on how it can be applied to wider groups of patients and in injury management. We have also included examples of new and evolving methods of analysis which may, in the future, further improve our understanding of the complexities of human movement. This book is targeted at physicians, physiotherapists, prosthetists, orthotists, podiatrists, sports rehabilitation specialists and anyone interested in human gait analysis.

We have also included examples of real gait data from a variety of clinical case studies which we hope will provide the reader with a greater opportunity to get a feel for this fascinating subject and its clinical impact. We are honoured to have been appointed editors of this textbook again.

Jim Richards and David Levine, 2022

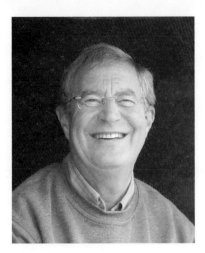

Michael Whittle was the sole author and editor of the first four editions of this textbook. Although a medical doctor, Mike was destined to become a research scientist with degrees in biomechanics and a PhD in human biology and health from the University of Surrey. As an exchange medical officer in the Royal Air Force, he was loaned to NASA to supervise six of the medical experiments on the Skylab space program in the 1970s. He later joined the faculty of the University of Oxford, and carried out pioneering work on the scientific measurement of gait analysis. Mike moved to the University of Tennessee at Chattanooga in 1989 and was a professor in the Department of Physical Therapy, and also in the Department of Orthopaedic Surgery of the University of Tennessee College of Medicine. He continued his research on gait analysis and established the H. Carey Hanlin Motion Analysis Laboratory (now called the UTC Motion Analysis Laboratory), which was one of the first motion analysis laboratories of its kind. Having had the privilege of working with Mike on a daily basis for 15 years (DL), I know him to be an exceptional researcher, teacher and scientist whose greatest asset is an inquisitive mind with a delightful personality to match. Now retired to the South of England, he enjoys travelling, sailing, hiking and spending time with his wife, Wendy, their children and their grandchildren. In his honour we have continued to title this book Whittle's Gait Analysis.

Richard Baker, PhD, CEng, CSci
Professor of Clinical Gait Analysis
University of Salford
Salford, UK

Cleveland Barnett, PhD, BSc (Hons)
Associate Professor of Biomechanics
School of Science and Technology
Nottingham Trent University
Nottingham, UK

Gabor Barton, MD, PhD, FHEA
Professor of Clinical Biomechanics
Research Institute for Sport and Exercise Sciences
Liverpool John Moores University
Liverpool, UK

Nancy Fell, PT, PhD
Board Certified Clinical Specialist in Neurologic Physical
    Therapy Emeritus
UC Foundation and Guerry Professor
Department Head, Physical Therapy
University of Tennessee at Chattanooga
Chattanooga, Tennessee, USA

June Hanks, PT, PhD, DPT, CLT
Associate Professor and Director of Anatomy Lab
Department of Physical Therapy
University of Tennessee at Chattanooga
Chattanooga, Tennessee, USA

Kim Hébert-Losier, PT, PhD
Senior Lecturer
Lead Biomechanics Researcher Adams Centre
    for High Performance
Division of Health, Engineering, Computing and Science
Te Huataki Waiora School of Health
University of Waikato
New Zealand

Max Jordon, PT, DPT, PhD
Assistant Professor
Department of Physical Therapy
University of Tennessee at Chattanooga
Chattanooga, Tennessee, USA

David Levine, PT, PhD, DPT, CCRP, FAPTA
Board-Certified Clinical Specialist in Orthopaedic
    Physical Therapy Emeritus
Professor and Walter M. Cline Chair of Excellence
    in Physical Therapy
Department of Physical Therapy
The University of Tennessee at Chattanooga
Chattanooga, Tennessee, USA

Derek Liuzzo, PT, DPT, PhD
Assistant Professor of Physical Therapy
Department of Physical Therapy
University of Tennessee at Chattanooga
Chattanooga, Tennessee, USA

Jim Richards, BEng, MSc, PhD
Faculty Director of Research and Innovation
Research Lead for the Allied Health Research Unit
Faculty of Allied Health and Well-being
University of Central Lancashire
Preston, UK

Ashley Schilling, PT, DPT
Board Certified Clinical Specialist in Pediatric Physical
    Therapy
Sharon Vanderbilt Professor of Physical Therapy
Department of Physical Therapy
University of Tennessee Chattanooga
Chattanooga, Tennessee, USA

Hannah Shepherd, PhD, MSc, BSc
Associate Lecturer in Clinical Biomechanics
School of Sport and Exercise Sciences
Liverpool John Moores University
Liverpool, UK

Komsak Sinsurin, PT, PhD, DPT
Assistant Professor
Biomechanics and Sports Research Unit
Faculty of Physical Therapy
Mahidol University
Thailand

Cathie Smith, PhD, DPT, PCS
ABPTS Board Certified in Pediatric Physical Therapy
Professor Emeritus and Adjunct Faculty
Department of Physical Therapy
University of Tennessee at Chattanooga
Chattanooga, Tennessee, USA

Frank Tudini, PT, DSc, OCS, FAAOMPT
Associate Professor
Board Certified Specialist in Orthopedic Physical Therapy
Department of Physical Therapy
University of Tennessee at Chattanooga
Chattanooga, Tennessee, USA

Natalie Vanicek, PhD, SFHEA
Professor of Clinical Biomechanics
Department of Sport, Health and Exercise Science
University of Hull
Hull, UK

Basic Sciences

Michael Whittle, David Levine and Jim Richards

INTRODUCTION

All voluntary movement, including walking, results from a complicated process involving the brain, spinal cord, peripheral nerves, muscles, bones and joints. Before considering in detail the process of walking, what can go wrong with it and how it can be studied, it is necessary to have a basic understanding of associated scientific disciplines including anatomy and biomechanics. This chapter will provide the rudiments of these subjects for those who are not already familiar with them, and will review the topic for those who are. Additional information included in the preceding edition of this book is available online at http://evolve.elsevier.com/Whittle/gait.

Anatomy

It is not the intention of this chapter to cover the anatomy of the locomotor system in detail. Rather, the chapter is intended to provide an outline of the subject which is sufficient for understanding the subsequent chapters in this book. This section starts by describing some basic anatomical terms including details on bones, joints, muscles and tendons.

Basic Anatomical Terms

The anatomical terms describing the relationships between different parts of the body are based on the *anatomical position* when a person is standing upright, with the feet together and the arms by the sides of the body, with the palms facing forward. This position, together with the reference planes and the terms describing the relationships between different parts of the body, is illustrated in Fig. 1.1.

Six terms are used to describe directions in relation to the centre of the body. These are best defined by example:
- The umbilicus is *anterior*.
- The buttocks are *posterior*.
- The head is *superior*.
- The feet are *inferior*.
- *Left* is self-evident.
- So is *right*.

The anterior surface of the body is referred to as *ventral* and the posterior surface as *dorsal*, although the word *dorsum* is also used for both the back of the hand and the upper surface of the foot. The terms *cephal* (towards the head) and *caudal* (towards the 'tail') are sometimes used in place of superior and inferior.

Within a single part of the body, six additional terms are used to describe relationships:
- *Medial* means towards the midline of the body: the big toe is on the medial side of the foot.
- *Lateral* means away from the midline of the body: the little toe is on the lateral side of the foot.
- *Proximal* means towards the rest of the body: the shoulder is the proximal part of the arm.
- *Distal* means away from the rest of the body: the fingers are the distal part of the arm.
- *Superficial* structures are close to the surface: the skin is superficial to the bones.
- *Deep* structures are far from the surface: the heart is deep to the sternum.

The motion of the limbs is described using three reference planes:

- The *sagittal* plane divides the body into right and left portions. The *median* plane is the midline sagittal plane, which divides the whole body into right and left halves.

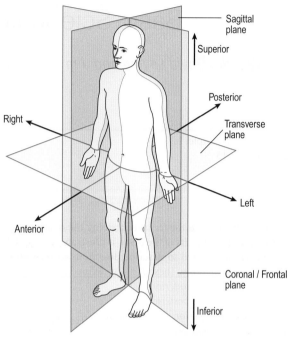

Fig. 1.1 The anatomical position, with the three reference planes and six fundamental directions.

- The *coronal* (or frontal) plane divides a body part into front and back portions.
- The *transverse* (or horizontal) plane divides a body part into upper and lower portions.

The term *coronal plane* is equivalent to frontal plane, and the transverse plane may also be called the *horizontal plane*. Most joints have their largest amount of movement in the sagittal plane, although the coronal and transverse planes can be very important clinically. The directions of these motions for the hip and knee shown in Fig. 1.2, and for the ankle and foot in Fig. 1.3.

The possible movements are:

- *Flexion* and *extension*, which take place in the sagittal plane. In the ankle these movements are called *dorsiflexion* and *plantarflexion*, where the foot (distal segment) moves up or down relative to the tibia (proximal segment), respectively.
- *Abduction* and *adduction*, which take place in the frontal/coronal plane, where the distal segment moves away or towards the midline of the body relative to the proximal segment, respectively.
- *Internal* and *external* rotation, which take place in the transverse plane. These movements, also called *medial* and *lateral* rotation, respectively, refer to the motion of the anterior surface of the distal segment relative to the proximal segment.

Other terms which are used to describe the motions of the joints or body segments are:

- *Varus* (adducted) and *valgus* (abducted), which describe an angulation of a joint towards or away from the midline, respectively, when viewed in the coronal plane.

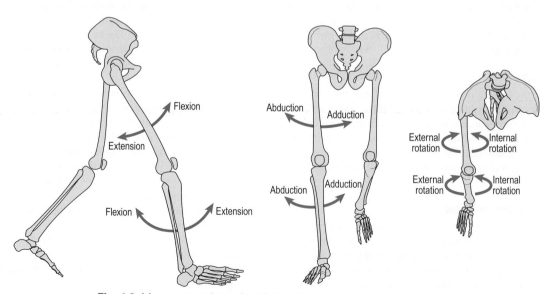

Fig. 1.2 Movements about the hip joint (above) and knee joint (below).

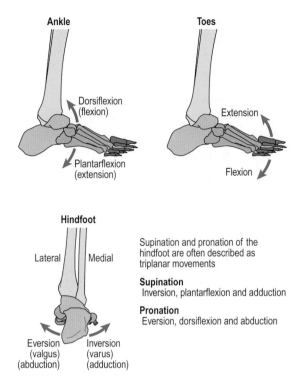

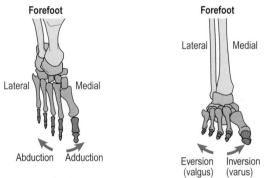

Supination and pronation of the hindfoot are often described as triplanar movements

Supination
Inversion, plantarflexion and adduction

Pronation
Eversion, dorsiflexion and abduction

Fig. 1.3 Movements of the ankle, toes, hindfoot and forefoot.

Therefore, knock knees are in valgus and bowlegs are in varus.

- *Pronation* and *supination*, which are internal and external rotations of the hand about the long axis of the forearm. Pronation of both hands brings the thumbs together; supination brings the little fingers together. Internal and external rotation of the foot about the long axis of the tibia has also been used to describe pronation and supination of the foot and ankle complex.
- *Inversion* (adduction) of the feet brings the soles together; *eversion* (abduction) causes the soles to point

away from the midline when viewed in the coronal plane.

Terminology in the foot is often confusing and lacking in standardisation. This book has adopted what is probably the commonest convention (Fig. 1.3), in which the term *pronation* is used for a combined movement which consists primarily of eversion but also includes some dorsiflexion and forefoot abduction. Similarly, *supination* is primarily inversion, but also includes some plantarflexion and forefoot adduction. These movements represent a 'twisting' of the forefoot (distal segment), relative to the hindfoot (proximal segment). However, some authorities regard pronation and supination as the basic movements and eversion and inversion as the combined movements. Increasingly, the foot is being modelled in multiple segments, most commonly into three or four segments although more have been used. This requires further referencing of the relative movement of the different segments, which will be dealt with later in this book.

Bones

It could be argued that almost every bone in the body is involved during walking. However, from a practical point of view, it is generally only necessary to consider the bones of the pelvis and legs. These are shown in Fig. 1.4.

The *pelvis* is composed of the sacrum, the coccyx and the two innominate bones. The *sacrum* consists of the five sacral vertebrae, fused together. The *coccyx* is the vestigial 'tail', made of three to five rudimentary vertebrae. The innominate bone on each side of the pelvis is formed by the fusion of three bones: the *ilium*, *ischium* and *pubis*. The only real movement between the bones of the pelvis occurs at the sacroiliac joint and this movement is generally very small in adults. It is thus reasonable, for the purposes of gait analysis, to regard the pelvis as being a single segment. The superior surface of the sacrum articulates with the fifth lumbar vertebra of the spine. On each side of the lower part of the pelvis is the acetabulum, which is the proximal part of the hip joint and the socket into which the head of the femur fits.

The *femur* is the longest bone in the body. The spherical femoral head articulates with the pelvic acetabulum to form the hip joint. The neck of the femur runs downwards and laterally from the femoral head to meet the shaft, which continues downwards to the knee joint. At the junction of the neck and the shaft are two bony protuberances; the greater trochanter on the lateral side, where a number of muscles are inserted which can be felt beneath the skin; and the lesser trochanter on the medial side. The bone widens at its lower end to form the medial and lateral condyles. These form the proximal part of the knee

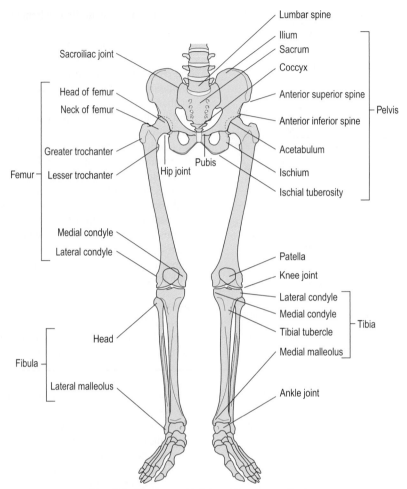

Fig. 1.4 Bones and joints of the lower limbs.

joint and have a groove between them anteriorly, which articulates with the patella.

The *patella* or kneecap is a sesamoid bone; that is to say, it is embedded within a tendon, in this case the massive quadriceps tendon, which below the patella is known as the patellar tendon. The anterior surface of the patella is subcutaneous (immediately below the skin); its posterior surface articulates with the anterior surface of the lower end of the femur to form the patellofemoral joint. The patella has an important mechanical function, which is to displace the quadriceps tendon forwards, thereby improving its leverage.

The *tibia* extends from the knee joint to the ankle joint. Its upper end is broadened into medial and lateral condyles, with an almost flat upper surface which articulates with the femur. The tibial tubercle is a small bony prominence on

the front of the tibia, where the patellar tendon is inserted. The anterior surface of the tibia is subcutaneous. The lower end of the tibia forms the upper and medial surfaces of the ankle joint, with a subcutaneous medial projection called the medial malleolus.

The *fibula* is next to the tibia on its lateral side. For most of its length it is a fairly slim bone, although it is broadened at both ends, the upper end being known as the head. The broadened lower end forms the lateral part of the ankle joint, with a subcutaneous lateral projection known as the lateral malleolus. The tibia and fibula are in contact with each other at their upper and lower ends, referred to as the tibiofibular joints. Movements at these joints are very small and will not be considered further. A layer of fibrous tissue, known as the interosseous membrane, lies between the bones.

The foot is a very complicated structure (Fig. 1.5), which is best thought of as having four parts:
- The *hindfoot or rearfoot*, which consists of two bones, one on top of the other
- The *midfoot*, which consists of five bones, packed closely together
- The *forefoot*, which consists of the five metatarsals
- The *toes*, which consist of the five sets of phalangeal bones

The *talus* or *astragalus* is the upper of the two bones in the hindfoot. Its superior surface forms the ankle joint, articulating above and medially with the tibia and laterally with the fibula. Below, the talus articulates with the calcaneus through the subtalar joint. It articulates anteriorly with the navicular which is the most medial and superior of the midfoot bones.

The *calcaneus* lies below the talus and articulates at the subtalar joint. Its lower surface transmits the body weight to the ground through a thick layer of fat, fibrous tissue and skin referred to as the heel pad. The anterior surface articulates with the cuboid, which is the most lateral and inferior of the midfoot bones.

The midfoot consists of five bones:
- The *navicular*, which is medial and superior
- The *cuboid*, which is lateral and inferior
- Three *cuneiform* bones (medial, intermediate and lateral), which lie in a row, distal to the navicular

The five *metatarsals* lie roughly parallel to each other, the lateral two articulating with the cuboid and the medial three articulating with the three cuneiform bones. The *phalanges* are the bones of the toes; there are two in the big toe and three in each of the other toes. The big toe is also referred to as the hallux.

Joints and Ligaments

A joint is the region where two bones come in contact with each other. From a practical point of view, they can be divided into synovial joints, in which significant movement can take place, and various other types of joint in which only small movements can occur. Since gait analysis is usually only concerned with fairly large movements, the description which follows deals only with synovial joints. In a *synovial joint*, the bone ends are covered in *cartilage* and the joint is surrounded by a *synovial capsule*, which secretes the lubricant *synovial fluid*. Most joints are stabilised by *ligaments*, which are bands of relatively inelastic fibrous tissue connecting one bone to another. The *fascia* is another type of connective tissue which is found throughout the human body, and can provide a functional role around joints, one example of this is the plantar fascia in the foot which provides dynamic support within the medial longitudinal arch during gait.

The *hip* joint is the only true ball-and-socket joint in the body, the ball being the head of the femur and the socket the acetabulum of the pelvis. Extremes of movement are prevented by a (1) number of ligaments running between the pelvis and the femur, (2) a capsule surrounding the joint and (3) the ligamentum teres, a small ligament which joins the centre of the head of the femur to the centre of the acetabulum. The joint is capable of flexion, extension, abduction adduction and internal and external rotation (Fig. 1.2).

The *knee* joint consists of the medial and lateral condyles of the femur, and the corresponding condyles of the tibia. The articular surfaces on the medial and lateral sides are separate, making the knee joint, in effect, two joints, side by side. The femoral condyles are curved both from front to back and from side to side, whereas the tibial condyles are almost flat. The 'gap' this would leave around the point of contact is filled on each side by the meniscus, which acts to spread the load and reduce the pressure at the points of contact. The motion of the joint is controlled by five structures which, between them, control the movements of the knee:

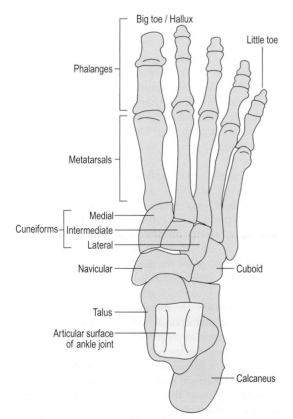

Fig. 1.5 Bones of the right foot, seen from above.

- The medial collateral ligament (MCL), which prevents the medial side of the joint from opening (i.e., it opposes abduction or valgus).
- The lateral collateral ligament (LCL), which similarly opposes adduction or varus.
- The posterior joint capsule, which prevents hyperextension (excessive extension) of the joint.
- The anterior cruciate ligament (ACL), which is located between the condyles in the centre of the joint and is attached to the tibia anteriorly and to the femur posteriorly. The ACL prevents the tibia from moving forwards relative to the femur, and helps prevent hyperextension of the knee and excessive internal rotation of the tibia.
- The posterior cruciate ligament (PCL), which is also in the centre of the joint and is attached to the tibia posteriorly and the femur anteriorly. The PCL prevents the tibia from moving backwards relative to the femur and helps limit external rotation of the tibia.

The anterior and posterior cruciate ligaments are named for the positions in which they are attached to the tibia. They appear to act together as what engineers call a 'four-bar linkage', which imposes a combination of sliding and rolling on the joint, moving the contact point forwards as the joint extends and backwards as it flexes. This means that the axis about which the joint flexes and extends is not fixed, but changes with the angle of flexion or extension. Pollo et al. (2003) challenged this description, saying that it only occurs in the unloaded knee and that during walking, the tibia moves backwards relative to the femur as the knee flexes.

The normal movements of the knee are flexion and extension, with a small amount of internal and external rotation. Significant amounts of abduction and adduction are only seen in damaged knees. As the knee comes to full extension, there is an external rotation of a few degrees which is sometimes referred to as the 'screw-home' mechanism.

The *patellofemoral* joint lies between the posterior surface of the patella and the anterior surface of the femur. The articular surface consists of a shallow V-shaped ridge on the patella, which fits into a shallow groove between the medial and lateral condyles. The principal movement is the patella gliding up and down in this groove during knee flexion and extension, respectively. This causes different areas of the patella to come into contact with different parts of the joint surfaces of the femur. There is also some medial-lateral movement of the patella.

The *ankle* or talocrural joint has three surfaces: upper, medial and lateral. The upper surface is the main articulation of the joint, which is cylindrical and formed by the tibia above and the talus below. The medial joint surface is between the talus and the inner aspect of the medial malleolus of the tibia. Correspondingly, the lateral joint surface is between the talus and the inner surface of the lateral malleolus of the fibula. The major ligaments of the ankle joint are those between the tibia and the fibula, preventing these two bones from moving apart; and the collateral ligaments on both sides, between the two malleoli and both the talus and calcaneus, which keep the joint stable. The ankle joint only has significant motion in the sagittal plane; this motion is referred to as dorsiflexion and plantarflexion.

The *subtalar* or talocalcaneal joint lies between the talus above and the calcaneus below. It has three articular surfaces: two anterior and medial and one posterior and lateral. Large numbers of ligaments join the two bones to each other and to all the adjacent bones. The axis of the joint is oblique, running primarily forwards but also upwards and medially. From a functional point of view, the importance of the subtalar joint is that it permits eversion/inversion (abduction and adduction or a valgus/varus motion) of the hindfoot. When performing gait analysis, it is usually impossible to distinguish between movement at the ankle joint and movement at the subtalar joint, and therefore it is reasonable to refer to such motion as taking place at the 'ankle/subtalar complex'. This motion in individuals with a normal gait includes dorsiflexion/plantarflexion, hindfoot abduction/adduction and internal/external rotation about the long axis of the tibia.

The *midtarsal* joints lie between each tarsal bone and its immediate neighbours, making for a very complicated structure. The movement of most of these joints is very small, as there are ligaments crossing the joints and the joint surfaces are not shaped for large movements. As a result, the midtarsal joints may be considered together to provide a flexible linkage between the hindfoot and the forefoot, which permits a small amount of movement in all planes.

The *tarsometatarsal* joints, between the cuboid and the cuneiforms proximally and the five metatarsals distally, are capable of only small gliding movements because of the relatively flat joint surfaces and the ligaments binding the metatarsals to each other and to the tarsal bones. There are also joint surfaces between adjacent metatarsals, except for the medial one.

The *metatarsophalangeal* and *interphalangeal* joints consist of a convex proximal surface fitting into a shallow concave distal surface. The metatarsophalangeal joints permit abduction and adduction as well as flexion and extension; the interphalangeal joints are restricted by their ligaments to flexion and extension, the range of flexion being greater than that of extension. In walking, the most important movement in this region is extension at the metatarsophalangeal joints.

No description of the anatomy of the foot is complete without a mention of the arches. The bones of the foot are bound together by ligamentous structures, reinforced by muscle tendons, to make a flexible structure which acts like two strong curved springs positioned side by side. These are the longitudinal arches of the foot, and they allow the body weight to be transmitted to the ground primarily through the calcaneus posteriorly and the metatarsal heads anteriorly. The midfoot transmits relatively little weight directly to the ground as it is lifted up on the medial side. The posterior end of both arches is the calcaneus. The *medial arch* (Fig. 1.6) goes upwards through the talus and then forwards and gradually down again through the navicular and cuneiforms to the medial three metatarsals, which form the distal end of the arch. The *lateral arch* (Fig. 1.7) passes forwards from the calcaneus through the cuboid to the two lateral metatarsals.

Muscles and Tendons

Muscles are responsible for movement at the joints. Most muscles are attached to different bones at their two ends and cross over either one joint (*monarticular* muscles), two joints (*biarticular* muscles) or several joints (*polyarticular* muscles). In many cases, the attachment to one of the

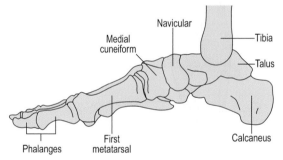

Fig. 1.6 Medial side of the right foot. The medial arch consists of the calcaneus, talus, navicular, cuneiforms and medial three metatarsals.

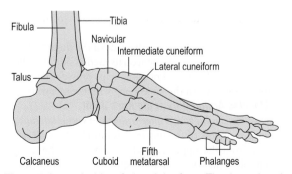

Fig. 1.7 Lateral side of the right foot. The lateral arch consists of the calcaneus, cuboid and lateral two metatarsals.

bones covers a broad area, whereas at the other end it narrows into a *tendon*, which is attached to the other bone. Ligaments and tendons are frequently confused; as a general rule, ligaments connect two bones together, whereas tendons connect muscles to bones. The following is a brief account of the muscles of the pelvis and lower limb, including their major actions. Most muscles also have secondary actions, which may vary according to the position of the joints, particularly with biarticular muscles. The larger and more superficial muscles are illustrated in Fig. 1.8.

Muscles Acting Only at the Hip Joint

- *Psoas major* originates from the anterolateral aspect of the lumbar vertebrae. *Iliacus* originates on the iliac fossa of the pelvis. The two tendons combine to form the *iliopsoas*, inserted at the lesser trochanter of the femur. The main action of these two muscles is to flex the hip.
- *Gluteus maximus* originates from the back of the pelvis and is inserted into the back of the shaft of the femur near its top. It serves to extend the hip.
- *Gluteus medius* and *gluteus minimus* originate from the side of the pelvis and are inserted into the greater trochanter of the femur. They primarily abduct the hip.
- *Adductor magnus*, *adductor brevis* and *adductor longus* originate from the ischium and pubis of the pelvis. They insert in a line down the medial side of the femur and adduct the hip.
- *Quadratus femoris*, *piriformis*, *obturator internus*, *obturator externus*, *gemellus superior* and *gemellus inferior* originate in the pelvis and insert close to the top of the femur. They all externally rotate the femur, although most also have secondary actions.
- *Pectineus* originates at the pubis of the pelvis running laterally and inserts on the front of the femur, near the lesser trochanter and flexes and adducts the hip.

Internal rotation of the femur was not mentioned in the preceding list, as this is achieved as a secondary action by the gluteus medius, gluteus minimus, psoas major, iliacus, pectineus and tensor fascia lata (described in the following lists).

Muscles Acting Across the Hip and Knee Joints

- *Rectus femoris* originates from around the anterior inferior iliac spine of the pelvis and inserts into the *quadriceps* tendon. It flexes the hip, and is part of the quadriceps, a group of four muscles which extend the knee.
- *Tensor fascia lata* originates from the pelvis close to the anterior superior iliac spine and inserts into the iliotibial tract, a broad band of fibrous tissue which runs down the outside of the thigh and attaches to the head of the fibula and abducts the hip and the knee.
- *Sartorius* is a strap-like muscle originating at the anterior superior iliac spine of the pelvis, winding around the front of the thigh and inserting on the front of the tibia

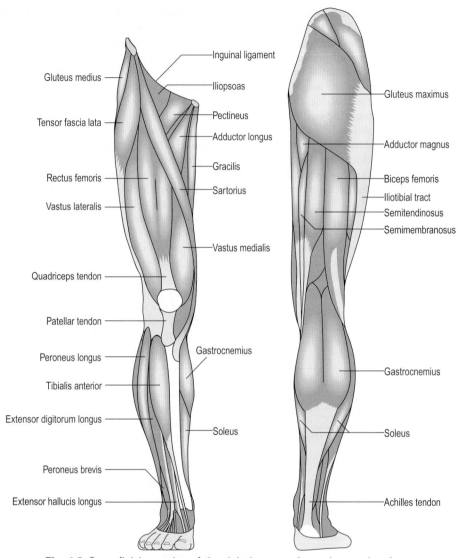

Fig. 1.8 Superficial muscles of the right leg: anterior and posterior views.

on its medial side. Its primary role is to act as a hip flexor and helps provide stability to the medial side of the knee along with the gracilis.

- *Semimembranosus* and *semitendinosus* are two of the *hamstrings*. Both originate at the ischial tuberosity of the pelvis and are inserted into the medial condyle of the tibia. They extend the hip and flex the knee.
- *Biceps femoris* is the third hamstring. It has two origins: the 'long head' comes from the ischial tuberosity and the 'short head' from the middle of the shaft of the femur. It inserts into the lateral condyle of the tibia and acts as a hip extensor and knee flexor.

- *Gracilis* runs down the medial side of the thigh from the pubis to the back of the tibia on its medial side. It adducts the hip and flexes the knee and helps provide stability to the medial side of the knee along with the sartorius.

Muscles Acting Only at the Knee Joint

- *Vastus medialis, vastus intermedius* and *vastus lateralis* are three elements of the quadriceps muscle. They all originate from the upper part of the femur, on the medial, anterior and lateral sides, respectively. The fourth element of the quadriceps is the rectus femoris, described in the preceding list. The four muscles combine and are attached via the quadriceps tendon, which surrounds the patella and continues beyond it as the patellar tendon, which inserts into the tibial tubercle. The quadriceps is the only muscle group which extends the knee.

- *Popliteus* is a small muscle behind the knee. It flexes and helps to unlock the knee by internally rotating the tibia at the beginning of flexion.

Muscles Acting Across the Knee and Ankle Joints

- *Gastrocnemius* originates from the back of the medial and lateral condyles of the femur, and its tendon joins with that of the soleus (and sometimes also the plantaris) to form the *Achilles tendon*, which inserts into the back of the calcaneus. The main action of these muscles is to plantarflex the ankle, although the gastrocnemius is also a flexor of the knee.
- *Plantaris* is a very slender muscle running deep to the gastrocnemius from the lateral condyle of the femur to the calcaneus and contributes to the plantarflexors of the ankle.

Muscles Acting Across the Ankle and Subtalar Joints

- *Soleus* arises from the posterior surface of the tibia, fibula and deep calf muscles. Its tendon joins with that of the gastrocnemius (and sometimes the plantaris) to plantarflex the ankle. The soleus and gastrocnemius together are called the *triceps surae*.
- *Extensor hallucis longus, extensor digitorum longus, tibialis anterior* and *peroneus tertius* form the anterior tibial group. They originate from the anterior aspect of the tibia and fibula and the interosseous membrane. The former two are inserted into the toes, which they extend; the latter two are inserted into the tarsal bones and raise the midfoot on the medial side (tibialis anterior) or lateral side (peroneus tertius). Tibialis anterior is the main ankle dorsiflexor, while the others are contributing dorsiflexors.
- *Flexor hallucis longus, flexor digitorum longus, tibialis posterior, peroneus longus* and *peroneus brevis* are the deep calf muscles, and all arise from the back of the tibia, fibula and interosseous membrane. The former two are flexors of the toes; the peronei are on the lateral side and evert the foot; and the tibialis posterior is on the medial side and inverts the foot. All five muscles are weak ankle plantarflexors.

Muscles Within the Foot

- *Extensor digitorum brevis* and the *dorsal interossei* are on the dorsum of the foot. The former muscle extends the toes, and the latter muscles abduct and flex the toes.
- *Flexor digitorum brevis, abductor hallucis* and *abductor digiti minimi* form the superficial layer of the sole of the foot. They flex the toes and abduct the big toe and little toe, respectively.
- *Flexor accessorius, flexor hallucis brevis* and *flexor digiti minimi brevis* form an intermediate layer in the sole of the foot. Between them, they flex all the toes.

- The *adductor hallucis* consists of two parts, the oblique head and the transverse head, and adducts the big toe.
- The *plantar interossei* and the *lumbricals* lie in the deepest layer of the sole of the foot. The former adduct and flex the toes, while the latter flex the proximal phalanges and extend the distal phalanges.

The five groups of muscles in the preceding lists are known together as the *intrinsic muscles* of the foot.

Biomechanics

Biomechanics is a scientific discipline which studies biological systems, such as the human body, through the methods of mechanical engineering. Since gait is a mechanical process which is performed by a biological system, it is appropriate to study it in this way. Mechanical engineering is a vast subject, but the descriptions which follow are limited to the aspects which are most relevant to gait analysis: centre of gravity, kinematics, kinetics, joint moments and power. Additional information included in the preceding edition of this book is available online at http://evolve.elsevier.com/Whittle/gait. The science of biomechanics uses mathematical principles. A useful text on the scientific basis is *The Comprehensive Textbook of Clinical Biomechanics* by Jim Richards (Elsevier 2018).

Centre of Gravity

Although the mass of any object is distributed throughout every part of the object, it is frequently convenient, as far as the effects of an applied force are concerned, to imagine that the entire mass is concentrated at a single point. This point, which should be called the centre of mass, is usually called the *centre of gravity*. For a regular shape, such as a cube, made of a uniform material, it is easy to see that the centre of gravity must be at the geometric centre. However, for irregular and changing shapes, such as the human body, it may be necessary to determine the centre of gravity by direct measurement. It is also possible to determine the centre of gravity of every part of the body separately and to find the centre of gravity of the whole body by adding these together. It is frequently stated that the centre of gravity of the body is just in front of the lumbosacral junction. This is approximately true for a person standing in the anatomical position, but any movement of the body will move the centre of gravity. It is not even necessary for the centre of gravity to remain within the body; the centre of gravity of someone bending down to touch their toes will usually be outside the body, in front of the top of the thigh (Fig. 1.9). An interesting example of this is the technique used by skilled high jumpers, who curve their body in such a way that although each part of the body in turn passes over the bar, the centre of gravity actually passes *under* it!

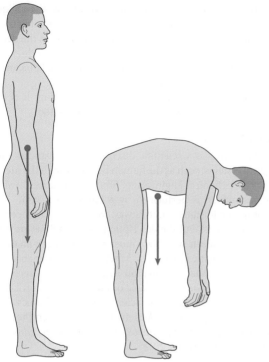

Fig. 1.9 Centre of gravity when standing and when bending.

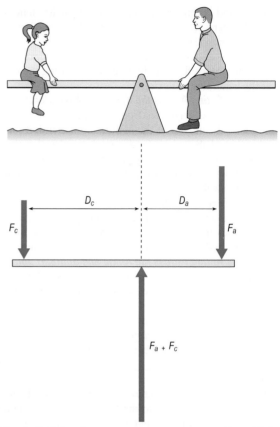

Fig. 1.10 Balancing moments on a seesaw. F_a multiplied by the distance D_a equals the force F_c multiplied by the distance D_c.

Kinematics

Kinematics describes motion, but without reference to the forces involved. An example of a kinematic instrument is a video camera, which can be used to observe the motion of the trunk and the limbs during walking, but which gives no information on the forces involved.

Kinetics

Kinetics is the study of forces, moments, masses and accelerations, but without any detailed knowledge of the position or orientation of the objects involved. For example, an instrument known as a force platform is used in gait analysis to measure the force beneath the foot during walking, but it gives no information on the position of the limb or the angle of the joints. For a complete quantitative description of an activity such as walking, both kinetic and kinematic data are needed.

Joint Moments

Moments, sometimes referred to as moments of force, can be considered similar to the moment of force involved in balancing a seesaw (Fig. 1.10). The moment about the pivot is calculated by multiplying the magnitude of the force by its perpendicular distance from the pivot point, this distance is commonly referred to as the *lever arm* or *moment arm*. The moment may also be referred to as the 'torque', the 'turning moment' or simply the 'moment'. The formula for calculating moments is:

$$\text{Moment (M)} = \text{Force (F)} \times \text{Distance (D)}$$

M is the moment (newton-metres, Nm), F is the force (newtons, N) and D is the distance (metres, m).

When considering the moments about the knee joint (Fig. 1.11) when standing with the knee flexed, the ground reaction force is acting at a perpendicular distance 'a' from the point of loadbearing. The quadriceps tendon is pulling at an oblique angle relative to the vertical, and the moment of force it provides is the product of the tension in the tendon and the perpendicular distance 'b'. The presence of the patella increases the value of b and hence reduces the

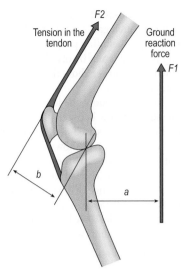

F2

Tension in the
tendon

Ground
reaction
force

F1

b

a

Fig. 1.11 The moment of force due to the ground reaction force, F_1 multiplied by a, is opposed by the contraction of the quadriceps, producing a moment of force F_2 multiplied by b.

muscle force needed to produce the given moment. For equilibrium, the two moments ($F_1 \times a$) and ($F_2 \times b$) must be equal (Fig. 1.11).

The measurement and interpretation of joint moments are essential for a full understanding of normal and pathological gait. 'Active' internal moments are generated by muscular contractions (concentric, isometric or eccentric), whereas 'passive' internal moments are generated by bone-on-bone forces and by tension in the soft tissues, in particular by ligaments; moments may also be transmitted from adjacent joints. Current gait analysis systems are able to measure the 'net moment' at the major joints during walking, which is the sum of all the active and passive moments present. This can be used to estimate the contraction force of a particular muscle, which is a technique sometimes used within research but is less common in clinical assessments.

There is sometimes confusion within the literature, with terms such as 'flexor moment' often being used without stipulating whether it refers to an internal or external moment. Contraction of a flexor muscle generates an *internal* flexor moment. In contrast, an *external* flexor moment attempts to flex the joint and is likely to be resisted by the contraction of extensor muscles. An example would be landing from a jump and the knee flexing from the force; the knee extensors would resist this external moment and prevent excessive knee flexion. To avoid such confusion, it is essential to make it clear whether an internal or external moment is being described.

Moments may be expressed in their original units (newton-metres, Nm), or they may be 'normalised' by dividing by body mass, changing the units to newton-metres per kilogram (Nm/kg), to make it easier to compare results between individuals of different body masses. It has also been suggested to normalise joint moments with reference to body mass and either height or limb length (Pierrynowski and Galea, 2001; Stansfield et al., 2003).

Work, Energy and Power

One of the remarkable features of normal gait is how energy is conserved by means of a number of optimisations. Abnormal gait patterns involve a loss of these optimisations, which may result in excessive energy expenditure, and hence, fatigue. The measurement, during walking, of energy transfers at individual joints and overall energy consumption is an important component of scientific gait analysis. There is a subtle difference in viewpoint between the physical scientist and the biologist as far as work, energy and power are concerned. To the physical scientist, work is done when a force moves an object a certain distance. It is calculated as the product of the force and the distance; if a force of 2 N moves an object 3 m, the work done is:

$$2N \times 3m = 6J \text{ (joules)}$$

The *joule* could also be called a newton-metre, but this would cause confusion with the identically named unit which is used to measure moments. *Energy* is the capacity to do work and is also measured in joules. It exists in two basic forms: *potential* or stored energy, and *kinetic* or movement energy. In walking, there are alternating transfers between potential and kinetic energy, with power being the rate at which work is done.

The reason biologists regard these matters slightly differently from physical scientists is that muscles can use energy without shortening—in other words, without doing any physical work. The potential energy stored in the muscles, in the form of ATP, is converted to mechanical energy in response to the muscle action potential. This energy is still used in an eccentric contraction, where the muscle actually gets longer while developing a force, which in physical terms is negative work. In other words, while everyone agrees that walking uphill involves doing work, the physicist might expect someone walking downhill to gain energy, whereas in reality the muscles are still activated and metabolic energy is still consumed. Even if a muscle shortens as it contracts, in a concentric contraction the conversion of metabolic energy to mechanical energy is relatively inefficient, with a typical efficiency of around 25%. The old unit for measuring metabolic energy was the Calorie (the capital C indicating 1000 calories or

1 kilocalorie); the conversion factor to Système International (SI) units , which are used in biomechanics, is is 4200 J or 4.2 kJ equals 1 Calorie (see Appendix 2).

The calculation of the mechanical power generated at the joints has become an important part of the biomechanical study of gait. In a rotary movement, when a joint flexes or extends the power is calculated as the product of the moment about that joint and its angular velocity, omega (ω):

$$P = M \,(\text{newton-metres}) \times \omega \,(\text{radians/second})$$

When a muscle is contracting concentrically (e.g., a flexor muscle contracting while a joint is flexing), power is generated. When a muscle is contracting eccentrically (e.g., a flexor muscle contracting while a joint is extending), it absorbs power. When a muscle is contracting isometrically (e.g., a flexor muscle contracting while the joint angle is unchanging), no power exchange takes place. Although in the gait cycle, power generation and absorption are often due to muscle contraction, it is important to realise that the stretching of ligaments and other soft tissues also involves power exchange. If a ligament is stretched, it absorbs power, with a resultant storage of potential energy. Some or all of this stored energy may be released later, with a resultant power generation. In gait analysis, it is a common practice to 'normalise' joint power by dividing it by body mass, giving a unit of watts per kilogram, in a similar way to the treatment of joint moments.

Worked Example

When an individual who is free of pain and pathology walks, the position of the ground reaction force in relation to the knee causes a muscular response. One common gait problem is that of crouch gait, which can affect several different patient groups, including people with cerebral palsy. By considering the mechanics involved, we are able to estimate the moments and power about the knee and the forces in the quadriceps muscles.

To find the moments about the knee we need to know the perpendicular distance between the ground reaction force and the knee joint, as well as the magnitude of the ground reaction force. Fig. 1.12 shows a point during loading of the front foot. In both cases the ground reaction force was 500 N. The individual who is free of pain and pathology had a distance to the knee of 0.08 m and the individual with crouch gait had a distance of 0.2 m. The moment may be found by multiplying the force by the perpendicular distance. Therefore, the moments will be:

- Moment for the pain and pathology free individual = 500 × 0.08 = 40 Nm
- Moment for the individual with crouch gait = 500 × 0.2 = 100 Nm

To find the eccentric power, we will need to know the angular velocity of the knee. If the pain and pathology free individual has angular velocity of 150° per second and the individual with crouch gait has a knee angular velocity of 40° per second, the eccentric power may be found by first converting degrees per second into radians per second:

- 150 degrees per second = 150 / 57.296 = 2.62 radians per second
- 40 degrees per second = 40 / 57.296 = 0.70 radians per second

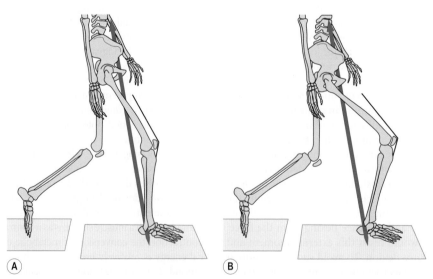

Fig. 1.12 Ground reaction forces in (A) normal gait and (B) crouch gait.

And then by using:

- Power = Moment × Angular velocity
- Eccentric power for the pain and pathology free individual = 40 × 2.62 = 104.8 Watts
- Eccentric power for the individual with crouch gait = 100 × 0.70 = 70.0 Watts

To find the muscle force we will need to know the knee moment and the perpendicular distance the muscle acts away from the knee joint. If in both cases the quadriceps tendon is only 0.06 m in front of the knee, the forces in the quadriceps may be found by:

- M = Force in quadriceps × 0.06
- Force in quadriceps = M / 0.06
- Force in the quadriceps for the pain and pathology free individual = 40 / 0.06 = 666.7 N or 1.3 times body weight
- Force in the quadriceps for the individual with crouch gait = 100 / 0.06 = 1666.7 N or 3.3 times body weight

Clearly, crouch gait changes the mechanics and loading patterns of the knee and surrounding structures. is more than two and The flexed position of the knee produces a much greater moment during crouch gait; however, individuals with crouch gait do not have the same eccentric control leading to a lower eccentric power. The increased moment at the knee has to be supported by the quadriceps, but this leads to a load in the knee that a half times that of individuals who are pain and pathology free.

REFERENCES

Pierrynowski, M.R., Galea, V., 2001. Enhancing the ability of gait analyses to differentiate between groups: scaling gait data to body size. Gait Posture 13, 193–201.

Pollo, F.E., Jackson, R.W., Komdeur, P., et al., 2003. Measuring dynamic knee motion with an instrumented spatial linkage device. In: Gait and Clinical Movement Analysis Society. Eighth Annual Meeting, Wilmington, Delaware, USA, pp. 15–16.

Richards, J., 2018. The Comprehensive Textbook of Clinical Biomechanics. Churchill Livingstone.

Stansfield, B.W., Hillman, S.J., Hazlewood, M.E., et al., 2003. Normalization of gait data in children. Gait Posture 17, 81–87.

2

Normal Gait

Michael Whittle, David Levine and Jim Richards

To understand pathological gait, it is necessary first to understand the gait of healthy, pain-free individuals, which for ease we will refer to as 'normal gait, within normal limits,' since this provides the standard against which the gait of a patient can be judged. However, there are pitfalls which need to be considered when using this approach. Firstly, the term *normal* covers both genders, a wide range of ages and an even wider range of extremes of body geometry, so an appropriate 'normal' standard needs to be chosen for the individual being studied. If results from an elderly female patient are compared with normal data obtained from physically fit young males, there will undoubtedly be large differences, whereas comparison with data from healthy elderly females may show the patient's gait to be well within normal limits appropriate for her gender and age. Another pitfall is that even though a patient's gait differs from normal, it may not be undesirable, and efforts to turn it into a normal gait should not be made. Many gait abnormalities are a compensation for some problem experienced by the patient and, although abnormal, are nonetheless useful. Having said this, it is very important to understand normal gait and the terminology used to describe it, before looking at pathological gait. This chapter starts with a brief historical review and then gives an overview of the gait cycle, before going on to study in detail how the different parts of the locomotor system are used in walking.

WALKING AND GAIT

Normal human walking and running can be defined as 'a method of locomotion involving the use of the two legs, alternately, to provide both support and propulsion'. In order to exclude running, we must add 'at least one foot being in contact with the ground at all times'. Unfortunately, this definition excludes some forms of pathological gait which are generally regarded as forms of walking, such as the three-point step-through gait (see Fig. 3.21), in which there is an alternate use of two crutches and either one or two legs. It is both unreasonable and pointless to attempt a definition of walking which will apply to all cases, at least in a single sentence!

Gait is no easier to define than walking, with many dictionaries regarding it as a word primarily for use in connection with horses! This is understandable, since quadruped animals have a repertoire of natural gaits (walking, trotting, pacing, galloping, etc.), as well as some artificial ones such as that learned by Tennessee Walking Horses in the area where one of the authors lives. Most people tend to use the words *gait* and *walking* interchangeably. However, there is a difference: the word *gait* describes the manner or style of walking rather than the walking process itself. It thus makes more sense to talk about a difference in gait between two individuals than about a difference in walking.

A BRIEF HISTORY

Walking has undoubtedly been observed since the dawn of humanity, but the systematic study of gait appears to date from the Renaissance when Leonardo da Vinci, Galileo and Newton gave useful descriptions of walking. The earliest account using a scientific approach was in the classic book *De Motu Animalium*, published in 1682 by Borelli, who worked in Italy and was a student of Galileo. Borelli measured the centre of gravity of the body and described how balance is maintained in walking by constant forward movement of the supporting area provided by the feet. The Weber brothers in Germany gave the first clear description of the gait cycle in 1836. They made accurate measurements of the timing of gait and of the pendulum-like swinging of the leg of a cadaver.

Kinematics

Two pioneers of kinematic measurement worked on opposite sides of the Atlantic in the 1870s. Marey, working in Paris, published a study of human limb movements in 1873. He made multiple photographic exposures, on a single plate, of a subject who was dressed in black, except for brightly illuminated stripes on the limbs. He also investigated the path of the centre of gravity of the body and the pressure beneath the foot. Eadweard Muybridge (born in England as Edward Muggeridge) became famous in California in 1878 by demonstrating that, when a horse is trotting, there are times when it has all four feet off the ground at once. The measurements were made using 24 cameras, triggered in quick succession as the horse ran into thin wires stretched across the track. In the next few years, Muybridge made a further series of studies, of naked human beings walking, running and performing a surprising variety of other activities!

The most serious application of the science of mechanics to human gait during the 19th century was the publication in Germany, in 1895, of *Der Gang des Menschen*, by Braune and Fischer. They employed a technique similar to Marey's, but using fluorescent striplights on the limbs instead of white stripes. The resultant photographs were used to determine the three-dimensional trajectories, velocities and accelerations of the body segments. Knowing the masses and accelerations of the body segments, they were then able to estimate the forces involved at all stages during the walking cycle.

Further valuable work on the dynamics of locomotion was done by Bernstein in Moscow in the 1930s. He developed a variety of photographic techniques for kinematic measurement, paying particular attention to the centre of gravity of the individual limb segments and of the body as a whole.

Force Platforms

Further progress followed the development of the *force platform* (also called the *force plate*). This instrument has contributed greatly to the scientific study of gait and is now standard equipment in gait laboratories. It measures the direction and magnitude of the ground reaction force beneath the foot. An early design was described by Amar in 1924 and an improved one by Elftman in 1938. Both were purely mechanical, with the force applied to the platform causing the movement of a pointer.

Muscle Activity

For a full understanding of normal gait, it is necessary to know which muscles are active during the different parts of the gait cycle. The role of the muscles was studied by

Scherb, in Switzerland, during the 1940s, initially by palpating the muscles as his subject walked on a treadmill, then later using electromyography (EMG). Further advances in the understanding of muscle activity and many other aspects of normal gait were made during the 1940s and 1950s by a group working at the University of California at San Francisco and the University of California at Berkeley, notable among whom was Verne Inman. This group wrote *Human Walking* (Inman et al., 1981), which was published just after Inman's death and to many is the definitive textbook on normal gait. *Human Walking* has gone through several editions, with the latest by Rose and Gamble (2005). Another classic text on EMG is *Muscles Alive: Their Functions Revealed by Electromyography*, by John Basmajian and Carlo De Luca (Basmajian and De Luca, 1985). Although this text has not been updated since 1985, *The Comprehensive Textbook of Clinical Biomechanics* (Richards, 2018) contains a useful summary chapter by De Luca and colleagues.

The use of EMG in gait analysis has received much attention, but perhaps the most influential paper published was 'The use of surface electromyography in biomechanics' by Carlo De Luca (De Luca, 1997), which gave a summary of recommendations but perhaps more importantly a summary of problems which at the time needed resolution. Further standardisation was achieved through the SENIAM (Surface ElectroMyoGraphy for the Non-Invasive Assessment of Muscles) project coordinated and managed by Hermie Hermens and Bart Freriks from Enschede, which is now considered by many to be the definitive recommendations for and sensor positioning for specific muscles.

Mechanical Analysis

A major contribution to the mechanical analysis of walking, also from the California group, was made by Bresler and Frankel (1950). They performed free-body calculations for the hip, knee and ankle joints, allowing for ground reaction forces, the effects of gravity on the limb segments and the inertial forces. The analytical techniques developed by these workers formed the basis of many current methods of modelling and analysis.

An important paper describing the possible mechanisms which the body uses to minimise energy consumption in walking was published by Saunders et al. (1953). Further important work on energy consumption and, in particular, the energy transfers between the body segments in walking was published by Cavagna and Margaria (1966). In the 1960s, research also began to concentrate on the variability of walking, the development of gait in children and the deterioration of gait in old age. Patricia Murray published a series of papers on these subjects, including a detailed review (Murray, 1967).

Mathematical Modelling

Once the motions of the body segments and the actions of the different muscles had been examined and documented, attention moved to the forces generated across the joints. Although limited calculations of this type had been made previously, the study by Paul (1965) was the first detailed analysis of hip joint forces during walking. A subsequent paper by Paul also included an analysis of the forces in the knee (Paul, 1966). Since then, there have been many mathematical studies of force generation and transmission across the hip, knee and ankle.

The 1970s and 1980s saw great improvements in methods of measurement. The development of more convenient kinematic systems, based on electronics rather than photography, meant that results could be produced in minutes rather than days. Reliable force platforms with high-frequency response became available, as well as convenient and reliable EMG systems. The availability of high-quality three-dimensional data on the kinetics and kinematics of walking, and the ease of access to powerful computers, made it possible to develop increasingly sophisticated mathematical models. Gait laboratories now routinely measure joint moments and powers for the hip, knee and ankle, and estimates can also be made of muscle, ligament and joint contact forces.

Recent decades have seen the emergence of increasingly powerful systems, higher-speed cameras, greater portability, smaller markers, a wide variety of marker sets and larger data collection volumes.

CLINICAL APPLICATION

In the 1960s, those working in the field of gait measurement started exploring the usefulness of gait analysis in the management of patients with walking disorders. Gait analysis has continuously advanced since that time, moving out of the research laboratory and into clinical settings. And with improvements in measurement and analytical techniques, today the major limitation is not an inability to produce high-quality data, but knowing how best to use these data for the benefit of patients. It is fair to say that in the early days, far more progress was made in scientific gait analysis, particularly as applied to normal subjects, than in the application of these techniques for the benefit of those with gait disorders. However, there has been a steady increase in the effective use of gait analysis in the clinical management of patients. Alongside this, there has also been a growing interest in the use of observational or visual gait analysis.

TERMINOLOGY USED IN GAIT ANALYSIS

The *gait cycle* is defined as the time interval between two successive occurrences of one of the repetitive events of walking. Although any event could be chosen to define the gait cycle, it is generally convenient to use the instant at which one foot contacts the ground (initial contact). If it is decided to start with initial contact of the right foot, as shown in Fig. 2.1, then the cycle will continue until the right foot contacts the ground again.

The following terms are used to identify major events during the gait cycle:

1. Initial contact
2. Opposite toe off
3. Heel rise
4. Opposite initial contact
5. Toe off
6. Feet adjacent
7. Tibia vertical

These seven events subdivide the gait cycle into seven periods—four of which occur in the stance phase, when the foot is on the ground, and three in the swing phase, when the foot is moving forwards through the air (Fig. 2.1). The stance phase, which is also called the *support phase* or *contact phase*, lasts from initial contact to toe off. It is subdivided into:

1. loading response,
2. mid-stance,
3. terminal stance, and
4. pre-swing.

The swing phase lasts from toe off to the next initial contact. It is subdivided into:

1. initial swing,
2. mid-swing, and
3. terminal swing.

The duration of a complete gait cycle is known as the *cycle time*, which is divided into *stance time* and *swing time*. Unfortunately, the nomenclature used to describe the gait cycle varies considerably from one publication to another. The present text attempts to use terms which will be understood by most people working in the field; alternative terminology will be given where appropriate. However, it should be noted that the usual terminology is inadequate to describe some severe pathological gaits which were highlighted in the paper by Wall et al. (1987), 'Two steps equals one stride equals what? The applicability of normal gait nomenclature to abnormal walking patterns'.

Gait Cycle Timing

Fig. 2.2 shows the timings of initial contact and toe off for both feet during a little more than one gait cycle.

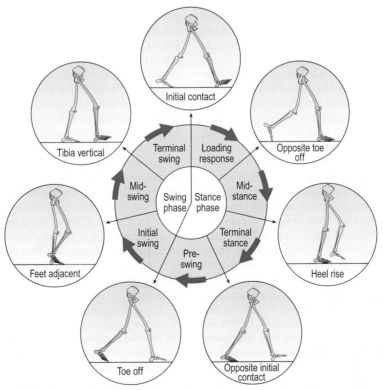

Fig. 2.1 Positions of the legs during a single gait cycle by the right leg *(blue leg)*.

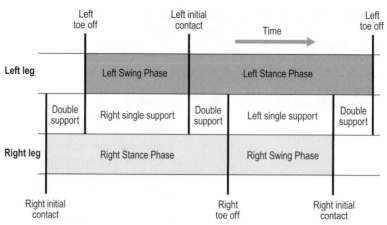

Fig. 2.2 Timing of single and double support during a little more than one gait cycle, starting with right initial contact.

Right initial contact occurs whilst the left foot is still on the ground and there is a period of *double support* (also known as *double limb stance*) between initial contact on the right and toe off on the left. During the swing phase on the left side, only the right foot is on the ground, giving a period of *right single support* (or single limb stance), which ends with initial contact by the left foot. There is then another period of double support, until toe off on the right side. *Left single support* corresponds to the right swing phase, and the cycle ends with the next initial contact on the right.

In each double support phase, one foot is forwards, having just landed on the ground, and the other one is backwards, being just about to leave the ground. When it is necessary to distinguish between the two legs in the double support phase, the leg in front is usually known as the *leading* leg and the leg behind as the *trailing* leg. The leading leg is in loading response, sometimes referred to as braking double support, initial double support or weight acceptance. The trailing leg is in *pre-swing*, also known as *second*, *terminal* or *thrusting double support*, or as *weight release*.

In each gait cycle, there are thus two periods of double support and two periods of single support. The stance phase usually lasts about 60% of the cycle, the swing phase about 40% and each period of double support about 10%. However, this varies with the speed of walking, with the swing phase becoming proportionately longer and the stance phase and double support phases shorter as the speed increases (Murray, 1967); see Blanc et al. (1999) for a detailed study of gait cycle timing. The final disappearance of the double support phase marks the transition from walking to running. Between successive steps in running there is a *flight phase*, also known as the *float*, *double-float* or *nonsupport* phase, when neither foot is on the ground.

For more detail, this book now includes a chapter considering gait analysis of running (Chapter 8, Gait Analysis in Running and the Management of Common Injuries).

Foot Placement

The terms used to describe the placement of the feet on the ground are shown in Fig. 2.3. The *stride length* is the distance between two successive placements of the same foot. It consists of two step lengths, left and right, each the distance by which the named foot moves forwards in front of the other. In pathological gait, it is common for the two *step lengths* to be different. If the left foot is moved forwards to take a step and the right one is brought up beside it rather than in front of it, the right step length will be zero. It is even possible for the step length on one side to be negative; for example, if the left foot never catches up with the right foot, the distance between the left and right feet will be negative. However, the *stride* length starting with the left heelstrike must always be the same as the stride length starting with the right heelstrike, unless the subject is walking around a curve where the inside leg will have a shorter stride length than the outside leg. This definition of a stride, consisting of one step by each foot, breaks down in some pathological gaits in which one foot makes a series of hopping movements whilst the other is in the air (Wall et al., 1987). There is no satisfactory nomenclature to deal with this situation.

The *walking base* (also known as the *stride width* or *base of support*) is the side-to-side distance between the line of the two feet, usually measured at the midpoint of the back of the heel but sometimes below the centre of the ankle joint. The preferred unit for stride length and step length is the metre and for the walking base, millimetres. The pattern of walking known as *tandem gait* involves walking with

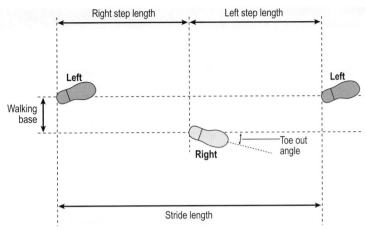

Fig. 2.3 Terms used to describe foot placement on the ground.

the heel of one foot placed directly in front of the toes of the other; that is, with a walking base close to zero. Although this pattern is not typically seen, even as a pathological gait it requires good balance and coordination.

The *toe out* (or, less commonly, *toe in*) is the angle in degrees between the direction of progression and a reference line on the sole of the foot. The reference line varies from one study to another; it may be defined anatomically but is commonly the midline of the foot, as judged by eye.

It is obvious that you need to walk more carefully on ice than on asphalt. Whether or not the foot slips during walking depends on two things: the coefficient of friction between the foot and the ground, and the relationship between the vertical force and the forces parallel to the walking surface (front to back and side to side). The ratio of the horizontal to the vertical force is known as the *utilised coefficient of friction*, and slippage will occur if this exceeds the actual coefficient of friction between the foot and the ground. In normal walking, a coefficient of friction of 0.35 to 0.40 is generally sufficient to prevent slippage; the most hazardous part of the gait cycle for slippage is initial contact. The literature on foot-to-ground friction and slippage is fairly extensive; examples include Cham and Redfern (2002) and Burnfield et al. (2005).

Cadence, Cycle Time and Speed

The *cadence* is the number of steps taken in a given time period, the usual unit being steps per minute. In most other types of scientific measurement, complete cycles are counted, but as there are two steps in a single gait cycle, the cadence is a measure of half-cycles. The normal ranges for both cadence and *cycle time* in both genders at different ages are shown in Table 2.1, where we consider the effect of age in more detail.

The *speed* of walking is the distance covered by the whole body in a given time, and should be measured in metres per second. Many authors use the term *velocity* in place of *speed*, but this is an incorrect usage of the term, unless the direction of walking is also stated, since velocity is a vector. The instantaneous speed varies from one instant to another during the walking cycle, but the average speed is the product of the cadence and the stride length, providing appropriate units are used. The cadence, in steps per minute, corresponds to half-strides per 60 seconds or full strides per 120 seconds. The speed can thus be calculated from cadence and stride length using the formula:

$$\text{speed (m/s)} = \text{stride length (m)} \times \text{cadence (steps/min)} / 120$$

If cycle time is used in place of cadence, the calculation becomes much more straightforward:

$$\text{speed (m/s)} = \text{stride length (m)} / \text{cycle time (s)}$$

The walking speed thus depends on the two step lengths, which in turn depend to a large extent on the duration of the swing phase on each side. The step length is the amount by which the foot can be moved forwards during the swing phase so that a short swing phase on one side will generally reduce the step length on that side. In pathological gait, the step length is often shortened, but it behaves in a way which is counterintuitive. When pathology affects one foot more than the other, an individual will usually try to spend a shorter time on the 'bad' foot and a correspondingly longer time on the 'good' one. Shortening the stance phase on the bad foot means bringing the good foot to the ground sooner, thereby shortening both the duration of the swing

TABLE 2.1   Normal ranges for gait parameters

Approximate range (95% limits) for general gait parameters in free-speed walking by normal female subjects of different ages.

Age (years)	Cadence (steps/min)	Cycle time (s)	Stride length (m)	Speed (m/s)
13–14	103–150	0.80–1.17	0.99–1.55	0.90–1.62
15–17	100–144	0.83–1.20	1.03–1.57	0.92–1.64
18–49	98–138	0.87–1.22	1.06–1.58	0.94–1.66
50–64	97–137	0.88–1.24	1.04–1.56	0.91–1.63
65–80	96–136	0.88–1.25	0.94–1.46	0.80–1.52

Approximate range (95% limits) for general gait parameters in free-speed walking by normal male subjects of different ages.

Age (years)	Cadence (steps/min)	Cycle time (s)	Stride length (m)	Speed (m/s)
13–14	100–149	0.81–1.20	1.06–1.64	0.95–1.67
15–17	96–142	0.85–1.25	1.15–1.75	1.03–1.75
18–49	91–135	0.89–1.32	1.25–1.85	1.10–1.82
50–64	82–126	0.95–1.46	1.22–1.82	0.96–1.68
65–80	81–125	0.96–1.48	1.11–1.71	0.81–1.61

Approximate range (95% limits) for general gait parameters in free-speed walking by normal children of different ages (ages 1–7 years based on Sutherland et al. [1988])

Age (years)	Cadence (steps/min)	Cycle time (s)	Stride length (m)	Speed (m/s)
1	127–223	0.54–0.94	0.29–0.58	0.32–0.96
1.5	126–212	0.57–0.95	0.33–0.66	0.39–1.03
2	125–201	0.60–0.96	0.37–0.73	0.45–1.09
2.5	124–190	0.63–0.97	0.42–0.81	0.52–1.16
3	123–188	0.64–0.98	0.46–0.89	0.58–1.22
3.5	122–186	0.65–0.98	0.50–0.96	0.65–1.29
4	121–184	0.65–0.99	0.54–1.04	0.67–1.32
5	119–180	0.67–1.01	0.59–1.10	0.71–1.37
6	117–176	0.68–1.03	0.64–1.16	0.75–1.43
7	115–172	0.70–1.04	0.69–1.22	0.80–1.48
8	113–169	0.71–1.06	0.75–1.30	0.82–1.50
9	111–166	0.72–1.08	0.82–1.37	0.83–1.53
10	109–162	0.74–1.10	0.88–1.45	0.85–1.55
11	107–159	0.75–1.12	0.92–1.49	0.86–1.57
12	105–156	0.77–1.14	0.96–1.54	0.88–1.60

phase and the step length on that side. Thus a short step length on one side generally means problems with single support on the *other* side.

When making comparisons among individuals, particularly children, it is useful to allow for differences in size. This is done by dividing a measurement by some aspect of body size, such as height (stature) or leg length, a procedure generally known as *normalisation*. It is thus fairly common to see walking speed expressed in statures per second or to see measures such as step factor, which is step length divided by leg length (Sutherland, 1997).

Since walking speed depends on both cadence and stride length, it follows that speed may be changed by altering only one of these variables—for instance, by increasing the cadence whilst keeping the stride length constant. In practice, however, people normally change their walking speed by adjusting both cadence and stride length. Sekiya and Nagasaki (1998) defined the walk ratio as step length (m) divided by step rate (steps/min) and found that it was fairly constant in both males and females over a range of walking speeds from very slow to very fast. Macellari et al. (1999) conducted a detailed study of the relationships among gender, body size, walking speed, gait timing and foot placement.

OVERVIEW OF THE GAIT CYCLE

The purpose of this section is to provide an overview of the gait cycle so that the detailed description which follows is easier to comprehend. The cycle is illustrated by Figs. 2.4 and 2.10–2.18, all of which are taken from a single walk by a 22-year-old healthy female, weight 540 N (55 kg, 121 lb), walking barefoot with a cycle time of 0.88 s (cadence 136 steps/min), a stride length of 1.50 m and a speed of 1.70 m/s. The individual measurements from this subject do not always correspond to 'average' values due to variability among individuals, although they are all close to the normal range. The measurements were made in the plane of progression, which is a vertical plane aligned to the direction of the walk; in normal walking it closely corresponds to the sagittal plane of the body. The data were obtained using a Vicon motion system and a Bertec force platform. It should be noted that different laboratories use different methods of measurement, so other publications may quote different values for some of the measured variables. The reader should thus concentrate on the changes in the variables during the gait cycle rather than on their absolute values.

When examining diagrams of the joint angles through the gait cycle, it is essential to understand how the angles are defined. Generally speaking, the knee angle is defined as the angle between the femur and the tibia, and there is usually no ambiguity. The ankle angle is usually defined as the angle between the tibia and an arbitrary line in the foot. Although this angle is normally around 90 degrees, it is conventional to define it as 0 degrees, with dorsiflexion and plantarflexion being movements in the positive and negative directions. In this book, dorsiflexion is a positive angle, but in some other publications it is negative. The hip angle may be measured in two different ways: the angle between the vertical and the femur, and the angle between the pelvis and the femur. The latter is the 'true' hip angle and is usually defined so that 0 degrees is close to the hip angle in the standing position. Forward flexion of the trunk appears as hip flexion when the hip angle is defined with reference to the pelvis, but not when it is defined with reference to the vertical.

The descriptions which follow assume that symmetry is present between the two sides of the body. This is approximately true for normal individuals, although detailed examination shows that everyone has some degree of asymmetry (Sadeghi, 2003). Such subtle asymmetries are negligible, especially when contrasted to the majority of pathological gaits.

In some gait studies the subject is barefoot, and in others the subject is wearing shoes. Oeffinger et al. (1999) found small differences in some of the gait parameters between these two conditions in children but did not consider them to be clinically important. It is usually at the discretion of the investigator whether or not shoes are worn, although in some cases this may be dictated by the presence of an intervention (e.g., when an ankle foot orthosis or an orthotic insole is used).

During gait, important movements occur in all three planes: sagittal, coronal and transverse. However, this chapter will concentrate on the sagittal plane, in which the largest movements occur. Fig. 2.4 shows the successive positions of the right leg at 40-ms intervals,

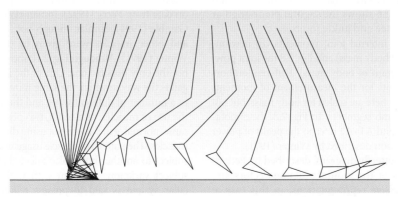

Fig. 2.4 Position of the right leg in the sagittal plane at 40-ms intervals during a single gait cycle.

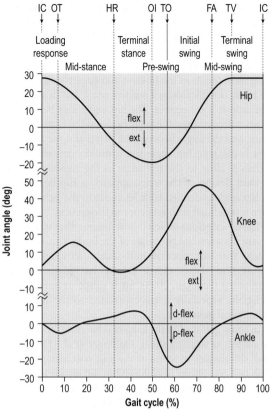

Fig. 2.5 Sagittal plane joint angles (degrees) during a single gait cycle of right hip (flexion positive), knee (flexion positive) and ankle (dorsiflexion positive). *FA*, Feet adjacent; *HR*, heel rise; *IC*, initial contact; *OI*, opposite initial contact; *OT*, opposite toe off; *TO*, toe off; *TV*, tibia vertical.

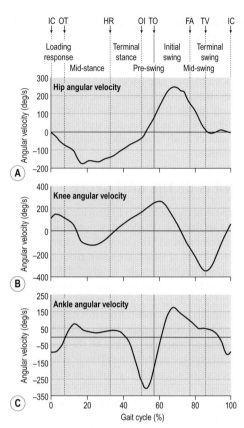

Fig. 2.6 (A–C) Sagittal plane joint angular velocities during a single gait cycle.

measured over a single gait cycle. Fig. 2.5 shows the corresponding sagittal plane angles at the hip, knee and ankle joints and Fig. 2.6 shows the sagittal plane angular velocity of the hip, knee and ankle joints.

Fig. 2.7 shows the internal joint moments (in newton-metres per kilogram of body mass) and Fig. 2.8 the joint powers (in watts per kilogram of body mass). Different authors have used different units for the measurement of moments and powers; those used here are scaled for body mass, but not for the length of the limb segments. In Fig. 2.8, the annotations H1–H3, K1–K4 and A1–A2 refer to the peaks of power absorption and generation described by Winter (1991).

Fig. 2.9 shows a 'butterfly diagram', described by Pedotti (1977). This is a plot of the ground reaction vectors and is made up of successive representations, in this case at 10-ms intervals, of the magnitude, direction and point of

application of the ground reaction force vector. The vectors move across the diagram from left to right and create a shape that resembles the wings of a butterfly.

Fig. 2.10 gives the typical activity of a number of key muscles or muscle groups during the gait cycle. This is based largely on data from Perry (1992), Inman et al. (1981) and Rose and Gamble (1994). Similar, though not identical, data for these and other muscles were given by Sutherland (1984) and Winter (1991). Although Fig. 2.10 shows a typical pattern, it is not the only possible one. One of the interesting things about gait is the way in which the same movement may be achieved in a number of different ways, and this particularly applies to the use of muscles; as a result, two people may walk with the same 'normal' gait pattern but using different combinations of muscles. The pattern of muscle usage not only varies from one subject to another but is also affected by fatigue, and within subject variations are seen with walking speed. The muscular system is said to possess *redundancy*, which means that if a particular muscle cannot be used, its functions may

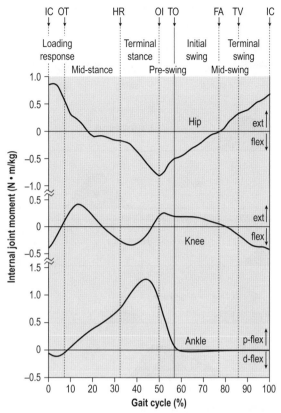

Fig. 2.7 Sagittal plane internal joint moments (newton-metres per kilogram of body mass) during a single gait cycle of right hip (extensor moment positive), knee (extensor moment positive) and ankle (plantarflexor moment positive). Abbreviations as in Fig. 2.5.

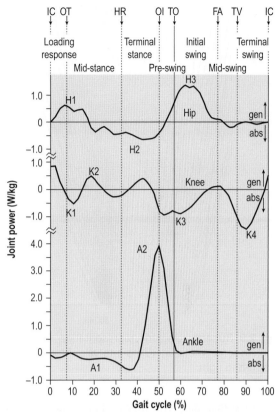

Fig. 2.8 Sagittal plane joint powers (watts per kilogram of body mass) during a single gait cycle of right hip, knee and ankle. Power generation is positive, absorption is negative. See text for meaning of H1, H2, etc. Other abbreviations as in Fig. 2.5.

be taken over by another muscle or group of muscles. A good review of muscle activity in gait was provided by Shiavi (1985).

Upper Body

The upper body moves forwards throughout the gait cycle. Its speed varies a little, being fastest during the double support phases and slowest in the middle of the stance and swing phases. The trunk twists about a vertical axis, with the shoulder girdle rotating in the opposite direction to the pelvis. The arms swing out of phase with the legs so that the left leg and the left side of the pelvis move forwards at the same time as the right arm and the right side of the shoulder girdle. Lamoth et al. (2002) made a detailed study of the relative motion between the pelvis and the trunk at different walking speeds. Murray (1967) found average total excursions of 7 degrees for the shoulder girdle and 12 degrees for the pelvis in adult males walking at free

speed. The fluidity and efficiency of walking depend to some extent on the motions of the trunk and arms, but these movements are commonly ignored in clinical gait analysis and have been relatively neglected in gait research. The whole trunk rises and falls twice during the cycle, through a total range of about 46 mm (Perry, 1992), being lowest during double support and highest in the middle of the stance and swing phases. An approximation to this vertical motion can be seen in the position of the hip joint in Fig. 2.4. The trunk also moves from side to side, once in each cycle, with the trunk being over each leg during its stance phase, as might be expected from the need for support. The total range of side-to-side movement is also about 46 mm (Perry, 1992). The pelvis twists about a vertical axis and tips slightly, both backwards and forwards (with an associated change in lumbar lordosis) and from side to side. The spinal muscles are selectively activated so that the head

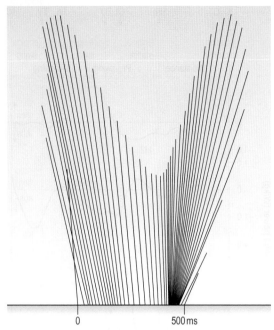

Fig. 2.9 Butterfly diagram representation of ground reaction force vector at 10-ms intervals. Progression is from left to right.

moves less than the pelvis, which is important for providing a stable platform for vision (Prince et al., 1994).

Hip

The hip flexes and extends once during the cycle (Fig. 2.5). The limit of flexion is reached around the middle of the swing phase, and the hip is then kept flexed until initial contact. The peak extension is reached before the end of the stance phase, after which the hip begins to flex again.

Knee

The knee shows two flexion and two extension peaks during each gait cycle. It is almost fully extended before initial contact, flexes during the loading response and the early part of mid-stance (stance phase knee flexion), extends again during the latter part of mid-stance, then starts flexing again, reaching a peak during initial swing (swing phase knee flexion). It extends again prior to the next initial contact.

Ankle and Foot

The ankle is usually within a few degrees of the neutral position for dorsiflexion/plantarflexion at the time of initial contact. After initial contact, the ankle plantarflexes, bringing the forefoot down onto the ground. During mid-stance, the tibia moves forwards over the foot, and the ankle joint

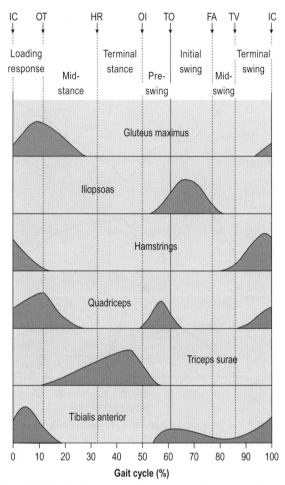

Fig. 2.10 Typical activity of major muscle groups during the gait cycle. Abbreviations as in Fig. 2.5. The timings of the events of the gait cycle are typical and not derived from a single subject.

becomes dorsiflexed. Before opposite initial contact, the ankle angle again changes, with a major plantarflexion taking place until just after toe off. During the swing phase, the ankle moves back into dorsiflexion until the forefoot has cleared the ground (around feet adjacent), after which something close to the neutral position is maintained until the next initial contact. In the frontal plane, the foot is slightly inverted (supinated, adducted or varus) at initial contact. The foot pronates as it contacts the ground, then moves back into supination as the ankle angle changes from plantarflexion to dorsiflexion; this supinated attitude is maintained as the heel rises and the ankle plantarflexes prior to toe off. Some degree of supination is retained throughout the swing phase.

THE GAIT CYCLE IN DETAIL

Each of the following sections begins with general remarks about the events surrounding a particular phase in the gait cycle and then describes what is happening in the upper body, hips, knees, ankles and feet, with particular reference to the activity of the muscles. These sections are very detailed and may be too much to comprehend in one pass. It is suggested that the reader should skip the sections on moments and powers on the first reading, but should go back to them later to gain a deeper understanding of the mechanical processes underlying the gait cycle. The figures shown in this section represent the normal positions of the lower limbs and pelvis at different events during gait and the ground reaction force vector expected. More detailed descriptions of the events of normal gait are given by Murray (1967), Perry (1992), Inman et al. (1981) and Rose and Gamble (1994).

Figs 2.11–2.19 show the positions of the two legs and the ground reaction force vector beneath the right foot (where present) at the seven major events of the gait cycle, and at two additional points: near the beginning of the loading response (Fig. 2.12) and halfway through mid-stance (Fig. 2.14). The description is based on a gait cycle from right initial contact to the next right initial contact.

Throughout the text, references will be made to the position of the ground reaction force vector relative to the axis of a joint and to the resultant joint moments. This approach, known as *vector projection*, is an approximation at best, since it neglects the mass of the leg below the joint in question (especially important at the hip) and also ignores the acceleration and deceleration of the limb segments (which primarily lead to errors in the swing phase). However, the authors have used this approach since it makes it much easier to understand joint moments. The graphs for joint moments (Fig. 2.7) and joint powers (Fig. 2.8) were calculated correctly using a method known as *inverse dynamics*, which is based on the kinematics, the ground reaction force and the subject's anthropometry.

Initial Contact (Fig. 2.11)

General

Initial contact is the beginning of the loading response and the first period of the stance phase. Initial contact is frequently called *heelstrike*, since in normal individuals there is often a distinct impact between the heel and the ground, known as the *heelstrike transient*. Other names for this event are *heel contact*, *footstrike* and *foot contact*. The direction of the ground reaction force changes from generally upwards during the heelstrike transient (Fig. 2.11) to upwards and backwards in the loading response immediately afterwards

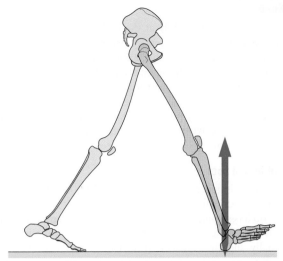

Fig. 2.11 Initial contact. Position of right leg *(blue)*, left leg *(grey)* and ground reaction force vector during the heelstrike transient. This illustration also applies to terminal foot contact.

(Fig. 2.12). This change in direction can also be seen in the butterfly diagram (Fig. 2.9), where the force vector changes direction immediately after initial contact.

Upper Body

The trunk is about half a stride length behind the leading (right) foot at the time of initial contact. In the side-to-side direction, the trunk is crossing the midline in its range of travel, moving towards the right as the foot on that side makes contact. The trunk is twisted, with the left shoulder and the right side of the pelvis each being at their furthest forwards and the left arm at its most advanced. The amount of arm swing varies greatly from one person to another, and it also increases with the speed of walking. At the time of initial contact, Murray (1967) found the mean elbow flexion to be 8 degrees and the shoulder flexion 45 degrees.

Hip

The attitude of the legs at the time of initial contact is shown in Fig. 2.11. The maximum flexion of the hip (generally around 30 degrees) is reached around the middle of the swing phase, after which it changes little until initial contact. The hamstrings are active during the latter part of the swing phase (since they act to prevent knee hyperextension), and the gluteus maximus begins to contract around the time of initial contact; together, these muscles start the extension of the hip, which will be complete around the time of opposite initial contact (Fig. 2.5).

Knee

The knee extends rapidly at the end of the swing phase, becoming nearly fully extended before initial contact, and then starts to flex again (Figs. 2.5 and 2.11). This extension is generally thought to be passive, although Perry (1992) states that it involves quadriceps contraction. Except in very slow walking, the hamstrings contract eccentrically at the end of the swing phase, to act as a braking mechanism to prevent knee hyperextension. This contraction continues into the beginning of the stance phase.

Ankle and Foot

The ankle is generally close to its neutral position in plantarflexion/dorsiflexion at the time of initial contact. Since the tibia is sloping backwards, the foot slopes upwards and only the heel contacts the ground (Fig. 2.11). The foot is usually slightly supinated (inverted, adducted or varus) at this time, and relatedly, most people show a wear pattern on the lateral side of the heel of the shoe. The tibialis anterior is active throughout the swing phase and in early stance, having maintained dorsiflexion during the swing and in preparation for the controlled movement into plantarflexion which occurs following initial contact.

Moments and Powers

At the time of initial contact, there is an internal extensor moment at the hip (Fig. 2.7), produced by contraction of the hip extensors (the gluteus maximus and the hamstrings, Fig. 2.10). As the hip joint moves in the direction of extension, these muscles contract concentrically and generate power (H1 in Fig. 2.8). The knee shows an internal flexor moment, due to contraction of the hamstrings (Fig. 2.10) as they prevent hyperextension at the end of the swing phase. As the knee starts to flex, concentric contraction of the hamstrings, as well as the release of energy stored in the ligaments of the extended knee, results in short-lived power generation (the unnamed peak in Fig. 2.8). Little moment or power exchange occurs at the ankle until just after initial contact. The heelstrike involves an absorption of energy by the elastic tissues of the heel and by compliant materials in footwear, very little of which could be recovered later in the stance phase. The amount of energy lost to the environment as sound and heat in this way is probably fairly small.

Loading Response (Fig. 2.12)

General

The loading response is the double support period between initial contact and opposite toe off. During this period, the foot is lowered to the ground by plantarflexion of the ankle. The ground reaction force increases rapidly in magnitude, its direction being upwards and backwards. In the subject

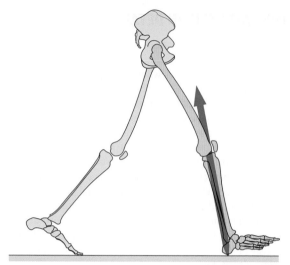

Fig. 2.12 Loading response. Position of right leg *(blue)*, left leg *(grey)* and ground reaction force vector 20 ms after initial contact.

used for illustration, loading response occupied the period from 0% to 7% of the cycle; this is unusually short, with loading response typically occupying the first 10% to 12% of the cycle. Fig. 2.12 represents 2% of the cycle.

Upper Body

During loading response, the trunk is at its lowest vertical position, about 20 mm below its average level for the whole cycle; its instantaneous forward speed is at its greatest, around 10% higher than the average speed for the whole cycle. It continues to move laterally towards the right foot. The arms, having reached their maximum forward (left) and backward (right) positions, begin to return.

Hip

During loading response, the hip begins to extend (Fig. 2.5) through concentric contraction of the hip extensors, the gluteus maximus and the hamstrings (Fig. 2.10).

Knee

From its nearly fully extended position at initial contact, the knee flexes during loading response (Fig. 2.5), initiating the stance phase flexion. This is accompanied by eccentric contraction of the quadriceps (Fig. 2.10) to control the speed and magnitude of flexion.

Ankle and Foot

The loading response period of the gait cycle, also called the *initial rocker*, *heel rocker* or *heel pivot*, involves plantarflexion at the ankle (Fig. 2.5). The plantarflexion is controlled by eccentric contraction of the tibialis anterior muscle. The movement into plantarflexion is accompanied by pronation of the foot and internal rotation of the tibia, as there is an automatic coupling between pronation/supination of the foot and internal/external rotation of the tibia (Inman et al., 1981; Rose and Gamble, 1994). The direction of the force vector changes from that shown in Fig. 2.11 to that shown in Fig. 2.12, within a 10- to 20-ms period.

Moments and Powers

As described earlier in 'Initial Contact', the hip shows an internal extensor moment with power generation during the loading response, and the knee shows an internal flexor moment with power generation. At the ankle, the posterior placement of the force vector (Fig. 2.12) produces an external plantarflexor moment. In the normal individual, this is resisted by an internal dorsiflexor moment (Fig. 2.7) produced by the tibialis anterior (Fig. 2.10), which contracts eccentrically, absorbs power (Fig. 2.8) and permits the foot to be lowered gently to the ground. Should the tibialis anterior fail to generate sufficient moment, the foot plantarflexes too rapidly, producing an audible 'foot slap'.

Opposite Toe Off (Fig. 2.13)
General

Opposite toe off, also known as *opposite foot off*, is the end of the double support period known as loading response and the beginning of mid-stance, the first period of single support. The forefoot, which was being lowered by plantarflexion

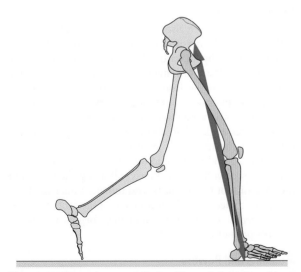

Fig. 2.13 Opposite toe off. Position of right leg *(blue)*, left leg *(grey)* and ground reaction force vector.

of the ankle, contacts the ground at *foot flat*, also known as *forefoot contact*, which generally occurs around the time of opposite toe off. On the opposite (left) side, it marks the end of the stance phase and the beginning of the swing phase. In the subject used for illustration, opposite toe off (Fig. 2.13) occurred at 7% and foot flat at 8% of the cycle.

Upper Body

At opposite toe off, the left shoulder and arm, having reached their most forward positions, are now moving posteriorly. Similarly, the pelvis on the right side now starts to twist back towards the neutral position. The trunk, having reached its lowest position during loading response, now begins to gain height but loses forward speed as a result of the backward and upward direction of the ground reaction force acting on the centre of gravity of the body. This represents a conversion of kinetic energy to potential energy, similar to a child's swing at its lowest point before it begins to climb up again.

Hip

The hip flexion angle is around 25 degrees at time of opposite toe off (Fig. 2.5). The hip continues to extend through the concentric contraction of the gluteus maximus and hamstrings.

Knee

At opposite toe off, the knee is continuing to flex, reaching peak stance phase knee flexion early in mid-stance, after which it begins to extend again (Fig. 2.5). The magnitude of the stance phase flexion is very sensitive to walking speed and can disappear during slow walking. Quadriceps contraction (eccentric, then concentric) permits the knee to act like a spring, preventing the vertical force from building up too rapidly (Perry, 1974).

Ankle and Foot

As soon as the foot is flat on the ground, around opposite toe off, the direction of ankle motion changes from plantarflexion to dorsiflexion, as the tibia moves over the now stationary foot (Fig. 2.5). Both foot pronation and internal tibial rotation reach a peak around opposite toe off and begin to reverse. These two motions are 'coupled'; that is, they always occur together, due in part to the geometry of the ankle and subtalar joints (Inman et al., 1981; Rose and Gamble, 1994). The tibialis anterior ceases to contract and is replaced by contraction of the triceps surae (Fig. 2.10).

Moments and Powers

At opposite toe off, the hip continues to have an internal extensor moment with power generation, as described earlier in 'Initial Contact'. At the knee, the force vector lies behind the joint (Fig. 2.13), producing an external flexor moment. This is opposed by an internal extensor moment (Fig. 2.7) generated by the quadriceps muscles (Fig. 2.10). These contract eccentrically, absorbing power (K1 in Fig. 2.8). The line of the ground reaction force begins to move forwards along the foot (Fig. 2.13), causing the internal dorsiflexor moment at the ankle to become smaller and then to reverse, to become a plantarflexor moment (Fig. 2.7). Little power exchange occurs at the ankle at this time.

Mid-stance (Fig. 2.14)
General
Mid-stance is the period of the gait cycle between opposite toe off and heel rise, although the term has been used in the past to describe an event in the gait cycle when the swing phase leg passes the stance phase leg, corresponding to the swing phase event of *feet adjacent*, or the point in time when the anterior posterior component of the ground reaction force is zero. In the subject used for illustration, mid-stance occupied the period from 7% to 32% of the cycle; Fig. 2.14A represents 18% of the cycle and Fig. 2.14B the event when the anterior posterior reaction force is zero.

Upper Body
The period of mid-stance sees the trunk climbing to its highest point, about 20 mm above the mean level, and slowing its forward speed as the kinetic energy of forward motion is converted to the potential energy of height. The side-to-side motion of the trunk also reaches its peak during mid-stance, with the trunk being displaced about 20 mm from its central position, towards the side of the stance (right) leg. Like the feet, the arms pass each other during mid-stance, as each follows the motion of the opposite leg. The twisting of the trunk has now disappeared, as both the shoulder girdle and pelvis pass through neutral before twisting the other way.

Hip
During the mid-stance period, the hip continues to extend, moving from a flexed attitude to an extended one (Fig. 2.5). Concentric contraction of the gluteus maximus and the hamstrings ceases during this period, as hip extension is achieved by inertia and gravity. Throughout mid-stance and terminal stance, significant muscle activity about the hip joint takes place in the frontal plane. As soon as the opposite foot has left the ground, the pelvis is supported only by the stance phase hip. It dips down slightly on the side of the swinging leg, but its position is maintained by contraction of the hip abductors, especially the gluteus medius and tensor fascia lata.

Knee
During mid-stance, the knee reaches its peak of stance phase flexion and starts to extend again (Fig. 2.5), initially through concentric contraction of the quadriceps. The peak generally occurs between 15% and 20% of the gait cycle. Its magnitude varies from one individual to another and with the speed of walking, but it is commonly between 10 degrees and 20 degrees.

Ankle and Foot
The *mid-stance rocker*, also called the *second rocker* or *ankle rocker*, occurs during mid-stance and terminal stance. It is characterised by forward rotation of the tibia about the ankle joint as the foot remains flat on the floor, with the ankle angle changing from plantarflexion to dorsiflexion and the triceps surae contracting eccentrically. The actual angles vary with the method of measurement; most authors report larger angles than those seen in Fig. 2.5. External rotation of the tibia and coupled supination of the foot occur during mid-stance and terminal stance. The ground reaction force vector moves forwards along the foot from the time of foot flat onwards, and moving under the forefoot prior to heel rise. The movement of the foot into supination peaks in mid-stance and then begins to reverse towards pronation.

Moments and Powers
During mid-stance, the internal extensor moment at the hip, generated by contraction of the extensor muscles,

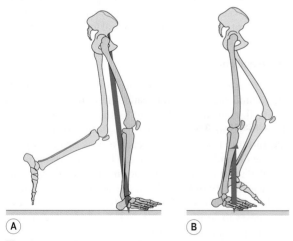

Fig. 2.14 (A) Mid-stance. Position of right leg *(blue)*, left leg *(grey)* and ground reaction force vector 100 ms after opposite toe off. (B) Mid-stance event when the anterior posterior component of the ground reaction force is zero.

declines and disappears, to be replaced by a moment in the opposite direction (Fig. 2.7). At the knee, the force vector remains behind the joint, producing an external flexor moment, opposed by an internal extensor moment (Fig. 2.7) due to quadriceps contraction (Fig. 2.10). According to Perry (1992), only the vasti, and not the rectus femoris, are active at this time. As the direction of knee motion changes from flexion to extension (Fig. 2.5), power generation takes place (K2 in Fig. 2.8). The ankle shows an increasing internal plantarflexor moment throughout mid-stance and into terminal stance (Fig. 2.7), as the force vector moves into the forefoot. This moment is generated by the triceps surae (Fig. 2.10), which are contracting eccentrically and absorbing power (A1 in Fig. 2.8).

Heel Rise (Fig. 2.15)

General

Heel rise, also called *heel off*, marks the transition from mid-stance to terminal stance. It is the time at which the heel begins to lift from the walking surface. Its timing varies considerably, both from one individual to another and with the speed of walking. The subject used for illustration shows heel rise at 32% of the gait cycle.

Upper Body

By heel rise, the trunk is falling from its highest point, reached during mid-stance. The lateral displacement over the supporting (right) leg also begins to diminish, in preparation

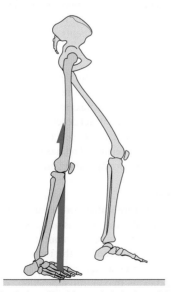

Fig. 2.15 Heel rise. Position of right leg *(blue)*, left leg *(grey)* and ground reaction force vector.

for the transfer of weight back to the left leg. As the right hip extends and the leg moves backwards, the right side of the pelvis twists backwards with it and the arm and shoulder girdle on the right move forwards.

Hip

At heel rise and into terminal stance, the hip continues to extend (Fig. 2.5). Peak hip extension is reached around the time of opposite initial contact. The activity of the hip abductors in the frontal plane is still required to stabilise the pelvis, although this activity ceases prior to initial contact by the other foot.

Knee

The knee has an extension peak close to the time of heel rise (Fig. 2.5). Around this time, active ankle plantarflexion brings the ground reaction force forwards, moving it under the forefoot and in front of the knee joint (barely visible in Fig. 2.15). This attempts to extend the knee, an effect known as the *plantarflexion/knee extension couple*, which becomes very important in some pathological gaits. Contraction of the gastrocnemius augments the action of the soleus as far as the ankle joint is concerned, but it also acts as a flexor at the knee, preventing hyperextension and subsequently initiating knee flexion.

Ankle and Foot

The peak of ankle dorsiflexion is reached some time after heel rise (Fig. 2.5). The triceps surae initially maintains the ankle angle as the knee begins to flex, with movement into plantarflexion beginning late in terminal stance. The tibia becomes increasingly externally rotated and the foot becomes increasingly supinated, the two being linked through coupled motion at the subtalar joint. As the heel rises, the toes remain flat on the ground and extension occurs at the metatarsophalangeal (MTP) joints, along an oblique line across the foot known as the *metatarsal break* or *toe break*. From the time the heel rises, hindfoot inversion (adduction or varus angulation) is seen.

Moments and Powers

At heel rise, there is a small but increasing internal hip flexor moment (Fig. 2.7). The source of this internal flexor moment does not appear to have been fully explained in the literature, although it could be due to a combination of adductor longus and rectus femoris contraction and the stretching of ligaments as the hip moves into extension, with a resultant power absorption (H2 in Fig. 2.8). At the knee, quadriceps contraction has ceased prior to heel rise and the internal knee moment has reversed to become a flexor moment. According to Perry (1992), this occurs because the upper body moves forwards faster than the tibia. If the ankle joint were totally free, the forward motion of the body would simply dorsiflex the ankle. However, contraction of the triceps surae (Fig. 2.10) slows down and controls the forward motion of the tibia so that as the femur moves forwards, an external extensor moment is generated at the knee, which is opposed by an internal flexor moment (Fig. 2.7). Only small and variable power exchanges occur at the knee around heel rise. At the ankle, the internal plantarflexor moment continues to increase, as first the soleus and then both the soleus and gastrocnemius together (triceps surae in Fig. 2.10) contract increasingly strongly. The contraction is initially eccentric, with power absorption (A1 in Fig. 2.8).

Opposite Initial Contact (Fig. 2.16)

General

As might be expected, opposite initial contact in symmetrical gait occurs at close to 50% of the cycle. It marks the end of the period of single support and the beginning of pre-swing, which is the second period of double support. At the time of opposite initial contact, also known as *opposite foot contact*, the hip begins to flex, the knee is already flexing and the ankle is plantarflexing. The period between heel rise and toe off (terminal stance followed by pre-swing) is sometimes called the *terminal rocker* phase. This is appropriate, since the leg is now rotating forwards about the forefoot rather than about the ankle joint. Another term for this period is the push off phase. Perry (1974) objected to this term, suggesting

instead the term roll-off, because 'the late floor-reaction peak is the result of leverage by body alignment, rather than an active downward thrust'. However, it is clear that the push off is not simply passive, since it is the period during which the generation of power at the ankle is greatest (Winter, 1983). What is not clear is whether this power is used to accelerate the whole body (as suggested by Winter) or merely the leg (as suggested by Perry) or (as seems most likely) some combination of the two. Buczek et al. (2003) showed that power generation at the ankle is necessary to sustain normal walking. Using terms borrowed from a study on posture control by Mueller et al. (1994), normal walking involves an 'ankle strategy' but may be replaced by a 'hip strategy' in which subjects 'decrease their push-off, pulling their leg forward from their hips'.

Upper Body

The attitude of the upper body at opposite initial contact resembles that described for initial contact, except that the trunk is now moving towards the left rather than the right, and the trunk is twisted so that the right shoulder and arm and the left side of the pelvis are forwards.

Hip

At opposite initial contact, the hip reaches its most extended position (typically between 10 degrees and 20 degrees of extension, depending on how it is measured), and motion reverses in the direction of flexion (Fig. 2.5). With the hip extended, the adductor longus acts as the primary hip flexor (Perry, 1992) and probably generates sufficient moment to initiate hip flexion, particularly when combined with tension in the stretched hip ligaments and the effects of gravity.

Knee

The knee is already moving into flexion by the time of opposite initial contact (Fig. 2.5). The force vector has moved behind the knee, aiding its flexion (Fig. 2.16), and the rectus femoris begins to contract eccentrically (included with the quadriceps in Fig. 2.10), to prevent flexion from occurring too rapidly. The term *pull off* has been used for the hip and knee flexion occurring during pre-swing.

Ankle and Foot

From before opposite initial contact until the foot leaves the ground at toe off, the ankle is moving into plantarflexion (Fig. 2.5), due to concentric contraction of the triceps surae (Fig. 2.10). Extension of the toes at the MTP joints continues and causes a tightening of the plantar fascia. The foot reaches its maximum supination, with hindfoot inversion (adduction or varus angulation) which is coupled with external tibial rotation. These various factors combine

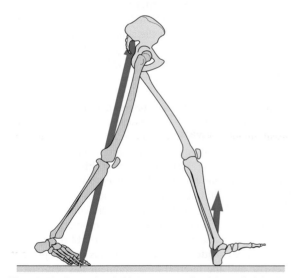

Fig. 2.16 Opposite initial contact. Position of right leg *(blue)*, left leg *(grey)* and ground reaction force vector.

to lock the midtarsal joints, resulting in high stability of the foot for loadbearing (Inman et al., 1981; Rose and Gamble, 1994).

Moments and Powers

A peak of hip internal flexor moment occurs around opposite initial contact (Fig. 2.7). As stated earlier in 'Opposite Initial Contact', this probably results from a combination of adductor longus contraction, passive tension in the hip ligaments and gravity. As the direction of hip motion reverses from extension to flexion, power absorption (H2 in Fig. 2.8) is replaced by power generation (H3 in Fig. 2.8). During terminal stance, flexion of the knee brings the joint in front of the force vector (Fig. 2.16), reversing the external moment from extensor to flexor and hence changing the internal moment from flexor to extensor (Fig. 2.7). The eccentric contraction of the rectus femoris (included with the quadriceps in Fig. 2.10) limits the rate of knee flexion and results in power absorption (K3 in Fig. 2.8). At the ankle, the force vector is well in front of the joint at opposite initial contact (Fig. 2.16). The resultant high external dorsiflexor moment is opposed by a correspondingly high internal plantarflexor moment (Fig. 2.7), produced by concentric contraction of the triceps surae (Fig. 2.10). The result is a large generation of power (A2 in Fig. 2.8), which is the highest power generation of the entire gait cycle. The immediate effect of this power generation is to accelerate the limb forwards into the swing phase.

Toe Off (Fig. 2.17)
General

Toe off generally occurs at about 60% of the gait cycle (57% in the subject used for illustration). It separates pre-swing from initial swing and is the point at which the stance phase ends and the swing phase begins. The name *terminal contact* has been proposed for this event, since in pathological gait the toe may not be the last part of the foot to leave the ground.

Upper Body

The extreme rotations of the shoulders, arms and trunk all begin to return towards the neutral position, as the trunk gains height and moves towards the front (left) supporting foot.

Hip

As the foot leaves the ground, the hip continues to flex (Fig. 2.5). This is achieved by gravity and tension in the hip ligaments, as well as by contraction of the rectus femoris (included with the quadriceps in Fig. 2.10) and adductor longus.

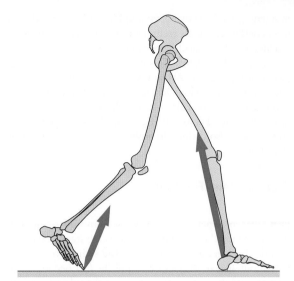

Fig. 2.17 Toe off. Position of right leg *(blue)*, left leg *(grey)* and ground reaction force vector.

Knee

By the time of toe off, the knee has flexed to around half of the angle it will achieve at the peak of swing phase flexion. This flexion is aided by the positioning of the ground reaction force vector well behind the knee (Fig. 2.17), although the magnitude of the force declines rapidly, reaching zero as the foot leaves the ground. The major part of knee flexion then results from hip flexion: the leg acts as a jointed 'double pendulum' so that as the hip flexes, the shank is 'left behind' due to its inertia, resulting in flexion of the knee. At the very beginning of the swing phase, the rectus femoris may contract eccentrically to prevent excessive knee flexion, particularly at faster walking speeds (Nene et al., 1999).

Ankle and Foot

The peak of ankle plantarflexion occurs just after toe off. The magnitude of plantarflexion depends on the method of measurement; it is 25 degrees in Fig. 2.5. Triceps surae contraction ceases prior to toe off and tibialis anterior contraction begins (Fig. 2.10), bringing the ankle up into a neutral or dorsiflexed attitude during the swing phase.

Moments and Powers

Around toe off, the hip still shows an internal flexor moment (Fig. 2.7), resulting from gravity, ligament elasticity and adductor longus and iliopsoas contraction. Since the hip is flexing at this time, power generation occurs (H3 in Fig. 2.8). During pre-swing and initial swing, hip flexion causes the knee to flex. This double pendulum motion results in an external flexor moment at the knee that is opposed by an internal extensor moment (Fig. 2.7) as the rectus femoris contracts eccentrically (included with the quadriceps in Fig. 2.10) to limit the speed at which the knee flexes. This eccentric contraction absorbs power (K3 in Fig. 2.8). At the ankle, the internal plantarflexor moment reduces rapidly during pre-swing as the magnitude of the ground reaction force declines, falling to zero as the foot leaves the ground at toe off (Fig. 2.7). The ankle power generation peak also declines to around zero during this period (Fig. 2.8).

Feet Adjacent (Fig. 2.18)
General

Feet adjacent separates initial swing from mid-swing. It is the time when the swinging leg passes the stance phase leg and the two feet are side by side. The swing phase occupies about 40% of the gait cycle and the feet become adjacent around the centre of this time; in the subject used for illustration, it occurred at 77% of the gait cycle. Alternative names for feet adjacent are foot clearance and mid-swing; the latter term is now applied to a period of the gait cycle rather than to a particular event.

Upper Body

When the feet are adjacent, the trunk is at its highest position and is maximally displaced over the stance phase leg (left). The arms are level with each other, with the left arm moving forwards and the right arm moving backwards.

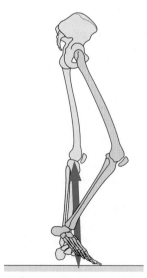

Fig. 2.18 Feet adjacent. Position of right leg *(blue)* and left leg *(grey)*.

Hip

The hip starts to flex prior to toe off, and by the time the feet are adjacent, it is well flexed (20 degrees in Fig. 2.5). This is achieved by a powerful contraction of the iliopsoas (Fig. 2.10), aided by gravity.

Knee

The flexion of the knee during the swing phase results largely from the flexion of the hip. As described earlier in 'Toe Off', the leg acts as a jointed pendulum, and no muscle contraction is necessary around the knee (thus enabling above-knee amputees to achieve swing phase knee flexion in their prosthetic limb). The peak swing phase knee flexion angle is usually between 60 degrees and 70 degrees (Fig. 2.5). It occurs before the feet are adjacent, by which time the knee has started to extend again. In fast walking, swing phase knee flexion is less than when walking at a natural speed, to shorten the swing phase. This is achieved by co-contraction of the rectus femoris and hamstrings (Gage, 2004).

Ankle and Foot

At the time the feet are adjacent, the ankle is moving from a plantarflexed attitude around toe off towards a neutral or dorsiflexed attitude in terminal swing (Fig. 2.5). Most of the shortening of the swing phase leg required to achieve toe clearance comes from flexion of the knee, but the ankle also needs to move out of plantarflexion. This movement requires contraction of the anterior tibial muscles, although the force of contraction is much less than that required (Fig. 2.10) to control foot lowering following initial contact. The closest approach of the toes to the ground occurs around the time the feet are adjacent. In normal walking, the toes clear the ground by very little; Murray (1967) found a mean clearance of 14 mm with a range of 1 to 38 mm. The degree of foot supination reduces following toe off, but the foot remains slightly supinated until the following initial contact.

Moments and Powers

As the hip moves into flexion, from opposite initial contact and through pre-swing and initial swing until the feet are adjacent, an internal flexor moment is present (Fig. 2.7). This is generated by gravity, the rectus femoris and the adductors, with the addition of ligament elasticity at the beginning of the movement and iliopsoas contraction towards its end (Fig. 2.10). Hip flexion, in response to this moment, results in the highest peak of power generation at the hip (H3 in Fig. 2.8), the power being used to accelerate the swinging leg forwards. The resultant kinetic energy is later transferred to the trunk, as the swinging leg is decelerated again at the end of the swing phase. Between toe off and feet adjacent, the knee continues to show a small internal extensor moment, as the rectus femoris (part of the quadriceps in Fig. 2.10) prevents the knee from flexing too rapidly in response to the external flexor moment transferred from the hip. Whilst the knee is still flexing, power absorption occurs (K3 in Fig. 2.8). Only very small moments and power exchanges are seen at the ankle, since only the weight of the foot is involved.

Tibia Vertical (Fig. 2.19)

General

The division between the periods of mid-swing and terminal swing is marked by the tibia of the swinging leg becoming vertical, which occurred at 86% of the gait cycle in the subject used for illustration. Terminal swing is also known as *reach*.

Upper Body

When the tibia is vertical on the swing phase leg (right), the trunk has begun to lose vertical height and to move from its maximum displacement over the supporting (left) leg back towards the midline. The left arm is now in front of the right and the right side of the pelvis is a little in front of the left side.

Hip

Tibia vertical marks approximately the time at which further hip flexion ceases; the subject used for illustration has a hip angle of about 27 degrees of flexion from tibia

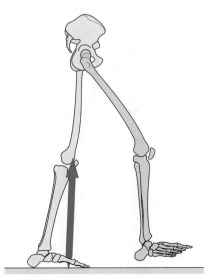

Fig. 2.19 Tibia vertical. Position of right leg *(blue)* and left leg *(grey)*.

vertical to the next initial contact (Fig. 2.5). The hamstrings contract increasingly strongly during terminal swing (Fig. 2.10) to limit the rate of knee extension whilst maintaining the hip joint in this flexed position.

Knee

Tibia vertical occurs during a period of rapid knee extension, as the knee goes from the peak of swing phase flexion prior to feet adjacent, to more or less full extension prior to the next initial contact (Fig. 2.5). This extension is largely passive, being the return swing of the lower (shank) segment of the double pendulum referred to earlier in 'Toe Off'. Eccentric contraction of the hamstrings prevents this motion from causing an abrupt hyperextension of the knee at the end of swing (Fig. 2.10).

Ankle and Foot

Once toe clearance has occurred, generally before the tibia becomes vertical, the ankle attitude becomes less important: it may be anywhere between a few degrees of plantarflexion and a few degrees of dorsiflexion, prior to the next initial contact (Fig. 2.5). The tibialis anterior continues to contract to hold the ankle in position, but its activity usually increases prior to initial contact in anticipation of the greater contraction forces which will be needed during the loading response (Fig. 2.10).

Moments and Powers

At the hip, by the time of tibia vertical, an increasing internal extensor moment is seen (Fig. 2.7); this is largely generated by the contraction of the hamstrings, although the gluteus maximus also begins to contract prior to the next initial contact (Fig. 2.10). This moment probably permits the transfer of momentum from the swinging leg to the trunk, recovering some of the kinetic energy imparted to the leg in initial swing (H3 in Fig. 2.8). Since the hip angle is essentially static during terminal swing, very little power exchange occurs at the joint itself. The knee demonstrates an increasing internal flexor moment (Fig. 2.7), which is generated by eccentric contraction of the hamstrings (Fig. 2.10), with power absorption (K4 in Fig. 2.8). This occurs in response to an external extensor moment generated by the inertia of the swinging shank, which would hyperextend the knee if it were not checked. The ankle moment remains negligible (Fig. 2.7), with very little power exchange (Fig. 2.8).

Terminal Foot Contact (Fig. 2.11)

The gait cycle ends at the next initial contact of the same foot (in this case, the right foot). Because it is confusing to refer to the *end* of the cycle as *initial* contact, it is sometimes known as *terminal foot contact*.

GROUND REACTION FORCES

The *force platform* (or force plate) is an instrument commonly used in gait analysis. It gives the total force applied by the foot to the ground, although it does not show the distribution of different parts of this force (e.g., heel and forefoot) on the walking surface. Some force platforms give only one component of the force (usually vertical), but most give a full three-dimensional description of the ground reaction force vector. The electrical output signals may be processed to produce three components of force (vertical or Fz, medial-lateral or Fy and fore-aft [anterior-posterior] or Fx). As force plates can be mounted in multiple directions, it is best to describe the forces as F_v, F_{A-P} and F_{M-L} to avoid confusion. The force plate also produces the two coordinates of the centre of pressure and the moments about the vertical axis. The *centre of pressure* is the point on the ground through which a single resultant force appears to act, although in reality the total force is made up of innumerable small force vectors, spread out across a finite area on the surface of the platform.

Since the ground reaction force is a three-dimensional vector, it would be preferable to display it as such for the purposes of interpretation. Unfortunately, this is seldom practical. The most common form of display is that shown in Fig. 2.20, where the three components of force are plotted against time for the walk shown in the previous figures. The sign convention used in Fig. 2.20 is the same as that used by Winter (1991), where the ground reaction force is positive upwards, forwards and to the right. Regrettably, there is no general agreement on sign conventions.

The vertical force shows a characteristic double hump, which results from an upward acceleration of the centre of gravity during early stance (F1), a reduction in downward force as the body 'flies' over the leg in mid-stance (F2) and a second peak due to deceleration (F3) as the downward motion is checked in late stance. The fore-aft (or antero-posterior) trace from the right foot shows braking during the first half of the stance phase (F4) and propulsion during the second half (F5). The left foot shows the same pattern, but with the direction of the lateral force reversed. The lateral component of force is generally very small; for most of the stance phase of the right foot, the ground reaction force accelerates the centre of gravity towards the left side of the body, and during the stance phase of the left foot, the acceleration is towards the right side.

Plots of this type are difficult to interpret and encourage consideration of the force vector as separate components rather than as a three-dimensional whole. The butterfly diagram shown in Fig. 2.9 is an improvement on this, since it combines two of the force components (vertical and fore-aft) with the centre of pressure in the fore-aft direction. It

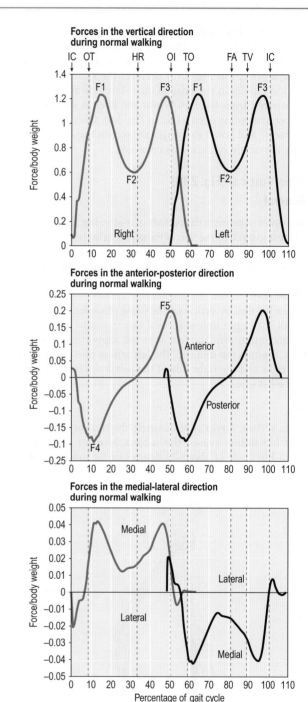

Fig. 2.20 Vertical, anterior-posterior and medial-lateral components of the ground reaction force, in newtons/ body weight, for right foot *(blue line)* and left foot *(black line)*. Abbreviations as in Fig. 2.5. See text for sign conventions.

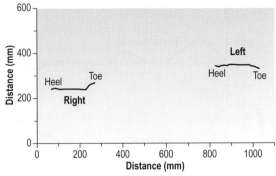

Fig. 2.21 View of the walking surface from above, showing the centre of pressure beneath the two feet, with the right heel contacting first and the subject walking towards the right of the diagram.

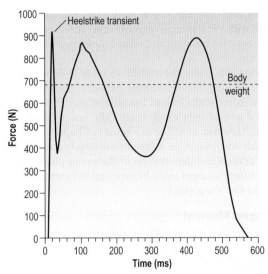

Fig. 2.23 Plot of vertical ground reaction force against time, showing the heelstrike transient in a particularly 'vigorous' walker wearing hard-heeled shoes. Unfiltered data from Bertec force platform, sampled at 1000 Hz.

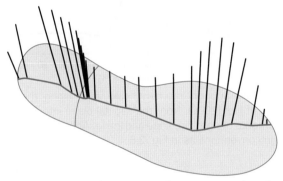

Fig. 2.22 Foot outline, centre of pressure and sagittal plane representation of ground reaction force vector; right foot of a normal male subject walking in shoes.

also preserves information on timing, since the lines representing the force vector are at regular intervals (10 ms in this case). Butterfly diagrams for the frontal and transverse planes are more difficult to interpret and are seldom used.

The other type of information commonly derived from the force platform is the position of the centre of pressure of the two feet on the ground, as shown in Fig. 2.21, again, for the same walk. This may be used to identify abnormal patterns of foot contact, including an abnormal toe-out or toe-in angle. The step length and walking base can also be measured from this type of display, provided there is an identifiable initial contact.

Should the pattern of foot contact be of particular interest, it is preferable to combine the data on the centre of pressure with an outline of the foot obtained by some other means (such as chalk or ink on the floor). This type of display, with the addition of a sagittal plane representation of

the ground reaction force vector, is shown in Fig. 2.22 for a normal male subject wearing shoes. The trace shows initial contact at the back of the heel on the lateral side, with progression of the centre of force along the middle of the foot to the metatarsal heads, where it moves medially, ending at the hallux. The spacing of the vectors shows how long the centre of pressure spends in any one area. It is worth noting that there is a cluster of vectors just in front of the edge of the heel where the shoe is not in contact with the ground, again pointing out the fact that the centre of pressure is merely the average of a number of forces acting beneath the foot.

There is considerable variation among individuals as to how much force is applied to the ground at initial contact. In some cases this leads to what is known as a heelstrike transient. This is caused by the swinging limb hitting the ground with a backward velocity, causing a rapid impact peak as the leg decelerates. Fig. 2.23 shows the vertical component of the ground reaction force from a fast walk, in hard-heeled shoes, by an individual with a marked heelstrike. The data were recorded at 1000 Hz from a Bertec force platform, which has a particularly high-frequency response. It has been suggested that transient forces in the joints, resulting from the heelstrike, may cause degenerative arthritis (Radin, 1987). The heelstrike transient represents the transfer of momentum from the moving leg to the ground. It is a fairly short event, typically lasting 10 to

20 ms, and can only be observed using measuring equipment with a fast enough response time. A review article on the heelstrike transient and related topics was published by Whittle (1999).

Moments about the vertical axis are seldom reported. In comparing these moments between normal children and children with clubfeet, Sawatzky et al. (1994) were surprised to find only small, statistically insignificant differences. However, as will be explained in Chapter 4, Methods of Gait Analysis, these moments are largely a result of the acceleration and deceleration of the swing phase leg, and only minor changes could be expected to be introduced by the foot on the ground.

Support Moment

Winter (1980) coined the term *support moment* to describe the sum of the sagittal plane moments about the hip, knee and ankle joints:

$$MS = MH + MK + MA \qquad \text{Winter (1980)}$$

where MS, MH, MK and MA are the support, hip, knee and ankle moments, respectively.

Winter noted that the support moment was far less variable than its individual components, suggesting that a decreased moment about one joint could be compensated for by an increased moment about one or both of the other joints. However, it was difficult to interpret this in biomechanical terms, since the sign convention was based on flexion and extension rather than on clockwise and anticlockwise moments, which caused the direction of the knee moment to be opposite to that of the hip and ankle moments. Hof (2000) published a justification for the support moment and suggested that it is responsible for preventing collapse of the knee. Based on his analysis, he suggested the following revised formula for its calculation:

$$MS = \tfrac{1}{2} MH + MK + \tfrac{1}{2} MA \quad \text{Hof (2000)}$$

Fig. 2.24 illustrates the support moment calculated from the sagittal plane hip, knee and ankle internal moments from the normal subject used for illustration throughout this chapter, using the formula suggested by Hof (2000). Anderson and Pandy (2003) suggested that a better alternative to the support moment would be the sum of the vertical components of force from individual muscles during walking.

ENERGY CONSUMPTION

It is relatively easy to measure the energy consumption of a vehicle, but much more difficult to make equivalent measurements of human walking, for two reasons. Firstly,

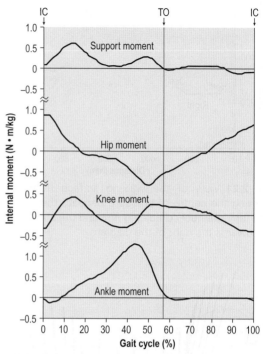

Fig. 2.24 Support moment, calculated using the formula of Hof (2000), from the sagittal plane internal joint moments of right hip, knee and ankle. Abbreviations and sign conventions as in Fig. 2.5.

there is a clear relationship between the fuel level in the tank of a vehicle and the amount of energy that has been used, whereas knowing how much food a person has eaten gives no information on the energy consumed in a particular activity. Secondly, a vehicle which is switched off uses no energy, whereas people use metabolic energy all the time, whether they are walking or not.

The first problem, that of measuring fuel consumption, can be solved by measuring not the fuel consumed but the oxygen which is used to oxidise it. Measurements of oxygen uptake, while not particularly pleasant for the subject (who has to wear a face mask or mouthpiece), are nonetheless perfectly practical and are used routinely to measure the metabolic cost of different activities.

The second problem, the lack of a suitable baseline for energy consumption measurements in humans, is not easy to solve and requires a different way of thinking about the topic. The energy used by a person who is walking can be divided into three parts:
1. The muscles used for walking consume energy, as they accelerate and decelerate the trunk and the limb segments in different directions.

2. There is an 'overhead' involved in walking, in that the expenditure of energy by the muscles involves increased activity by the heart and the muscles used in breathing, which themselves use energy. Energy is also expended in maintaining the upright posture.

3. The basal metabolic rate (BMR) is the energy expended by the body at rest to maintain normal body functions. This continual work makes up about 60% to 70% of the energy we use and includes respiration, cardiovascular function and the maintenance of body temperature.

The relationship between metabolic energy and physical energy is very complicated. As explained in Chapter 1, Basic Sciences, if a muscle undergoes an isometric contraction, it still uses energy, although its length does not change and the physical work it does is zero. In an eccentric contraction, when it lengthens under tension it uses metabolic energy, when in physical terms one would expect it to gain energy rather than to lose it.

In the past it has been usual to estimate the mechanical efficiency of walking by looking at the difference in oxygen consumption between the basal state and walking at a given speed. Inman et al. (1981) and Rose and Gamble (1994) suggested that it is more realistic to use standing or very slow walking as the baseline for measurements of faster walking. Despite these uncertainties, a figure of 25% is often quoted for the efficiency of the conversion of metabolic energy into mechanical energy in a wide range of activities, including walking. A comprehensive review of the energy expenditure of normal and pathological gait was given by Waters and Mulroy (1999).

The energy requirements of walking can be expressed in two ways: the energy used per unit time and the energy used per unit distance. Since energy expenditure is usually inferred from the oxygen used, these are generally known as *oxygen consumption* and *oxygen cost*, respectively.

Energy Consumption per Unit Time (Oxygen Consumption)

Inman et al. (1981) and Rose and Gamble (1994) quoted an equation, based on several studies, for the relationship between walking speed and energy consumption per unit time. Energy consumption included both the basal metabolism and the overheads. They showed, not surprisingly, that energy consumption per unit time is less for slow walking than for fast walking. Translating their equation into SI units, it becomes:

$$E_w = 2.23 + 1.26\,v^2$$

where E_w is the energy consumption in watts per kilogram of body mass and v is the speed in m/s.

As an example of the application of this equation, a 70-kg person walking at 1.4 m/s, which is a typical speed for adults, would consume energy at a rate of 330 W. The term v^2 in the equation shows that energy consumption increases as the square of the walking speed.

Energy Consumption per Unit Distance (Oxygen Cost)

The energy consumption per metre walked, also known as *energy cost*, has a less straightforward relationship with walking speed, as both very slow and very fast walking speeds use more energy per metre than intermediate walking speeds. The equation describing this relationship, again converted into SI units, is:

$$E_m = 2.23\,/\,v + 1.26\,v$$

where E_m is the energy consumption in joules per metre per kilogram of body mass and v is the speed in m/s. The energy cost of walking is higher in children and decreases steadily with age up to adulthood.

Minimum energy usage is predicted by this equation at a speed of 1.33 m/s. A 70-kg person walking at this speed would use 235 J/m, or 235 kJ/km. A typical candy bar contains around 1000 kJ and would thus supply enough energy to walk 4.26 km, or more than 2.5 miles!

The preceding equations merely give average values for adults, which may be modified by age, gender, walking surface, footwear and so on. Pathological gait is frequently associated with an energy consumption which is considerably above average values, due to some combination of abnormal movements, muscle spasticity and co-contraction of antagonistic muscles. To provide a baseline for studies of pathological gait, Waters et al. (1988) made a detailed study of the energy consumption of 260 normal children and adults of both genders, walking at a variety of speeds.

Optimisation of Energy Usage

If people were fitted with wheels, very little energy would be needed for locomotion on a level surface, and some of the energy expended in going uphill would be recovered when coming down again. For this reason, both wheelchairs and bicycles are remarkably efficient forms of transport, although much less versatile than legs. During walking, each leg in turn has to be started and stopped, and the body's centre of gravity rises, falls and moves from side to side. All of these movements use energy. Despite this, walking is not as inefficient as it might be due to two forms of optimisation: those involving transfers of energy and those which minimise the displacement of the centre of gravity.

Energy Transfers

Two types of energy transfer occur during walking: an exchange between potential and kinetic energy and the transfer of energy between one limb segment and another. The most obvious exchange between potential and kinetic energy is in the movement of the trunk. During the double support phase, the trunk is at its lowest vertical position with its highest forward speed. During the first half of the single support phase, the trunk is lifted up by the supporting leg, converting some of its kinetic energy into potential energy as its speed reduces. During the latter part of the single support phase, the trunk drops down again in front of the supporting leg and reduces its height whilst picking up speed again. These exchanges between potential and kinetic energy are the same as in a child's swing, in which the potential energy at the highest point in its travel is converted into kinetic energy as it swings downwards, then back into potential energy again as it swings up the other side.

As well as the vertical motion of the trunk, there are other exchanges between potential and kinetic energy in walking. The twisting of the shoulder girdle and pelvis in opposite directions stores potential energy as tension in the elastic structures, which is converted to kinetic energy as the trunk untwists and then back to potential energy again as the trunk twists the other way.

Winter et al. (1976) studied the energy levels of the limb segments and of the quaintly named HAT (head, arms and trunk). These authors criticised some earlier studies that had included the kinetic energy of linear motion but had neglected the kinetic energy due to rotation, which is responsible for about 10% of the total energy of the shank. Winter et al. studied only the sagittal plane, regarding energy exchanges in the other planes as negligible. They confirmed the exchange between potential and kinetic energy, described earlier, and estimated that roughly half of the energy of the HAT segment was conserved in this way. The thigh conserved about one-third of its energy by exchanges of this sort and the shank virtually none. They also noted that the changes in total body energy were less than the changes in energy of the individual segments, indicating a transfer of energy from one segment to another. In one subject, during a single gait cycle, the energy changes were shank 16 J, thigh 6 J and HAT 10 J, for a total of 32 J. However, the total body energy change was only 22 J, indicating a saving of 10 J by intersegment transfers. Siegel et al. (2004) performed a detailed analysis on the relationship between lower limb joint moments and mechanical energy during gait.

THE SIX DETERMINANTS OF GAIT

The six optimisations used to minimise the excursions of the centre of gravity were called the *determinants of gait* by Saunders et al. (1953) in a classic paper, the main points of which were reiterated, with slight changes, by Inman et al. (1981) and Rose and Gamble (1994). A brief description is given here, but one of these sources should be consulted for a detailed and well-illustrated account. The fourth and fifth determinants were combined in the original descriptions, but for the purposes of clarity, the present authors have separated them and made other minor changes.

For more than 50 years after their first publication, the determinants of gait were generally accepted and have been redescribed in numerous publications, including previous editions of the present book. However, it has more recently been suggested in a series of publications (e.g., Della Croce et al., 2001; Gard and Childress, 1997) that although these motions certainly occur, some of them may play little or no part in reducing energy expenditure. Kerrigan (2003) suggested that only the fifth determinant of gait, foot mechanism, significantly reduces the vertical excursions of the centre of mass. Baker et al. (2004) rejected the notion that energy is conserved by restricting the vertical movements of the centre of gravity and proposed instead that energy is mainly conserved by a backward-and-forward exchange between potential energy and kinetic energy, as described earlier. However, having provided these warnings, we will nonetheless reiterate the original descriptions by Saunders et al. (1953)! The six determinants of gait are as follows.

1. Pelvic Rotation

If the knee is kept straight, a movement of the hip from a flexed position to an extended one, such as occurs in the stance phase of gait, will result in the centre of mass of the body moving forwards, but also in its rising and then falling again. The amount of forward movement and the amount of rising and falling both depend on the total angle through which the hip joint moves from flexion to extension (Fig. 2.25A). Since the forward movement is equal to the stride length, it follows that the greater the stride length, the greater will be the angles of flexion and extension of the hip and the more the centre of mass will move vertically between its highest and lowest positions. The first determinant of gait is the way in which the pelvis twists about a vertical axis during the gait cycle, bringing each hip joint forwards as that hip flexes and backwards as it extends. This means that for a given stride length, the hip joint itself moves forwards through a smaller distance than the foot so that less flexion and extension of the hip is required. A proportion of the stride length thus comes from the forward-and-backward movement of the hip joint. The reduction in the range of hip flexion and extension leads to a reduction in the vertical movement of the hip (Fig. 2.25B).

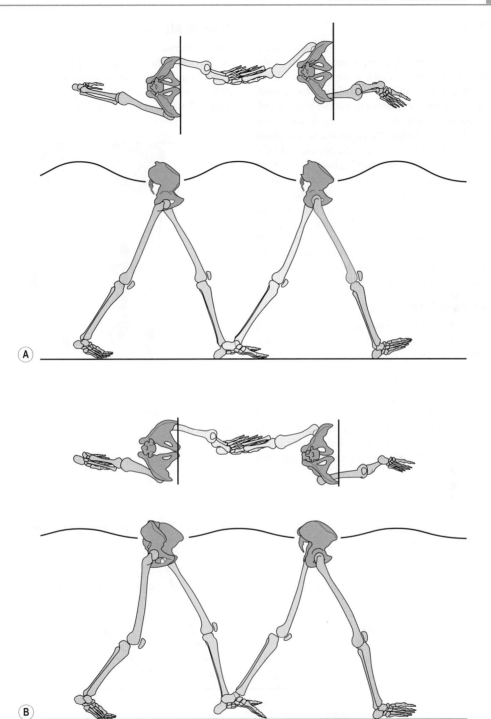

Fig. 2.25 The first determinant of gait. Pelvic rotation and vertical movement of the centre of mass; if the pelvis did not rotate, the whole of the stride length would come from hip flexion and extension (A). Pelvic rotation about a vertical axis or transverse plane reduces the angle of hip flexion and extension, which in turn reduces the vertical movement of the hip (B).

2. Pelvic Obliquity

As described in the preceding section, flexion and extension of the hip are accompanied by a rise and fall in the height of the hip joint. If the pelvis were to remain level, the trunk would follow this up-and-down movement. However, the second determinant of gait is the way the pelvis tips about an anteroposterior axis, raising first one side and then the other so that when the hip of the stance phase leg is at its highest point, the pelvis slopes downwards, resulting in the hip of the swing phase leg being lower than that of the stance phase leg. Since the height of the trunk does not depend on the height of either hip joint alone but on the average of the two of them, this pelvic obliquity reduces the total vertical excursion of the trunk (Fig. 2.26). However, it can only be achieved if the swing phase leg can be shortened sufficiently to clear the ground (normally by both flexing the knee and dorsiflexing the ankle), when the height of its hip joint is reduced.

3. Knee Flexion in Stance Phase

The third, fourth and fifth determinants of gait (Fig. 2.27) are concerned with adjusting the effective length of the leg, by lengthening it at the beginning and end of the stance phase and shortening it in the middle, to keep the hip height as constant as possible. The third determinant is the stance phase flexion of the knee. As the femur passes from flexion of the hip into extension, if the leg remained straight, the hip joint would rise and then fall, as described earlier. However, flexion of the knee shortens the leg in the middle of this movement, reducing the height of the apex of the curve.

4. Ankle Mechanism

Complementary to the way in which the apex of the curve is lowered by shortening the leg in the middle of the movement from hip flexion to extension, the beginning of the curve is elevated by lengthening the leg at the start of the stance phase, or initial contact. This is achieved by the fourth

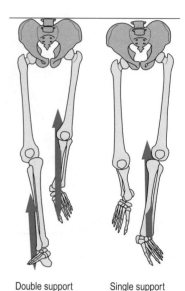

Double support   Single support

Fig. 2.26 Second determinant of gait. The vertical movement of the trunk is less than that of the hip, due to pelvic obliquity in the coronal plane, about an anteroposterior axis.

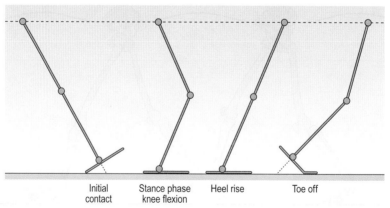

Initial contact   Stance phase knee flexion   Heel rise   Toe off

Fig. 2.27 Third, fourth and fifth determinants of gait. Stance phase knee flexion shortens the leg in mid-stance (third determinant); backward projection of the heel at initial contact lengthens the leg (fourth determinant), as does forward projection of the forefoot during pre-swing (fifth determinant).

determinant of gait, or the ankle mechanism. Because the heel sticks out behind the ankle joint, it effectively lengthens the leg during the loading response (Fig. 2.27).

5. Foot Mechanism

In the same way that the heel lengthens the leg at the start of the stance phase, the forefoot lengthens it at the end of the stance phase, in the fifth determinant, or the terminal rocker (Fig. 2.27). From the time of heel rise, the effective length of the lower leg increases as the ankle moves from dorsiflexion into plantarflexion.

6. Lateral Displacement of the Body

The first five determinants of gait are all concerned with reducing the vertical excursions of the centre of gravity. The sixth is concerned with side-to-side movement. If the feet were as far apart as the hips, the body would need to tip from side to side to maintain balance during walking (Fig. 2.28A). By keeping the walking base narrow, little lateral movement is needed to preserve balance (Fig. 2.28B). The reduction in lateral acceleration and deceleration leads to a reduction in the use of muscular energy. The main adaptation which allows the walking

base to be narrow is a slight valgus angulation of the knee, which permits the tibia to be vertical whilst the femur inclines inwards, from a slightly adducted hip.

It should be obvious that although the six determinants of gait have been described separately, they are integrated during each gait cycle. The combined effect is a much smoother trajectory for the centre of gravity and (according to the original description) a much lower energy expenditure. According to Perry (1992), the determinants of gait reduce the vertical excursions of the trunk by about 50% and the horizontal excursions by about 40%.

STARTING AND STOPPING

To this point, only steady-state continuous walking has been considered. In order to achieve that state, the individual has to start off, and when they reach their destination, they have to stop. Winter (1995) gave a good description of gait initiation and gait termination. In gait initiation, from standing on both feet, the body weight is shifted to one foot, thus permitting the other foot to be lifted off the ground and moved forwards. As an example, suppose the left foot was going to move forwards first (swing limb), whilst the body

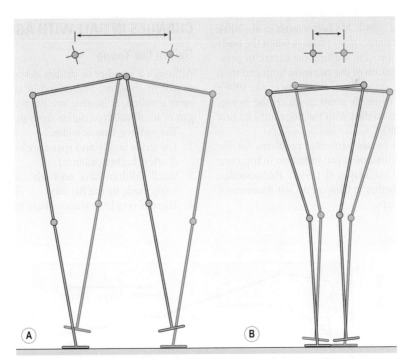

Fig. 2.28 Sixth determinant of gait. If the feet are placed on the ground far apart (A), large side-to-side movements of the centre of gravity would be necessary to maintain balance; having them closer together (B) reduces the size of these movements.

weight is supported by the right foot (stance limb). The shifting of weight over the right foot is achieved by a brief initial push, backwards and to the left, by the left foot. This moves the centre of gravity of the body forwards and to the right. Once the centre of gravity is over the right foot, it is safe to lift the left foot off the ground and move it forwards. At the same time, the trunk has started to move forwards. The left foot lands on the ground in front of the subject, with a step that is almost exactly the same as in steady-state gait. Body weight is transferred to the left leg, the right foot leaves the ground with a normal toe off, and the subject is walking. By the time the left foot has contacted the ground, the trunk is moving forwards at around 85% of the final walking speed and only one or two more steps are needed before the steady-state speed and pattern are achieved. Probably the slowest adjustment is that of side-to-side balance, which may need several steps to stabilise.

One way gait initiation has been assessed is by considering the mechanical process by which the body's centre of mass decouples, or separates from, the centre of pressure, causing the body to fall forwards about the ankle joint (Halliday et al., 1998; Henriksson and Hirschfeld, 2005; Martin et al., 2002; Viton et al., 2000). The process of gait initiation has been generally accepted to consist of two phases, the first of these being the preparatory (postural) phase and the second being a stepping (monopodal) phase (Fiolkowski et al., 2002; Mickelborough et al., 2004; Viton et al., 2000). The preparatory phase is when the body begins the decoupling process, shifting the centre of pressure initially in the direction of the swinging limb and then in the direction of the stance limb (Halliday et al., 1998). The stepping phase is from the point at which the swinging limb is no longer in contact with the floor until its first initial contact (Fig. 2.29).

A pathology which causes particular problems for the initiation of gait is parkinsonism; gait initiation in this condition was reviewed by Halliday et al. (1998). Parkinsonian gait will be discussed further in Chapter 6, Gait Assessment in Neurological Disorders.

Less research has been done on gait termination, although it appears to present a greater challenge to the neural control system. Gait termination involves a stance phase on one side, which is not followed by a swing phase, and a shortened swing phase on the other, with the moving foot being placed beside the stationary one. If the left foot is the swinging one, the forces to terminate gait are provided by the right foot, which directs the ground reaction force forwards and to the right, thus applying a backward and leftward force to the body's centre of gravity, arresting its forward motion and bringing it to the midpoint between the feet. The left foot is then planted on the ground beside the right one and the walk has terminated.

OTHER VARIETIES OF GAIT

As well as normal walking, humans walk backwards, skip, run, ascend and descend slopes and stairs, step over obstacles and carry loads in their hands, on their backs or on their heads. These other types of locomotion have been studied to a greater or lesser extent, particularly because patients with abnormal neuromuscular systems frequently have greater problems with some of these activities than they do with walking. However, such considerations are beyond the scope of the present text.

CHANGES IN GAIT WITH AGE

Gait in the Young

Although a number of studies described the development of gait in children, Sutherland et al. (1988) is one of the most detailed. Following are the main ways in which the gait of small children differs from that of adults:
1. The walking base is wider.
2. The stride length and speed are lower and the cycle time shorter (higher cadence).
3. Small children have no heelstrike, with initial contact being made by the flat foot.
4. There is very little stance phase knee flexion.

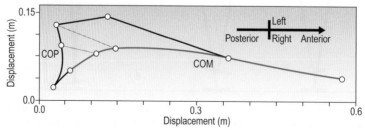

Fig. 2.29 Centre of mass (COM) and centre of pressure (COP) during gait initiation.

5. The whole leg is externally rotated during the swing phase.
6. There is an absence of reciprocal arm swinging.

These differences in gait mature at different rates. The characteristics numbered (3), (4) and (5) in the preceding list have changed to the adult pattern by the age of 2, and (1) and (6) by the age of 4. The cycle time, stride length and speed continue to change with growth, reaching normal adult values around the age of 15.

Most children commence walking within 3 months of their first birthday. Prior to this, even young babies will make reciprocal stepping motions if they are moved slowly forwards whilst held in the standing position with their feet on the ground. However, this is not true walking, as there is little attempt to take any weight on the legs.

Fig. 2.30, which is based on data from Sutherland et al. (1988), shows the average sagittal plane motion at the hip, knee and ankle joints in 49 children between 11 and 13 months of age. It should be compared with Fig. 2.5, which shows the same parameters for a normal adult female. Sutherland et al. only gave the timing of initial contact and toe off on the two sides and used a different definition of hip angle; the data in Fig. 2.30 have been adjusted into extension by 15 degrees to make them comparable with the other figures in this book.

The pattern of hip flexion and extension differs from that in adults in that the degree of extension is reduced and the hip does not remain flexed for so long at the end of the swing phase. The knee never fully extends, but this is seen at all ages in Sutherland's data and may reflect the method of measurement. There is some stance phase knee flexion in infants, but it is both smaller in magnitude and earlier than in adults. The flexion of the knee in the swing phase is also somewhat reduced at the age of 1, and most adults have more swing phase flexion than is seen in Fig. 2.5.

Initial contact in small children is by the whole foot, with heelstrike being replaced by foot flat. The ankle is plantarflexed at initial contact and remains so into the early stance phase, in contrast to the adult pattern, in which the ankle is approximately neutral at initial contact but moves rapidly into plantarflexion. The pattern of dorsiflexion followed by plantarflexion through the remainder of the stance phase is essentially the same at all ages.

Since children are smaller than adults, it is not surprising that they walk with a shorter stride length and at a slower speed. Sutherland et al. (1988) showed that stride length is closely related to height and that the ratio of stride length to stature is similar to that found in adults. The change in stride length with age mirrors the change in height, showing a rapid increase up to age 4 and a slower increase thereafter. Todd et al. (1989) detailed the relationships between the height of children and their general

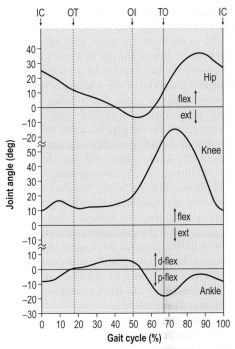

Fig. 2.30 Sagittal plane hip, knee and ankle angles in 1-year-old children. The hip angle has been moved into extension by 15 degrees to allow for a difference in measurement methods. Sign conventions and abbreviations as in Fig. 2.5. (Based on data from Sutherland et al., 1988.)

gait parameters. Small children walk with a short cycle time (rapid cadence), the mean at the age of 1 being about 0.70 s (171 steps/min). Cycle time increases with age but is still around 0.85 s (141 steps/min) at age 7, which is well below the typical adult values of 1.06 s (113 steps/min) for males and 1.02 s (118 steps/min) for females. The shorter cycle time partly compensates for the short stride length and the speed ranges from 0.64 m/s at age 1 to 1.14 m/s at age 7, compared with the typical adult values of 1.46 m/s for males and 1.30 m/s for females. Sutherland did not report on the gait of children beyond the age of 7 and did not distinguish between the results from male and female children. Table 2.1 gives the normal ranges for the general gait parameters in children, derived in part from Sutherland's data. However, values based on age alone may be misleading; stride length depends on height and walking speed, both of which may be lower in children with a disability than in normal children of the same age.

As can be seen in Fig. 2.30, the swing phase occupies a smaller proportion of the gait cycle in very small children than in adults, thus minimising the time spent in the less stable condition of single-legged stance. The relative duration of the swing phase increases with age, reaching the adult proportion around the age of 4 years. There is symmetry between the two sides at all ages. Sutherland et al. (1988) related the width of the walking base to the width of the body at the top of the pelvis, using the somewhat confusing 'pelvic-span/ankle-spread' ratio. Changing the measurement units for the sake of clarity, the walking base is about 70% of the pelvic width at the age of 1 year, falling to about 45% by the age of 3 1/2 years, at which level it remains until the age of 7. An average value for adults is not readily available, but it is probably less than 30%.

At the very youngest ages, the EMG patterns showed that there is a tendency to activate most muscles for a higher proportion of the gait cycle than in adults. With the exception of the triceps surae, adult patterns are established for most muscles by the age of 2. Sutherland et al. (1988) found that children could be divided into two groups depending on whether the triceps surae was activated in a prolonged (infant) pattern or the normal (adult) pattern. More than 60% of the children younger than 2 years of age showed the infant pattern; the proportion dropped to less than 30% by the age of 7. The authors speculated that this might relate to delayed myelination of the sensory branches of the peripheral nerves.

An excellent review of the main changes in gait occurring during childhood was given by Sutherland (1997). The gait of children younger than 2 was examined in detail by Grimshaw et al. (1998). The joint moments and powers of this same group were studied by Hallemans et al. (2005).

Gait in the Elderly

Cunha (1988) discussed the gait of the elderly and pointed out that many pathological gait disorders are incorrectly thought to be part of the normal ageing process. Identification of an underlying cause, which may be treatable, could result in improved quality of life for the patient and a reduced risk of falls and fractures. Cunha classified the causes of the gait disorders of old age as follows: neurological, psychological, orthopaedic, endocrinological, general, drugs, senile gait and associated conditions. He described the features of the gait in many conditions affecting the elderly and suggested a plan for the investigation and management of these patients.

A number of investigations have been made of the changes in gait which occur with advancing age, especially by Murray et al. (1969), who studied the gait of males up to the age of 87. The description which follows is confined to the effects of age on free-speed walking, although Murray et al. also examined fast walking. A companion paper

(Murray et al., 1970) studied the gait of females up to age 70. It did not provide as much information on the effects of age, but generally confirmed the observations made on males.

The gait of elderly people is subject to two influences: the effects of age itself and the effects of pathological conditions, such as osteoarthritis and parkinsonism, which become more common with advancing age. Provided patients with pathological conditions are carefully excluded, the gait of elderly people appears to be simply a 'slowed down' version of the gait of younger adults. Murray et al. (1969) were careful to point out that 'the walking performance of older men did not resemble a pathological gait'.

Typically, the onset of age-related changes in gait takes place in the decade from 60 to 70 years of age. There is a decreased stride length, a variable but generally increased cycle time (decreased cadence) and an increase in the walking base. Many other changes can also be observed, such as a relative increase in the duration of the stance phase as a percentage of the gait cycle, but most of them are secondary to the changes in stride length, cycle time and walking base. The speed (stride length divided by cycle time) is almost always reduced in elderly people. Table 2.1 gives normal ranges for the general gait parameters up to the age of 80.

Some of the differences between the gait of the young and the elderly are apparent in Fig. 2.31, which is taken from Murray et al. (1969). These authors suggested that

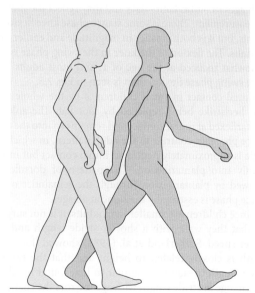

Fig. 2.31 Body position at right initial contact in older males *(left)* and younger males *(right)* (Murray et al., 1969).

the purpose of gait changes in the elderly is to improve the security of walking. Both decreasing the stride length and increasing the walking base make it easier to maintain balance whilst walking. Increasing the cycle time (reducing the cadence) leads to a reduction in the percentage of the gait cycle for which there is only single-limb support, since the increase in cycle length is largely achieved by lengthening the stance phase and hence the double support time.

Changes in the angular excursions of the joints in the elderly include a reduction in the total range of hip flexion and extension, a reduction in swing phase knee flexion and a reduction in ankle plantarflexion during the push off phase. However, all of these depend on both cycle time and stride length and are probably within normal limits if these factors are taken into account. Nigg et al. (1994) confirmed these observations in a detailed study on three-dimensional joint ranges of motion in walking, in male and female subjects from 20 to 79 years of age. The vertical movement of the head is reduced and its lateral movement increased, probably secondary to the changes in stride length and walking base, respectively.

The trajectory of the toe over the ground is modified in old age, giving an improved ground clearance during the first half of the swing phase. This is probably another mechanism for improving security. The heel rises less during pre-swing and the foot attitude is closer to the horizontal at initial contact, both of these changes being related to the reduction in stride length. There is also an increase in the angle of toe out in elderly people and changes in the posture and movements of the arms, the elbows being more flexed and the shoulders more extended. The reasons for these differences are not known.

The dividing line between normal and abnormal may be difficult to define in elderly people. A condition known as *idiopathic gait disorder of the elderly* has been described, which is essentially an exaggeration of the gait changes which normally occur with age and is characterised by a cautious attitude to walking, with a prolonged cycle time (low cadence), a short stride length and an increased step-to-step variability. For a comprehensive review of the changes in gait with advancing age, see Prince et al. (1997).

REFERENCES

Anderson, F.C., Pandy, M.G., 2003. Individual muscle contributions to support in normal walking. Gait Posture 17, 159–169.

Baker, R., Kirkwood, C., Pandy, M., 2004. Minimizing the vertical excursion of the center of mass is not the primary aim of walking. In: Eighth International Symposium on the 3-D Analysis of Human Movement. Tampa, Florida, USA, March 31–April 2, pp. 101–104.

Basmajian, J.V., De Luca, C.J., 1985. Muscles Alive: Their Functions Revealed by Electromyography. Lippincott Williams & Wilkins, Baltimore, MD.

Blanc, Y., Balmer, C., Landis, T., Vingerhoets, F., 1999. Temporal parameters and patterns of foot roll over during walking: normative data for healthy adults. Gait Posture 10, 97–108.

Bresler, B., Frankel, J.P., 1950. The forces and moments in the leg during level walking. American Society of Mechanical Engineers Transactions 72, 27–36.

Buczek, F.L., Sanders, J.O., Concha, M.C., et al., 2003. Inadequacy of an inverted pendulum model of human gait. In: Gait and Clinical Movement Analysis Society. Eighth Annual Meeting, Wilmington, Delaware, USA, pp. 185–186.

Burnfield, J.M., Tsai, Y.J., Powers, C.M., 2005. Comparison of utilized coefficient of friction during different walking tasks in persons with and without a disability. Gait Posture 22, 82–88.

Cavagna, G.A., Margaria, R., 1966. Mechanics of walking. J. Appl. Physiol. 21, 271–278.

Cham, R., Redfern, M.S., 2002. Changes in gait when anticipating slippery floors. Gait Posture 15, 159–171.

Cunha, U.V., 1988. Differential diagnosis of gait disorders in the elderly. Geriatrics 43, 33–42.

De Luca, C.J., 1997. The use of surface electromyography in biomechanics. J. Appl. Biomech. 13 (2), 135–163.

Della Croce, U., Riley, P.O., Lelas, J.L., et al., 2001. A refined view of the determinants of gait. Gait Posture 14, 79–84.

Fiolkowski, P., Brunt, D., Bishop, M., Woo, R., 2002. Does postural instability affect the initiation of human gait? Neurosci. Lett. 323 (3), 167–170.

Gage, J.R. (Ed.), 2004. The Treatment of Gait Problems in Cerebral Palsy. MacKeith Press, London.

Gard, S.A., Childress, D.S., 1997. The effect of pelvic list on the vertical displacement of the trunk during normal walking. Gait Posture 5, 233–238.

Grimshaw, P.N., Marques-Bruna, P., Salo, A., et al., 1998. The 3-dimensional kinematics of the walking gait cycle of children aged between 10 and 24 months: cross sectional and repeated measures. Gait Posture 7, 7–15.

Hallemans, A., De Clercq, D., Otten, B., et al., 2005. 3D joint dynamics of walking in toddlers. A cross- sectional study spanning the first rapid development phase of walking. Gait Posture 22, 107–118.

Halliday, S.E., Winter, D.A., Frank, J.S., et al., 1998. The initiation of gait in young, elderly and Parkinson's disease subjects. Gait Posture 8, 8–14.

Henriksson, M., Hirschfeld, H., 2005. Physically active older adults display alterations in gait initiation. Gait Posture 21 (3), 289–296.

Hof, A.L., 2000. On the interpretation of the support moment. Gait Posture 12, 196–199.

Inman, V.T., Ralston, H.J., Todd, F., 1981. Human Walking. Williams & Wilkins, Baltimore, MD.

Kerrigan, C.D., 2003. Discoveries from quantitative gait analysis. Gait Posture 18 (Suppl. 1), S13.

Lamoth, C.J.C., Beek, P.J., Meijer, O.G., 2002. Pelvis-thorax coordination in the transverse plane during gait. Gait Posture 16, 101–114.

Macellari, V., Giacomozzi, C., Saggini, R., 1999. Spatial-temporal parameters of gait: reference data and a statistical method for normality assessment. Gait Posture 10, 171–181.

Martin, M., Shinberg, M., Kuchibhatla, M., Ray, L., Carollo, J.J., Schenkman, M.L., 2002. Gait initiation in community-dwelling adults with Parkinson disease: comparison with older and younger adults without the disease. Phys. Ther. 82 (6), 566–577.

Mickelborough, J., van der Linden, M.L., Tallis, R.C., Ennos, A.R., 2004. Muscle activity during gait initiation in normal elderly people. Gait Posture 19 (1), 50–57.

Mueller, M.J., Sinacore, D.R., Hoogstrate, S., et al., 1994. Hip and ankle walking strategies: effect on peak plantar pressures and implications for neuropathic ulceration. Arch. Phys. Med. Rehabil. 75, 1196–1200.

Murray, M.P., 1967. Gait as a total pattern of movement. Am. J. Phys. Med. 46, 290–333.

Murray, M.P., Kory, R.C., Clarkson, B.H., 1969. Walking patterns in healthy old men. J. Gerontol. 24, 169–178.

Murray, M.P., Kory, R.C., Sepic, S.B., 1970. Walking patterns of normal women. Arch. Phys. Med. Rehabil. 51, 637–650.

Nene, A., Mayagoitia, R., Veltink, P., 1999. Assessment of rectus femoris function during initial swing phase. Gait Posture 9, 1–9.

Nigg, B.M., Fisher, V., Ronsky, J.L., 1994. Gait characteristics as a function of age and gender. Gait Posture 2, 213–220.

Oeffinger, D., Brauch, B., Cranfill, S., et al., 1999. Comparison of gait with and without shoes in children. Gait Posture 9, 95–100.

Paul, J.P., 1965. Bio-engineering studies of the forces transmitted by joints. (II) Engineering analysis. In: Kenedi, J.P. (Ed.), Biomechanics and Related Bioengineering Topics. Pergamon, Oxford, pp. 369–380.

Paul, J.P., 1966. Forces transmitted by joints in the human body. Proceedings of the Institute of Mechanical Engineers 181, 8–15.

Pedotti, A., 1977. Simple equipment used in clinical practice for the evaluation of locomotion. IEEE Transactions on Biomedical Engineering BME-24 456–461 BME-24.

Perry, J., 1974. Kinesiology of lower extremity bracing. Clin. Orthop. Relat. Res. 102, 18–31.

Perry, J., 1992. Gait Analysis: Normal and Pathological Function. Slack Incorporated, Thorofare, NJ.

Prince, F., Winter, D.A., Stergiou, P., et al., 1994. Anticipatory control of upper body balance during human locomotion. Gait Posture 2, 19–25.

Prince, F., Corriveau, H., Hébert, R., et al., 1997. Gait in the elderly. Gait Posture 5, 128–135.

Radin, E.L., 1987. Osteoarthrosis: what is known about its prevention. Clin. Orthop. Relat. Res. 222, 60–65.

Richards, J., 2018. The Comprehensive Textbook of Clinical Biomechanics. Churchill Livingstone.

Rose, J., Gamble, J.G., 1994. Human Walking, second ed. Williams & Wilkins, Baltimore, MD.

Rose, J., Gamble, J.G., 2005. Human Walking, third ed. Lippincott Williams Wilkins.

Sadeghi, H., 2003. Local or global asymmetry in gait of people without impairments. Gait Posture 17, 197–204.

Saunders, J.B.D.M., Inman, V.T., Eberhart, H.S., 1953. The major determinants in normal and pathological gait. J. Bone Joint Surg. Am. 35, 543–558.

Sawatzky, B.J., Sanderson, D.J., Beauchamp, R.D., et al., 1994. Ground reaction forces in gait in children with clubfeet – a preliminary study. Gait Posture 2, 123–127.

Sekiya, N., Nagasaki, H., 1998. Reproducibility of the walking patterns of normal young adults: test-retest reliability of the walk ratio (step-length/step-rate). Gait Posture 7, 225–227.

Shiavi, R., 1985. Electromyographic patterns in adult locomotion: a comprehensive review. J. Rehabil. Res. Dev. 22, 85–98.

Siegel, K.L., Kepple, T.M., Stanhope, S.J., 2004. Joint moment control of mechanical energy flow during normal gait. Gait Posture 19, 69–75.

Sutherland, D.H., 1984. Gait Disorders in Childhood and Adolescence. Williams & Wilkins, Baltimore, MD.

Sutherland, D.H., 1997. The development of mature gait. Gait Posture 6, 163–170.

Sutherland, D.H., Olshen, R.A., Biden, E.N., et al., 1988. The Development of Mature Walking. MacKeith Press, London.

Todd, F.N., Lamoreux, L.W., Skinner, S.R., et al., 1989. Variations in the gait of normal children. J. Bone Joint Surg. Am. 71, 196–204.

Viton, J.M., Timsit, M., Mesure, S., Massion, J., Franceschi, J.P., Delarque, A., 2000. Asymmetry of gait initiation in patients with unilateral knee arthritis. Arch. Phys. Med. Rehabil. 81 (2), 194–200.

Wall, J.C., Charteris, J., Turnbull, G.I., 1987. Two steps equals one stride equals what? The applicability of normal gait nomenclature to abnormal walking patterns. Clin. Biomech. (Bristol, Avon) 2, 119–125.

Waters, R.L., Mulroy, S., 1999. The energy expenditure of normal and pathological gait. Gait Posture 9, 207–231.

Waters, R.L., Lunsford, B.R., Perry, J., et al., 1988. Energyspeed relationship of walking: standard tables. J. Orthop. Res. 6, 215–222.

Whittle, M.W., 1999. Generation and attenuation of transient impulsive forces beneath the foot: a review. Gait Posture 10, 264–275.

Winter, D.A., 1980. Overall principle of lower limb support during stance phase of gait. J. Biomech. 13, 923–927.

Winter, D.A., 1983. Energy generation and absorption at the ankle and knee during fast, natural and slow cadences. Clin. Orthop. Relat. Res. 175, 147–154.

Winter, D.A., 1991. The Biomechanics and Motor Control of Human Gait, second ed. University of Waterloo Press, Waterloo, Ontario.

Winter, D.A., 1995. Human balance and posture control during standing and walking. Gait Posture 3, 193–214.

Winter, D.A., Quanbury, A.O., Reimer, G.D., 1976. Analysis of instantaneous energy of normal gait. J. Biomech. 9, 253–257.

3

Pathological and Other Abnormal Gaits

Michael Whittle, David Levine and Jim Richards

Although some variability is present in normal gait, particularly in the use of the muscles, there is an identifiable 'normal pattern' of walking, and a 'normal range' can be defined for all the variables which can be measured. Pathology of the locomotor system frequently produces gait patterns which are clearly 'abnormal'. Some of these abnormalities can be identified by eye, but others can only be identified by the use of appropriate measurement systems.

In order for a person to walk, the locomotor system must be able to accomplish four things:

- Each leg in turn must be able to support the body weight without collapsing.
- Balance must be maintained, either statically or dynamically, during single leg stance.
- The swinging leg must be able to advance to a position where it can take over the supporting role.
- Sufficient power must be provided to make the necessary limb movements and to advance the trunk.

In normal walking, all of these are achieved without any apparent difficulty and with modest energy consumption.

However, in many forms of pathological gait, they can be accomplished only by means of abnormal movements, which usually increase energy consumption, or by the use of walking aids such as canes, crutches, orthoses or braces. If even one of these four requirements cannot be met, the subject is unable to walk.

The pattern of gait is the outcome of a complex interaction between the many neuromuscular and structural elements of the locomotor system. Abnormal gait may result from a disorder in any part of this system, including the brain, spinal cord, nerves, muscles, joints and skeleton. Abnormal gait may also result from the presence of pain, so although a person is physically capable of walking normally, they find it more comfortable to walk in some other way.

The term *limp* is commonly used to describe a wide variety of abnormal gait patterns. However, dictionary definitions are unhelpful, with a typical one being 'to walk lamely'. Since the word has no clearly defined scientific meaning, it should only be used with caution in the context of gait analysis. The most appropriate use of the word

47

is probably for a gait abnormality involving some degree of asymmetry which is readily apparent to an untrained observer.

Since gait is the end result of a complicated process, a number of different original problems may manifest themselves in the same gait abnormality. For this reason, we will describe the abnormal gait patterns separately from the pathological conditions which cause them. This chapter begins with a detailed description of the most common abnormal gait patterns. This is followed by a description of the use of walking aids such as canes and orthotic walkers, and a description of treadmill gait.

SPECIFIC GAIT ABNORMALITIES

The following sections are based on a manual of lecture notes for student orthotists published by New York University (1986). Despite being almost 40 years old, the manual includes a very useful list of common gait abnormalities, all of which can be identified by eye. The manual criticises the common practice of identifying gait abnormalities by their pathological cause—for example, 'hemiplegic gait', which immediately suggests that all hemiplegics walk in the same way, which is far from true—and also neglects the changes in gait which may occur with the passage of time or as the result of treatment. The manual suggests that it is preferable to use purely descriptive terms, such as 'excessive medial foot contact'. This practice will be adopted in the following sections. Some of the gait abnormalities described in the New York University publication apply only to the gait of subjects wearing orthoses; these descriptions have been omitted from the present text.

The pathological gait patterns described may occur either alone or in combination. If in combination, they may interact, so the individual gait modifications may not exactly fit the descriptions. The list that follows is not exhaustive; a subject may use a variation of one of the general patterns or may use other gait patterns not listed here. When studying a pathological gait, particularly one which does not appear to fit into one of the standard patterns, it is helpful to remember that an abnormal movement may be performed for one of two reasons:

- The subject has no choice, as the movement is being 'forced' on them by weakness, spasticity or deformity.
- The movement is a compensation the subject is using to correct for some other problem which therefore needs to be identified.

Lateral Trunk Bending

Bending the trunk towards the side of the supporting limb during the stance phase is known as *lateral trunk bending*, *ipsilateral lean* or, more commonly, a *Trendelenburg gait*.

The purpose of the manoeuvre is generally to reduce the forces in the abductor muscles and hip joint during single leg stance.

Lateral trunk bending is best observed from the front (coronal plane) view. During the double support phase, the trunk is generally upright. But as soon as the swing leg leaves the ground, the trunk leans over towards the side of the stance phase leg, returning to the upright attitude again at the beginning of the next double support phase. The bending of the trunk may be *unilateral* (i.e., restricted to the stance phase of one leg) or it may be *bilateral* (i.e., with the trunk swaying from one side to the other) to produce a gait pattern known as *waddling*. In the examples which follow, the weight of the trunk is 452 N, corresponding to a mass of 46 kg, and the weight of the right leg is 147 N, corresponding to a mass of 15 kg.

Fig. 3.1 shows a schematic of the trunk, pelvis and hip joints when standing on both legs. The abductor muscles

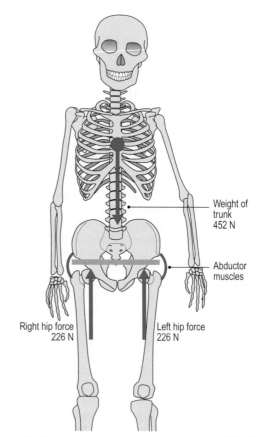

Weight of trunk 452 N

Abductor muscles

Right hip force 226 N

Left hip force 226 N

Fig. 3.1 Schematic of double legged stance. The force in each hip joint (226 N) is half the weight of the trunk (452 N). The abductors are not contracting.

are inactive and the weight of the trunk is divided equally between the two hip joints. Fig. 3.2 shows what happens in a normal individual when the right foot is lifted off the ground: the force through the left hip joint increases by a factor of six, from 226 N (23 kg or 51 lb) to 1510 N (154 kg or 339 lb). This increase in force is made up of three components:

1. The whole of the weight of the trunk is now supported by the left hip joint instead of being shared between the two hips, which produces an anticlockwise moment.
2. The weight of the right leg is now taken by the left hip instead of by the ground, which also produces an anticlockwise moment.
3. The left hip abductors (primarily the gluteus medius) contract, producing a clockwise moment to keep the pelvis from dropping on the unsupported side. The reaction force to this contraction passes through the left hip.

These three components contribute to the increased force in the left hip as follows:

1. The force from the trunk increases from 226 N to 452 N (23 kg or 51 lb) as this is now not shared.
2. The weight of the right leg increases to 147 N (15 kg or 33 lb).
3. The contraction of the abductors increases to 911 N (93 kg or 204 lb).

The result is a total increase of 1284 N (131 kg or 288 lb).

It should be noted that this example was invented for the purposes of illustration and the actual numbers should not be taken too seriously!

The four conditions which must be met if this mechanism is to operate satisfactorily are:

1. the absence of significant pain on loading,
2. adequate power in the hip abductors,
3. a sufficiently long lever arm for the hip abductors, and
4. a solid and stable fulcrum in or around the hip joint.

Should one or more of these conditions not be met, the subject may adopt lateral trunk bending in an attempt to compensate. The effect of lateral trunk bending on the joint force is shown in Fig. 3.3. There is no effect on components (1) and (2) of the increased force, but if the centre of gravity of the trunk is moved directly above the left hip, this eliminates the anticlockwise moment produced by the mass of the trunk. The abductors are now only required to contract with a force of 363 N (37 kg or 81 lb) to balance the anticlockwise moment provided by the weight of the right leg. There is thus a reduction of 548 N (56 kg or 123 lb) in the abductor contraction force and a corresponding reduction in the total joint force, from 1501 N down to 962 N. The numbers in the illustrations refer to standing; during the stance phase of walking, higher forces are to be expected due to the vertical accelerations of the centre of gravity, which cause the force transmitted through the leg to fluctuate above and below the body weight (see Fig. 2.20). However, these fluctuations tend to be less in pathological than in normal gait, since the vertical accelerations are less in someone walking with a shorter stride length. The numbers also suppose that the bending of the trunk brings its centre of gravity exactly above the hip joint. This is unlikely to happen in practice, but the principles remain the same, whether the centre of gravity is not deviated as far as the hip joint or even if it passes lateral to it. There are a number of conditions in which this gait abnormality is adopted. They are discussed in the following sections.

Painful Hip

If the hip joint is painful, as in osteoarthritis and rheumatoid arthritis, the amount of pain experienced usually depends to a very large extent on the force being transmitted through the joint. Since lateral trunk bending reduces the total joint force, Trendelenburg gait is extremely

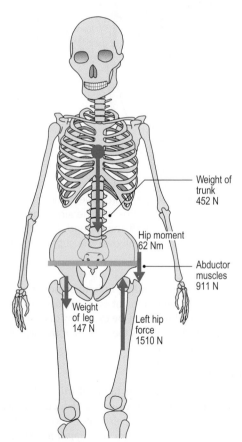

Fig. 3.2 Schematic of single legged stance on the left (the right leg is held up). The force in the left hip (1510 N) is the sum of (i) weight of trunk (452 N), (ii) weight of right leg (147 N) and (iii) contraction force of abductor muscles (911 N).

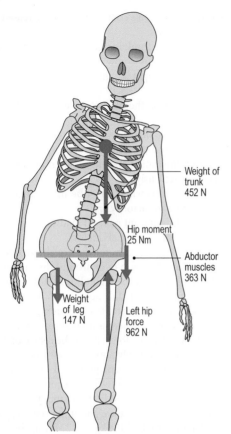

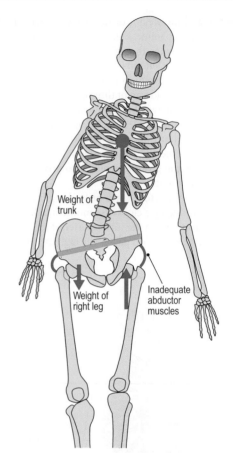

Fig. 3.3 Lateral trunk bending. Bringing the trunk across the supporting hip reduces the anti-clockwise moments about the left hip from 62 Nm to 25 Nm, permitting the pelvis to be stabilised by a smaller abductor force. The force in the left hip (962 N) is the sum of (i) weight of trunk (452 N), (ii) weight of right leg (147 N) and (iii) contraction force of abductor muscles (363 N).

Fig. 3.4 Trendelenburg's sign. Due to inadequate hip abductors, the pelvis drops on the unsupported side when one foot is lifted off the ground. To compensate, the subject bends the trunk over the supporting hip.

common in people with arthritis of the hip. Although it produces a useful reduction in force and hence in pain, the forces still remain substantial (962 N in Fig. 3.3), and these compensations can lead to overload of other parts of the musculoskeletal system. Therefore some form of definitive treatment is usually required.

Hip Abductor Weakness

If the hip abductors are weak, they may be unable to contract with sufficient force to stabilise the pelvis during single leg stance. In this case, the pelvis will dip on the side of the foot which is off the ground (Trendelenburg's sign, as opposed to Trendelenburg gait). In order to reduce the demands on the weakened muscles, the subject will usually

employ lateral trunk bending in both standing and walking to reduce the joint moment as far as possible (Fig. 3.4). Hip abductor weakness may be caused by disease or injury affecting either the muscles themselves or the nervous system which controls them.

Abnormal Hip Joint

Three conditions around the hip joint will lead to difficulties in stabilising the pelvis using the abductors: *congenital dislocation of the hip* (CHD, also known as *developmental dysplasia of the hip*), *coxa vara* and *slipped femoral epiphysis*. In all three, the effective length of the gluteus medius is reduced because the greater trochanter of the femur moves proximally, towards the pelvic brim. Since the muscle is shortened, it is unable to function efficiently and thus contracts with a reduced tension. In CHD and in severe cases of slipped femoral epiphysis, a further problem exists in that the normal hip joint is effectively lost and is replaced by a false hip joint, or pseudarthrosis. This abnormal joint is more laterally placed, giving a reduced lever arm for the abductor muscles, and it may fail to provide the solid and stable fulcrum required. The combination of reduced lever arm and reduced muscle force gives these subjects a powerful incentive to walk with lateral trunk bending (Fig. 3.5). In many cases, particularly in older people with CHD, the false hip joint becomes arthritic and they add a painful hip to their other problems. Pain is frequently also a factor in slipped femoral epiphysis.

Wide Walking Base

If the walking base is abnormally wide, there is a problem with balance during single leg stance. Rather than tip the whole body to maintain balance, as in Fig. 2.28A, lateral bending

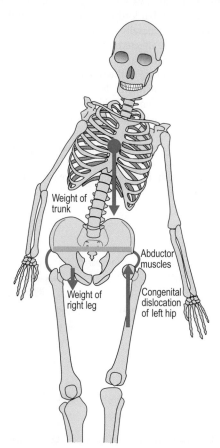

Fig. 3.5 Congenital dislocation of the hip. Both the working length and the lever arm of the hip abductors are reduced. To compensate, the subject bends the trunk over the supporting hip.

of the trunk may be used to keep the body's centre of gravity roughly over the supporting leg. In most cases, this will need to be done during the stance phase on both sides, leading to bilateral trunk bending and a waddling gait.

Unequal Leg Length

When walking with an unequal leg length, the pelvis tips downwards on the side of the shortened limb as the body weight is transferred to it. This is sometimes described as 'stepping into a hole'. The pelvic tilt is often accompanied by a compensatory lateral bend of the trunk.

Other Causes

Perry (2010) gives a number of other causes for lateral bending of the trunk, including adductor contracture, scoliosis and an impaired body image, typically following a stroke.

Anterior Trunk Bending

In anterior trunk bending, the subject flexes their trunk forwards early in the stance phase. If only one leg is affected, the trunk is straightened again around the time of opposite initial contact. But if both sides are affected, the trunk may be kept flexed throughout the gait cycle. This gait abnormality is best seen from the side (sagittal plane view).

One important purpose of this gait pattern is to compensate for an inadequacy (weakness) of the knee extensors. The left image in Fig. 3.6 shows that early in the stance phase, the line of action of the ground reaction force vector normally passes behind the axis of the knee joint and generates an

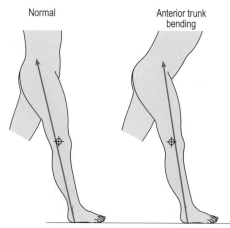

Fig. 3.6 Anterior trunk bending. In normal walking, the line of force early in the stance phase passes behind the knee; anterior trunk bending brings the line of force in front of the knee, to compensate for weak knee extensors.

external moment which attempts to flex it. This is opposed by the contraction of the quadriceps, to generate an internal extension moment. If the quadriceps are weak or paralysed, they cannot generate this internal moment, and the knee will tend to collapse. As shown in the right image in Fig. 3.6, anterior trunk bending is used to move the centre of gravity of the body forwards, which results in the line of force passing in front of the axis of the knee, producing an external extension (or hyperextension) moment. In addition to anterior trunk bending, subjects will sometimes keep one hand on the affected thigh whilst walking, to provide further stabilisation for the knee. Other causes for anterior trunk bending are equinus deformity of the foot, hip extensor weakness and hip flexion contracture (Perry, 2010).

Posterior Trunk Bending

One form of posterior trunk bending is essentially a reversed version of anterior trunk bending, in that early in the stance phase, the whole trunk moves in the sagittal plane, but this time backwards instead of forwards. Again, it is most easily observed from the sagittal plane view. The purpose of this is to compensate for ineffective (weak) hip extensors. The line of the ground reaction force early in the stance phase normally passes in front of the hip joint. This produces an external moment which attempts to flex the trunk forwards on the thigh and is opposed by contraction of the hip extensors, particularly the gluteus maximus. Should these muscles be weak or paralysed, the subject may compensate by moving the trunk backwards at this time, bringing the line of action of the external force behind the axis of the hip joint (Fig. 3.7).

A different type of posterior trunk bending may occur early in the swing phase, where the subject may throw the trunk backwards in order to propel the swinging leg forwards. This is most often used to compensate for weakness of the hip flexors or spasticity of the hip extensors, either of which makes it difficult to accelerate the femur forwards at the beginning of the swing. This manoeuvre may also be used if the knee is unable to flex, since the whole leg must be accelerated forwards as one unit, which greatly increases the demands on the hip flexors. Posterior trunk bending may also occur when the hip is ankylosed (fused), with the trunk moving backwards as the thigh moves forwards.

Increased Lumbar Lordosis

Many people have an exaggerated lumbar lordosis, but it is regarded as a gait abnormality only if the lordosis is used to aid walking in some way, which generally means the degree of lordosis varies during the course of the gait cycle. Increased lumbar lordosis is observed from the sagittal plane view and generally reaches a peak at the end of the stance phase on the affected side.

The most common cause of increased lumbar lordosis is a flexion contracture of the hip. It is also seen if the hip joint is immobile due to ankylosis. Both of these deformities cause the stride length to be very short, by preventing the femur from moving backwards from its flexed position. This difficulty can be overcome if the femur can be brought into the vertical (or even extended) position, not through movement at the hip joint but by extension of the lumbar spine, with a consequent increase in the lumbar lordosis (Fig. 3.8).

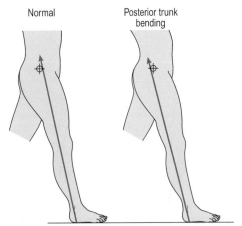

Fig. 3.7 Posterior trunk bending. In normal walking, the line of force early in the stance phase passes in front of the hip; posterior trunk bending brings the line of force behind the hip, to compensate for weak hip extensors.

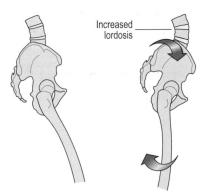

Fig. 3.8 Increased lumbar lordosis. When there is a fixed flexion deformity of the hip (left), the whole pelvis must rotate forwards for the femur to move into a vertical position (right), with a resultant increase in lumbar lordosis.

The orientation of the pelvis in the sagittal plane is maintained by the opposing pulls of the trunk muscles above and the limb muscles below. If there is muscle imbalance, for example, a weakness of the muscles of the anterior abdominal wall, weakness of the hip extensors or spasticity of the hip flexors, the subject may develop an excessive *anterior pelvic tilt*, again with an increase in the lumbar lordosis.

Functional Leg Length Discrepancy

Four gait abnormalities, circumduction, hip hiking, steppage and vaulting, are closely related in that they are designed to overcome the problem of a functional leg length discrepancy. A review on the topic of leg length discrepancy was published by Gurney (2002). An *anatomical* leg length discrepancy occurs when the legs are actually different lengths, as measured with a tape measure or, more accurately, by long-leg X-rays. A *functional* leg length discrepancy means the legs are not necessarily different lengths (although they may be) but that one or both are unable to adjust to the appropriate length for a particular phase of the gait cycle. In order for natural walking to occur, the stance phase leg needs to be 'functionally longer' than the swing phase leg. If it is not, the swinging leg collides with the ground and is unable to pass the stance leg. The way in which a leg is functionally lengthened (for the stance phase) is to extend at the hip and knee and to plantarflex at the ankle. Conversely, the way in which a leg is functionally shortened (for the swing phase) is to flex at the hip and knee and to dorsiflex at the ankle. Failure to achieve all the necessary flexions and extensions is likely to lead to a functional leg length discrepancy and hence to one of these gait abnormalities. This usually occurs as the result of a neurological problem. Spasticity of any of the extensors or weakness of any of the flexors tends to make a leg too long in the swing phase, as does the mechanical locking of a joint in extension. Conversely, spasticity of the flexors, weakness of the extensors or a flexion contracture in a joint makes the limb too short for the stance phase. Other causes of functional leg length discrepancy include musculoskeletal problems such as sacroiliac joint dysfunction.

An increase in functional leg length is particularly common following a stroke, where a foot drop (due to anterior tibial weakness or paralysis) may be accompanied by an increase in tone in the hip and knee extensor muscles.

The gait modifications designed to overcome the problem may either lengthen the stance phase leg or shorten the swing phase leg, thus allowing a normal swing to occur. They are not mutually exclusive, and a subject may use them in combination. The gait modification employed by a particular person may have been forced on them by the underlying pathology or it may have been a matter of chance. Two people with apparently identical clinical conditions may have found different solutions to the problem.

Circumduction

Ground contact by the swinging leg can be avoided if it is swung outwards, in a movement known as circumduction (Fig. 3.9). The swing phase of the other leg will usually be normal. The movement of circumduction is best seen from the coronal plane view. Circumduction may also be used to advance the swinging leg in the presence of weak hip flexors, by improving the ability of the adductor muscles to act as hip flexors whilst the hip joint is extended.

Hip Hiking

Hip hiking is a gait modification in which the pelvis is lifted on the side of the swinging leg (Fig. 3.10) by contraction of the spinal muscles and the lateral abdominal wall. The movement is best seen from the coronal plane view.

By tipping the pelvis up on the side of the swinging leg, hip hiking involves a reversal of the second determinant of gait (pelvic obliquity about an anteroposterior axis). It may also involve an exaggeration of the first determinant (pelvic rotation about a vertical axis), to assist with leg advancement. Leg advancement may also be helped by posterior trunk bending at the beginning of the swing phase.

According to the New York University manual (1986), hip hiking is commonly used in slow walking with weak hamstrings, since the knee tends to extend prematurely and thus to make the leg too long towards the end of the swing phase. It is seldom employed for limb lengthening due to plantarflexion of the ankle.

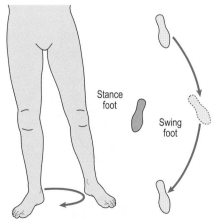

Stance foot

Swing foot

Fig. 3.9 Circumduction. The swinging leg moves in an arc rather than straightforwards, to increase the ground clearance for the swing foot.

Steppage

Steppage is a very simple swing phase modification consisting of exaggerated knee and hip flexion to lift the foot higher than usual for increased ground clearance (Fig. 3.11). It is best observed from the sagittal plane view. It is particularly used to compensate for a plantarflexed ankle,

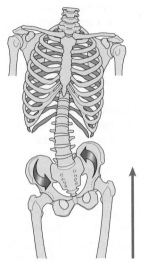

Fig. 3.10 Hip hiking. The swing phase leg is lifted by raising the pelvis on that side.

commonly known as *foot drop*, due to inadequate dorsiflexion control and/or strength, which will be described later.

Vaulting

The ground clearance for the swinging leg will be increased if the subject goes up on the toes of the stance phase leg, a movement known as vaulting (Fig. 3.12). This causes an exaggerated vertical movement of the trunk, which is both ungainly in appearance and wasteful of energy. It may be observed from either the sagittal or coronal plane view.

Vaulting is a stance phase modification, whereas the related gait abnormalities (circumduction, hip hiking and steppage) are swing phase modifications. For this reason, vaulting may be a more appropriate solution for problems involving the swing phase leg. As with hip hiking, it is commonly used in slow walking with hamstring weakness, when the knee tends to extend too early in the swing phase. It may also be used on the normal side of an above-knee amputee whose prosthetic knee fails to flex adequately during swing phase.

Abnormal Hip Rotation

As the hip is able to make large rotations in the transverse plane for which the knee and ankle cannot compensate, an abnormal rotation at the hip involves the whole leg, with the foot showing an abnormal toe-in or toe-out alignment. The gait pattern may involve both stance and swing phases and is best observed from the coronal plane view.

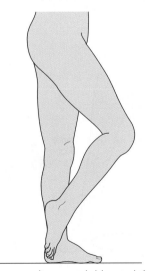

Fig. 3.11 Steppage. Increased hip and knee flexion improve ground clearance for the swing phase leg, in this case necessitated by a foot drop.

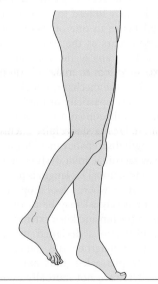

Fig. 3.12 Vaulting. The subject goes up on the toes of the stance phase leg to increase ground clearance for the swing phase leg.

Abnormal hip rotation may result from one of three causes:

- A problem with the muscles producing hip rotation
- A fault in the way the foot makes contact with the ground
- As a compensatory movement to overcome some other problem such as femoral anteversion or retroversion

Problems with the muscles producing hip rotation usually involve spasticity or weakness of the muscles which rotate the femur about the hip joint. For example, over-activity of the medial hamstrings in cerebral palsy may include an element of internal rotation. Imbalance between the medial and lateral hamstrings is a common cause of rotation; and weakness of the biceps femoris or spasticity of the medial hamstrings will cause internal rotation of the leg. Conversely, spasticity of the biceps femoris or weakness of the medial hamstrings will result in an external rotation.

A number of foot disorders will produce an abnormal rotation at the hip. Inversion of the foot, whether due to a fixed inversion (pes varus) or to weakness of the peroneal muscles, will internally rotate the whole limb when weight is taken on it. A corresponding eversion of the foot, whether fixed (pes valgus) or due to weakness of the anterior and posterior tibial muscles, will result in an external rotation of the hip.

External rotation may be used as a compensation for quadriceps weakness, to alter the direction of the line of force through the knee. This could be used as an alternative to, or in addition to, anterior trunk bending. External rotation may also be used to facilitate hip flexion, using the adductors as flexors, if the true hip flexors are weak. Subjects with weakness of the triceps surae may also externally rotate the leg to permit the use of the peroneal muscles as plantar flexors. Femoral anteversion or retroversion could cause excessive hip internal or external rotation, respectively.

Excessive Knee Extension

In the gait abnormality of excessive knee extension, the normal stance phase flexion of the knee is lost, to be replaced by full extension or even hyperextension, in which the knee is angulated backwards. This is best seen from the sagittal plane view.

A few causes of knee hyperextension have already been described: quadriceps weakness can be compensated for by keeping the leg fully extended using anterior trunk bending (Fig. 3.6), external rotation of the leg, or both, to keep the line of the ground reaction force from passing behind the axis of the knee joint. Other means of keeping the knee fully extended are pushing the thigh back by keeping one hand on it whilst walking, and using the hip extensors to snap the thigh sharply back at the time of initial contact.

Hyperextension of the knee, accompanied by anterior trunk bending, is seen quite frequently in people with paralysis of the quadriceps following poliomyelitis. The gait abnormality is clearly of great value to the subject, since without it they would be unable to walk. However, the external hyperextension moment is resisted by tension in the posterior joint capsule, which gradually stretches, allowing the knee to develop a hyperextension deformity known as *genu recurvatum*. As a result of this deformity, the joint frequently develops osteoarthritis in later life. This is illustrated in Fig. 3.13, which shows the left sagittal plane hip, knee and ankle angles during walking in a 41-year-old female whose quadriceps were paralysed on both sides by poliomyelitis at the age of 12. She walked very slowly, using two forearm crutches (cycle time 1.9 s; cadence 63 steps/min; stride length 1.00 m; speed 0.52 m/s). The knee hyperextended to 32 degrees during weightbearing but flexed

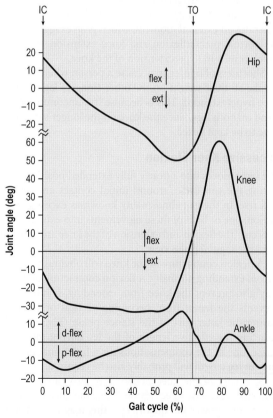

Fig. 3.13 Excessive knee extension. Sagittal plane hip, knee and ankle angles in a subject with paralysed quadriceps, showing gross hyperextension of the knee and increased extension of the hip. Abbreviations as in Fig. 2.5.

normally to 63 degrees during the swing phase. The hip extended more than in normal individuals, since hyperextension of the knee places the knee joint more posteriorly than usual, thus altering the angle of the femur.

In normal walking, an external moment attempts to hyperextend the knee during terminal stance. This is resisted by an internal flexor moment (see Fig. 2.7), generated primarily by the gastrocnemius. Should the gastrocnemius be weak, the knee may be pushed backwards into hyperextension. This may help with walking, since the leg lengthening required during pre-swing can be provided by extending the knee rather than by plantarflexing the ankle. However, there is a risk that the knee will go beyond full extension into hyperextension, with consequent damage to the posterior capsule.

Hyperextension of the knee is common in spasticity. One typical cause is overactivity of the quadriceps, which extends the knee directly. Another is spasticity of the triceps surae, which plantarflexes the ankle and causes the body weight to be taken through the forefoot. The resultant forward movement of the ground reaction force vector generates an external moment, which is an exaggeration of the normal plantarflexion and knee extension moments, which results in hyperextension of the knee.

Shortness of one leg may cause a person when standing to take all their weight on the other (longer) leg, with the knee hyperextended. This is because it is uncomfortable to stand on both legs, since the knee on the longer side would have to be kept flexed.

Excessive Knee Flexion

The knee moves into a nearly fully extended position twice during the gait cycle: around initial contact and around heel rise. In the gait abnormality known as excessive knee flexion, one or both of these movements into extension fail to occur. The flexion and extension of the knee are best seen from the sagittal plane view.

A flexion contracture of the knee will obviously prevent it from extending normally. A flexion contracture of the hip may also prevent the knee from extending, if hip flexion prevents the femur from becoming vertical or extended during the latter part of the stance phase (Fig. 3.14). By reducing the effective length of the leg during the stance phase, one of the compensations for a functional discrepancy in leg length will probably also be required.

Spasticity of the knee flexors may also cause the gait pattern of excessive knee flexion. Since the knee flexors are able to overpower the quadriceps, this may lead to other gait modifications, such as anterior trunk bending, to compensate for a relative weakness of the quadriceps. The knee may flex excessively following initial contact if the normal plantarflexion of the foot during loading response is

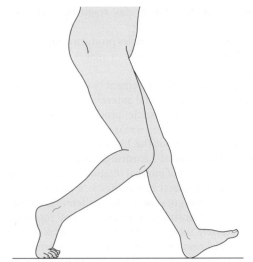

Fig. 3.14 Excessive knee flexion. In the late stance phase, there is increased knee flexion, caused by a flexion contracture of the hip.

prevented, through immobility of the ankle joint or a calcaneus deformity of the foot, preventing the force vector from moving forwards under the foot. Increased flexion of the knee may also be part of a compensatory movement, either to reduce the effective limb length in functional leg length discrepancy or as part of a pattern of exaggerated hip, knee and arm movements to make up for a lack of plantarflexor power in push off.

Inadequate Dorsiflexion Control

The dorsiflexors are active at two different times during the gait cycle; therefore, inadequate dorsiflexion control may give rise to two different gait abnormalities. During loading response, the dorsiflexors resist the external plantarflexion moment, thus permitting the foot to be lowered to the ground gently. If they are weak, the foot is lowered abruptly resulting in a *foot slap*. The dorsiflexors are also active during the swing phase, when they are used to raise the foot and achieve ground clearance. Failure to raise the foot sufficiently during initial swing may cause *toe drag*, where the foot catches on the ground. Both problems are best observed from the sagittal plane view and both make a distinctive noise. A subject with inadequate dorsiflexion control can often be diagnosed by ear, before they have come into view!

Inadequate dorsiflexion control may result from weakness or paralysis of the anterior tibial muscles or from these muscles being overpowered by spasticity of the triceps surae. An inability to dorsiflex the foot during the swing phase causes a functional leg length discrepancy, for which a number of compensations were described previously. Toe drag will only be observed if the subject fails to compensate. Toe drag may also occur if there is delayed flexion of the hip or knee in initial swing despite adequate dorsiflexion at the ankle.

Even if they suffer from inadequate dorsiflexion control, subjects with spasticity are frequently able to achieve dorsiflexion during swing phase, as flexion of the hip and knee are often accompanied by reflex dorsiflexion of the ankle in a primitive movement pattern related to the flexor withdrawal reflex.

Abnormal Foot Contact

The foot may be abnormally loaded so that the weight is primarily borne on only one of its four quadrants. Loading on the heel or forefoot is best observed from the side, and loading on the medial or lateral side is best observed from the coronal plane view, although some authorities state that the foot should always be observed from behind. Where a glass walkway is available, viewing the foot from below gives an excellent idea of the pattern of foot loading.

Loading of the heel occurs in the deformity known as *talipes calcaneus* (also known as *pes calcaneus*), where the forefoot is pulled up into extreme dorsiflexion (Fig. 3.15), usually as a result of muscle imbalance such as spasticity of the anterior tibial muscles or weakness of the triceps surae. Except in mild cases, weight is never taken by the forefoot and the stance phase duration is reduced by the loss of the terminal rocker. The reduced stance phase duration on the affected side reduces the swing phase duration on the opposite side, which in turn reduces the opposite step length and the overall stride length. The ground reaction force vector remains posterior, producing an increased external flexion moment at the knee.

In the deformity known as *talipes equinus* (or *pes equinus*) (Fig. 3.16), the forefoot is fixed in plantarflexion, usually through spasticity of the plantarflexors. In a mild equinus deformity, the foot may be placed onto the ground flat; in more severe cases, the heel never contacts the ground at all, and initial contact is made by the metatarsal heads in a gait pattern known as *primary toestrike*. Because the line of force from the ground reaction is displaced anteriorly, an increased external moment tending to extend the knee is present (plantarflexion/knee extension couple). The loss of the initial rocker shortens the stride length.

Excessive medial contact occurs in a number of foot deformities. Weakness of the inverters or spasticity of the evertors will cause the medial side of the foot to drop and to take most of the weight. In *pes valgus*, the medial arch is lowered, permitting weightbearing on the medial border of the foot. Increased medial foot contact may also be due to a valgus deformity of the knee accompanied by an increased walking base.

Excessive lateral foot contact may also result from a foot deformity, when the medial border of the foot is elevated or the lateral border is depressed due to spasticity or weakness. The foot deformity known as *talipes equinovarus* (Fig. 3.17) combines equinus with varus, producing a curved foot where all the load is borne by the outer border of the forefoot. Although the term *club foot* may be applied to any foot deformity, it is most commonly applied to talipes equinovarus.

Another form of abnormal foot contact is the *stamping* (walking with forcible steps) that commonly accompanies a loss of sensation in the foot, such as occurs in tabes dorsalis, the final stage of syphilis. The subject receives feedback on ground contact from the vibration caused by the impact of the foot on the ground.

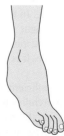

Fig. 3.16 Talipes equinus.

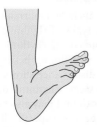

Fig. 3.15 Talipes calcaneus.

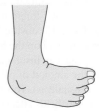

Fig. 3.17 Talipes equinovarus.

Abnormal Foot Rotation

Normal individuals place their foot on the ground approximately in line with the direction of their walk, typically with a few degrees of toe out. Pathological toe-in or toe-out angles may be produced by internal or external hip rotation, torsion (twisting) of the femur or tibia or deformity of the foot itself. An important consequence of an abnormal foot rotation is that it causes the ground reaction force to be in an abnormal position relative to the rest of the leg. For example, if the foot is internally rotated, the ground reaction force is more medial than normal, which will generate external adductor moments at the ankle and knee. In either internal or external foot rotation, the effective length of the foot is reduced in the direction of progression so that the ground reaction force during terminal stance and pre-swing is likely to be more posterior than normal. This reduces the lever arm for the triceps surae to generate an internal plantarflexion moment.

This is one example of a problem known as *lever arm disease* or *lever arm deficiency*, in which individuals with normal muscle strength are unable to generate sufficient internal joint moments due to a reduction in the length of a muscle's lever arm. This is particularly seen in individuals with cerebral palsy who have a severe degree of internal or external foot rotation; the resultant posterior placement of the ground reaction force increases the external moment flexing the knee.

Insufficient Push Off

In normal walking, weight is borne on the forefoot during the push off in pre-swing. In the gait pattern known as insufficient push off, the weight is taken primarily on the heel and there is no push off phase, as the whole foot is lifted off the ground at once. It is best observed from the sagittal plane view.

The main cause of insufficient push off is a problem with the triceps surae or Achilles tendon, which prevents adequate weightbearing on the forefoot. Rupture of the Achilles tendon and weakness of the soleus and gastrocnemius are typical causes. Weakness or paralysis of the intrinsic muscles of the foot may also prevent the foot from taking load through the forefoot. Insufficient push off may also result from any foot deformity if the anatomy is so distorted that it prevents normal forefoot loading. A talipes calcaneus deformity (Fig. 3.15) obviously makes it impossible to put any significant load on the forefoot.

Another important cause of insufficient push off is pain under the forefoot, if the amount of pain is affected by the degree of loading (as it usually is). This may occur in metatarsalgia and also when arthritis affects the metatarsophalangeal joints. The loss of the terminal rocker causes the foot to leave the ground prematurely, before the hip has fully extended. This reduces the stance phase duration on the affected side and hence the swing phase duration and step length on the opposite side, producing an asymmetry in gait timing.

Abnormal Walking Base

The walking base is usually in the range of 50 to 130 mm. In pathological gait, it may be either increased or decreased beyond this range. Although ideally determined by actual measurement, changes in the walking base may be estimated by eye, preferably from behind the subject.

An increased walking base may be caused by any deformity, such as an abducted hip or valgus knee, which causes the feet to be placed on the ground wider apart than usual. A consequence of an increased walking base is that increased lateral movement of the trunk is required to maintain balance, as shown in Fig. 2.28.

The other important cause of an increased walking base is instability and a fear of falling, which leads to the feet being placed wide apart to increase the area of support. This allows a margin of error in the positioning of the centre of gravity over the feet. This gait abnormality is likely to be present when there is a deficiency in the sensation or proprioception of the legs so that the subject is not quite sure where the feet are relative to the trunk. It is also used in cerebellar ataxia to increase the level of security in an uncoordinated gait pattern. Another effective way to improve stability is to walk with one or two canes.

A narrow walking base usually results from an adduction deformity at the hip or a varus deformity at the knee. Hip adduction may cause the swing phase leg to cross the midline in a gait pattern known as *scissoring*, which is commonly seen in cerebral palsy. In milder cases, the swing phase leg is able to pass the stance phase leg, but then moves across and in front of it. In more severe cases, the swinging leg is unable to pass the stance leg: it stops behind it, with the side-to-side positions of the two feet reversed. This is clearly a very disabling gait pattern, with a very short stride length and negative values for the walking base and for the step length on one side.

Rhythmic Disturbances

Gait disorders may include abnormalities in the timing of the gait cycle. Two types of rhythmic disturbance can be identified: an *asymmetrical* rhythmic disturbance shows a difference in the gait timing between the two legs; an *irregular* rhythmic disturbance shows differences between one stride and the next. Rhythmic disturbances are best observed from the side and may also be audible.

An *antalgic* gait pattern is specifically a gait modification that reduces the amount of pain a person is experiencing.

The term is usually applied to a rhythmic disturbance, in which as short a time as possible is spent on the painful limb and a correspondingly longer time is spent on the pain-free side. The pattern is *asymmetrical* between the two legs but is generally *regular* from one cycle to the next. A marked difference in leg length between the two sides may also produce a regular gait asymmetry of this type, as may a number of other differences between the two sides, such as joint contractures or ankylosis.

Irregular gait rhythmic disturbances, where the timing alters from one step to the next, are seen in a number of neurological conditions. In particular, cerebellar ataxia leads to loss of the pattern generator, which is responsible for a regular, coordinated sequence of footsteps. Loss of sensation or proprioception may also cause a rhythmic disturbance due to a general uncertainty about limb position and orientation.

Other Gait Abnormalities

A number of other gait abnormalities may be observed, either alone or in combination with some of the gait patterns described earlier. These include:

- abnormal movements such as intention tremors and athetoid movements;
- abnormal attitude or movements of the upper limb, including a failure to swing the arms;
- abnormal attitude or movements of the head and neck;
- sideways rotation of the foot following heelstrike;
- excessive external rotation of the foot during swing, sometimes called a whip; and
- rapid fatigue.

This account has concentrated on gait abnormalities which may be observed visually. However, a number of gait abnormalities can only be detected using kinetic/kinematic gait analysis systems. An example is the presence of an abnormal moment, such as the excessive internal varus moment which may be present in the knee of children with myelomeningocoele and which may predispose them to the development of osteoarthritis (Lim et al., 1998).

WALKING AIDS

The use of walking aids may modify the gait pattern considerably. While some people choose to use a walking aid to make it easier to walk (e.g., to reduce the pain in a painful joint), others are unable to walk without some form of aid. Although there are many detailed variations in design, walking aids, also called *assistive devices*, can be classified into three basic types: *canes*, *crutches* and *frames*. All three operate by supporting part of the body weight through the arm rather than the leg. While this is an effective way of coping with inadequacies of the legs, it frequently leads to

problems with the wrist and shoulder joints, which are simply not designed for the transmission of large forces. There is considerable variability in the way in which walking aids are used, and people will often use them in ways which do not quite fit the typical patterns described in the following sections.

Canes

The simplest form of walking aid is the cane, also known as a *walking stick*, by means of which force can be transmitted to the ground through the wrist and hand. Since the forearm muscles are relatively weak and the joints of the wrist fairly small, it is impossible to transmit large forces through a cane for any length of time. The moment which can be applied to the upper end of the cane is limited by the grip strength and the shape of the handle, since the hand tends to slip. For this reason, the major direction of force transmission is along the axis of the cane. Canes may be used for three purposes, which are often combined:

- To improve stability
- To generate a moment
- To take part of the load away from one of the legs

Improve Stability

Canes are frequently used by elderly and infirm people to improve their stability. This is achieved by increasing the size of the area of support, thus removing the need to position the centre of gravity over the relatively small supporting area provided by the feet. In those with only minor stability problems, a single cane may be used. This will not provide a secure supporting area during single limb support, but it does make it easier to correct for small imbalances. Since the cane is usually placed on the ground some distance away from the feet, giving a relatively long lever arm, a modest force through the cane will produce a substantial moment to correct for any positioning error. For maximum security, a person will need to use two canes so that a triangular supporting area is always available. This is provided by two canes and one foot during single limb support and by one cane and two feet during double limb support. If only a single cane is used, it will usually be advanced during the stance phase of the more secure leg. If two canes are used, they are usually advanced separately, during double limb support, to provide maximum stability at all times.

Generate a Moment

The use of a cane to generate a moment is illustrated in Fig. 3.18. A vertical force of 100 N (10 kg or 22 lb) is applied through the cane, which generates a clockwise moment, applied to the shoulder girdle and hence to the pelvis. This reduces the size of the moment which the hip muscles (463 N), less (iv) the force through the cane (100 N). Compare with Fig. 3.2 (force in left hip of 1510 N during single leg stance).

Reduce Limb Loading

When using a cane to remove some of the load from the leg, it is usually held in the same hand as the affected leg and placed on the ground close to the foot. In this way, load sharing can be achieved between the leg and the cane, even to the extent of removing the load entirely from the leg. The cane follows the movements of the affected leg, being advanced during the swing phase on that side. The person will normally lean sideways over the cane, in a lateral lurch, to increase the vertical loading on it and hence to reduce the load on the leg. A cane may be used in this way to relieve pain in the hip, knee, ankle or foot. If the cane is held in the opposite hand, as is often recommended, the lateral lurching can be avoided but the degree of off-loading is reduced.

Whichever of these three reasons a person has for using a cane, the degree of disability will determine whether one or two canes are used. It may be observed that a subject uses a cane in the opposite hand from what might have been expected. In some cases, they have simply not discovered that they would benefit more from using the cane in the other hand, but more often, the observer has failed to appreciate fully all the compensations which the subject has adopted.

There are a number of ways in which the simple cane can be modified, including many different types of handgrip. A particularly important variant on the simple cane is the *broad-based cane*, also known as a *Hemi* or *crab cane*, which may have three feet (*tripod*) or four feet (*tetrapod* or *quad cane*). This differs from the simple cane in that it will stand up by itself and will tolerate small horizontal force components, so long as the overall force vector remains within the area of its base. It is particularly helpful when standing up from the sitting position. The increased stability is gained at the expense of an increase in weight and particularly bulk, which may cause difficulties when going through doorways.

Crutches

The main difference in function between a crutch and a cane is that a crutch is able to transmit significant forces in the horizontal plane. This is because, unlike the cane, which is effectively fixed to the body at only a single point, the crutch has two points of attachment, one at the hand and one higher up the arm, which provide a lever arm for the transmission of a moment. Although there are many different designs of crutch, they fall into two categories: axillary crutches and forearm crutches. As with the cane,

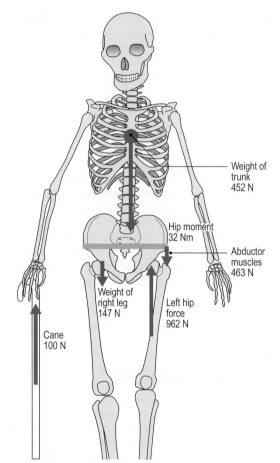

Fig. 3.18 The use of a cane to generate a clockwise moment reduces the contraction force of the hip abductors and hence the force in the hip joint, during right leg swing phase.

abductor muscles need to generate to keep the pelvis level. The contraction of these muscles is reduced from 911 N (93 kg or 204 lb) to 463 N (47 kg or 104 lb), a reduction of 448 N (56 kg or 123 lb). The total force in the hip joint is reduced by the sum of this amount and the force applied by the cane to the ground. For this mechanism to work, the cane must be held in the hand opposite the painful hip. A cane may also be used to generate a lateral moment at the knee and reduce the loading on one side of the joint. The cane is advanced during the swing phase of the leg it is protecting.

The force in the left hip (962 N) is the sum of (i) the weight of the trunk (452 N), (ii) the weight of the right leg (147 N) and (iii) the contraction force of the abductor it is also possible to have a broad-based crutch, ending in three or four feet.

Axillary crutches (Fig. 3.19, left), as their name suggests, fit under the axilla (armpit). They are usually of simple design, with a padded top surface and a handhold in the appropriate position. The lever arm between the axilla and the hand is fairly long and enough horizontal force can be generated to permit walking when both legs are straight and nonfunctional. A disadvantage of this type of crutch is that the axilla is not an ideal area for weightbearing and incorrect fitting or prolonged use may damage the blood vessels or nerves. Although some people use axillary crutches for many years, they are more suitable for short-term use—for instance, whilst a patient has a broken leg set in plaster.

There are many different types of *forearm crutches*, also called *elbow*, *Lofstrand* or *Canadian crutches* (Fig. 3.19, centre). They differ from axillary crutches in that the upper point of contact between the body and the crutch is provided by either the forearm or the upper arm rather than by the axilla. The lever arm is thus shorter than for an axillary crutch, although this is seldom a problem, and they usually run less risk of tissue damage and are lighter and more acceptable cosmetically. In the normal forearm crutch, most of the vertical force is transmitted through the hand, but the use of a gutter or platform permits more load to be taken by the forearm itself (Fig. 3.19, right).

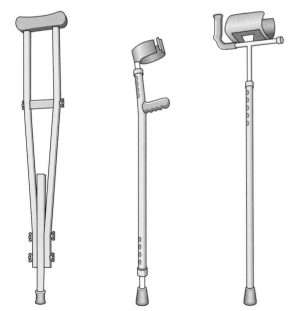

Fig. 3.19 Three types of crutches: axillary *(left),* forearm *(centre)* and gutter *(right).*

Walking Frames

The most stable walking aid is the *frame*, also called a *walker* or *Zimmer frame*, which enables the subject to stand and walk within the area of support provided by its base. Considerable force can be applied to the frame vertically and moderate forces can be applied horizontally, provided that the overall force vector remains within the area of support. The usual method of walking is first to move the frame forwards, then to take a short step with each foot, then to move the frame again, and so on. Walking is thus extremely slow, with a start-stop pattern. Although the subject is encouraged to lift the frame forwards at each step, they more often simply slide the frame along the ground.

A *rolling walker* is a variant on the walking frame in which the front feet are replaced by wheels. This makes it easier to advance, at the expense of a slight reduction in stability in the direction of progression. The mode of walking is very similar to that with the frame, except that it is easier to move forwards, since tipping the rolling walker lifts the back feet clear of the ground. Commonly, patients misuse the rolling walker by sliding it forwards rather than tipping it, and tennis balls are now frequently placed on the rear legs to facilitate sliding it due to its frequent occurrence. A further variant on the design is a *rollator*, which is a walking frame that has four wheels on all four legs and is equipped with hand-operated brakes. These devices also often have a seat in the middle, which the operator can use if they need to quickly sit, but the operator must turn around and face the opposite direction before sitting in most models. There are many other designs of frames and walkers, including those which fold, those with gutters to support the body weight through the forearms, and those in which the two sides are connected at the back rather than at the front. The stop-start gait pattern seen with some walking aids (especially frames) is known as an *arrest gait*.

Gait Patterns With Walking Aids

There are a number of different ways of walking when using walking aids. The terminology varies somewhat from one author to another; the descriptions which follow are based on the well-illustrated text by Pierson (1994). Gait patterns 1 through 4 involve the greatest support from the upper limbs, by means of a walking frame, two crutches or two canes. Gait patterns 5 and 6 require less support, with a crutch or cane held in only one hand.

1. Four-point gait can be employed with canes or crutches. Also known as *reciprocal gait*, it involves the separate and alternate movement of each of the two legs and the two walking aids; for example, left crutch – right leg – right crutch – left leg (Fig. 3.20). This pattern is very stable and requires little energy, but it is very slow, so

the oxygen cost (oxygen consumption per unit distance) may be higher than for the three-point gait, described next.

2. Three-point gait is used when only one leg can take weight or when the two legs move together as a single unit. It is only used with crutches or a walking frame. Two main forms of three-point gait are recognised: *step-through* and *step-to*. These terms are used when the lower limb musculature is able to provide the movement of the legs. If the legs are paralysed and their movement is provided by the upper limbs and trunk, the terms *swing-through* and *swing-to* are used (Pierson, 1994). In step-through gait, the foot or feet move from behind the line of the two crutches to in front of them (Fig. 3.21). This gait pattern requires a lot of energy and good control of balance but it can be fairly fast. In step-to gait, the foot or feet are advanced to just behind the line of the crutches, which are then moved further forwards and the process repeated (Fig. 3.22). Since the stride length is short, walking speed is slow but energy and stability requirements are not as high as for step-through gait.

3. Modified three-point gait (also known as *three-one gait*) may be used when one leg is able to take full body weight but the other is not. This may be employed with a walking frame or with two crutches or canes. The walking aids and the affected leg move forwards together, whilst weight is taken on the sound leg. That leg is then advanced, whilst weight is taken on the affected leg and the walking aids. This makes for a stable gait pattern requiring little strength or energy, but the speed is fairly low.

4. Two-point gait resembles four-point gait, except that the crutch or cane on one side is moved forwards at the same time as the leg on the other; for example, left crutch/right leg – right crutch/left leg. This is faster than four-point gait, yet is still fairly stable and requires little energy. However, it demands good coordination by the subject.

5. Modified four-point gait is performed when the walking aid is carried in the hand opposite the affected leg. This gait pattern is typically used in hemiplegia, where there is paralysis of an arm and a leg on the same side.

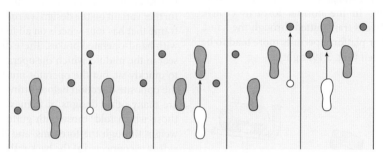

Fig. 3.20 Four-point gait. One crutch or leg is moved at a time in the pattern: left crutch – right leg – right crutch – left leg.

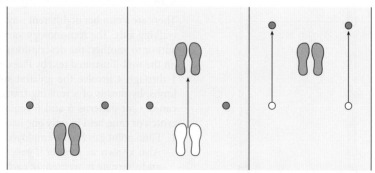

Fig. 3.21 Three-point step-through gait in a person taking weight on both legs. The legs are advanced together, in front of the line of the crutches, then the crutches are advanced together, in front of the line of the legs.

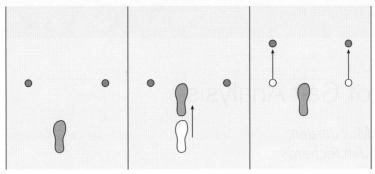

Fig. 3.22 Three-point step-to gait in a person taking weight on only one leg. The leg is advanced to behind the line of the crutches, which are then moved forwards again.

A typical walking sequence would be right crutch – left leg – right leg.

6. Modified two-point gait also involves the use of a walking aid on the opposite side to the affected leg, but the walking aid and the affected leg are moved forwards together; for example, right crutch/left leg – right leg. It clearly needs better strength and coordination than modified four-point gait, but gives better speed.

TREADMILL GAIT

It is often more convenient to study gait whilst the subject walks on a treadmill rather than over the ground, since the volume in which measurements need to be made is much smaller and the subject can conveniently be connected to wires or breathing tubes. However, there are subtle differences between treadmill and overground gait, particularly with regard to joint angles. The reduced airflow over the body is unlikely to be a significant factor, but the subject's awareness of the limited length of the treadmill belt may cause them to shorten their stride. However, the most important differences are probably due to changes in the speed of the treadmill belt, as the subject's feet decelerate the belt at initial contact and accelerate the belt at push off, effectively storing energy in the treadmill motor. This effect is minimised by using a large treadmill with a powerful motor (Savelberg et al., 1998). Treadmills

instrumented with force plates have been used to examine potential differences between overground and treadmill walking and running. In general, these studies have found minimal differences in treadmill walking/running versus overground walking/running in both kinetic and kinematic parameters, provided the treadmill belt was sufficiently stiff and the subjects were habituated to treadmill use (Riley et al., 2008).

REFERENCES

Gurney, B., 2002. Leg length discrepancy. Gait Posture 15, 195–206.

Lim, R., Dias, L., Vankoski, S., et al., 1998. Valgus knee stress in lumbosacral myelomeningocele: a gait-analysis evaluation. J. Pediatr. Orthop. 18, 428–433.

New York University, 1986. Lower Limb Orthotics. New York University Postgraduate Medical School, New York, NY.

Perry, J., 2010. Gait Analysis: Normal and Pathological Function. Slack Incorporated, Thorofare, NJ.

Pierson, F.M., 1994. Principles and Techniques of Patient Care. WB Saunders, Philadelphia, PA.

Riley, P.O., Paolini, G., Croce, U.D., et al., 2008. A kinematics and kinetic comparison of overground and treadmill running. Med. Sci. Sports Exerc. 40 (6), 1093–1100.

Savelberg, H.H.C.M., Vorstenbosch, M.A.T.M., Kamman, E.H., et al., 1998. Intra-stride belt-speed variation affects treadmill locomotion. Gait Posture 7, 26–34.

4

Methods of Gait Analysis

Michael Whittle, Max Jordon,
David Levine and Jim Richards

Walking is often impaired by neurological and musculoskeletal pathology and is one of the health domains of the International Classification of Functioning, Disability and Health (ICF). Walking is also a key aspect in the activities and participation component of mobility and is often adopted as the underlying framework for assessment of mobility in clinical practice. Therefore, it is very important for members of an interdisciplinary team to assess a patient for any loss of function in gait.

Gait analysis is used to aid directly in the treatment of individual patients. It is also used to improve our understanding of gait through research; that is, the fundamental studies of walking and clinical research, topics which we will explore in Chapter 5, Applications of Gait Analysis. Clearly, no single method of analysis is suitable for such a wide range of uses. Consequently, a number of different analysis methodologies have been developed.

When considering analysis methodologies used in gait analysis, it is helpful to regard them as being in a spectrum or continuum ranging from the absence of technological aids at one extreme to the use of complicated and expensive equipment at the other. This chapter begins with discussion of a gait analysis method which requires no equipment, and goes on to describe progressively more elaborate systems. As a general rule, the more elaborate the system, the higher the cost, but the better the quality of objective data that can be provided. However, this does not mean some of the simpler techniques are not worth using. It has often been found, particularly in a clinical setting, that the use of high-technology gait analysis is inappropriate because of its high cost in terms of money, space and time, and because some clinical problems can be adequately assessed using simpler techniques.

OBSERVATIONAL GAIT ANALYSIS

Observational gait analysis has advantages in some environments, and in others it may be the only form of assessment available. It is tempting to say that this is the simplest form of gait analysis, but this, of course, neglects the remarkable abilities of the human brain to process the data received by the eye. Although observational gait analysis is, in reality, the most versatile form of analysis available, it does suffer from limitations:

- It is transitory, giving no permanent record.
- The eye cannot observe high-speed events.
- It is only possible to observe movements, not forces.
- It depends entirely on the skill of the individual observer.
- It is subjective, and it can be difficult to avoid assessor bias if the patient is undergoing treatment.
- Subjects may act differently when they know they are being watched, a situation sometimes referred to as the *Hawthorne effect*.
- A clinic or laboratory environment may be very different from the real world.

The reproducibility of observational gait analysis has been the subject of considerable research, and when systematic observations are taken using checklists, such as in Fig. 4.1, agreement among observers can be seen when a movement pattern is noted as being either *present* or *absent*, or when a simple 3-point Likert scale with options such as *present, maybe present* or *absent* is used. It is also possible, with specific targeted questions, for assessors to accurately infer the presence or absence of impaired performance of a specific joint (McGinley et al., 2003). This shows the value

	Stance phase					Swing phase		
	IC	LR	MSt	Tst	PSw	ISw	MSw	TSw
Trunk								
Forward lean								
Backward lean								
Lateral lean (R/L)								
Pelvis								
No forward rotation (R/L)								
No contralateral drop (R/L)								
Hiking (R/L)								
Hip								
Inadequate extension								
Circumduction/abduction								
Knee								
Excessive flexion								
Uncontrolled extension								
Inadequate flexion								
Ankle/foot								
Foot slap								
Forefoot contact								
Foot Flat contact								
Late heel off								
Contralateral vaulting								

Fig. 4.1 Gait analysis checklist. *IC*, initial contact; *LR*, loading response; *MSt*, mid-stance; *Tst*, terminal stance; *PSw*, pre-swing; *ISw*, initial swing; *MSw*, mid-swing; *TSw*, terminal swing. © 2006 LAREI, Rancho Los Amigos National Rehabilitation Center, Downey, CA 90242.

of a 0–10 rating scale specific to a question focused on one aspect of movement push-off after stroke, with a score of 0 representing a person with a severe functional deficit and 10 representing a person with no functional deficit (Fig. 4.2). Historically, this has been very useful in the clinical assessment and classification of patients with a variety of pathological gait patterns, however it is not possible to gain any reliable assessments of joint angles.

THE GAIT ANALYSIS ENVIRONMENT

The minimum length required for a gait analysis walkway is a hotly debated subject. The authors believe that 8 metres (26 feet) is about the minimum for use with fit young people, but that at least 12 metres (39 feet) is preferable, since it permits fast walkers to hit their stride before any measurements are made. However, shorter walkways are satisfactory for people who walk more slowly, such as those with a pathological gait. The width required for a walkway depends on what equipment, if any, is being used

to make measurements. For observational gait analysis, as little as 3 metres (10 feet) may be sufficient. If video recording is being used, the camera needs to be positioned a little farther from the subject, and about 4 metres (13 feet) is needed. A kinematic system making simultaneous measurements from both sides of the body normally requires a width of at least 6 metres (20 feet). Fig. 4.3 shows the layout of a small gait laboratory used for observational gait analysis and video recording to measure basic gait parameters.

Some investigators permit subjects to choose their own walking speed, whereas others control the cycle time or cadence by asking them to walk in time with a metronome. The rationale for controlling the cadence is that many of the measurable parameters of gait vary with walking speed, and controlling this provides one means of reducing variability. However, subjects are unlikely to walk naturally when trying to keep pace with a metronome, and patients with motor control problems may find it difficult or even impossible to walk at an imposed cadence. The resolution to this dilemma is probably to accept the fact that subjects need to walk at different speeds and to interpret the data appropriately.

GAIT ASSESSMENT

Simply observing the gait and noting abnormalities is of little value by itself. This needs to be followed by *gait assessment*, which is the synthesis of these observations with information about the subject obtained from the history and physical examination, combined with the intelligence and experience of the observer (Rose, 1983). Observational gait analysis is entirely subjective and the quality of the analysis depends on the skill of the person performing it. It can be an interesting exercise to perform observational gait analysis on people

```
                     ABNORMAL
   0   1   2   3   4   5   6   7   8   9   10
  No                                      Just
  push off                                abnormal

                     NORMAL
   0   1   2   3   4   5   6   7   8   9   10
  Just                                    Upper
  normal                                  limit of
                                          normal
```

Fig. 4.2 Rating scale provided for observer judgments. Adapted from McGinley et al. (2003).

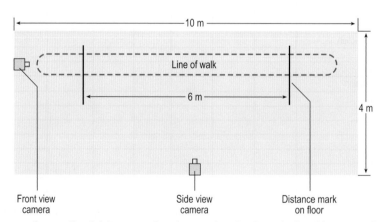

Fig. 4.3 Layout of a small gait laboratory for observational gait analysis, video recording and measurement of the general gait parameters.

walking by in the street, but without knowing their clinical details, it is easy to misinterpret what is wrong with them.

When performing any type of gait analysis, one thing that must constantly be kept in mind is that you are observing effects and not causes. Putting it another way, the observed gait pattern is not the direct result of a pathological process but the net result of a pathological process and the subject's attempts to compensate for it. The observed gait pattern is 'what is left after the available mechanisms for compensation have been exhausted' (Rose, 1983).

Examination by Video Recording

Historically, the use of videotape for examining a patient's gait was widespread in the 1990s, although today, this is achieved by direct recording to a memory card or computer. This has provided one of the most useful enhancements to gait analysis in the clinical setting in recent years, as it helps overcome two of the limitations of observational gait analysis: the lack of a permanent record, and the difficulty of observing high-speed events. In addition, it confers the following advantages:

- The number of repeated walks needed for analysis is reduced.
- Events, positions and movements can be analysed frame by frame and in slow motion.
- Gait can be compared over time and in different situations.
- Objective data such as cadence, joint angles and timings of movements from the recordings can be gathered.
- The recordings can be shared with others for their opinions.
- It produces a permanent record of a person's gait.
- The recordings can be used as a tool when teaching or learning the art of gait analysis.
- You can zoom in and study a joint or other feature of interest in detail.

Important features to consider when selecting a device with which to capture video recordings for use in gait analysis include automatic focus, a zoom lens and a high-speed mode that eliminates blurring due to movement. Many gait laboratories record video data directly to a computer. This enables the data to be synchronised with data collected from other motion analysis systems, and allows playback and analysis using freeze-frame, frame-by-frame advance and variable slow-speed play, which facilitates the observation of movements which are too fast for the unaided eye to determine.

A number of studies have reported the importance of the angle of the camera relative to the subject (Toro et al., 2007; Larsen et al., 2008; Birch et al., 2013). Two camera positions are commonly used; they can be adjusted to show the whole body from head to feet, with one camera viewing the subject from the side of the walkway and capturing a sagittal plane view and the other viewing the subject from the end of the walkway and capturing a frontal plane view (Fig. 4.3). The subject is recorded as they walk the length of the walkway, then turn and walk back to their starting position. In this way, footage is captured from both sides and from the front and back of the subject. The use of video recording permits the subject to do a much smaller number of walks, as the person performing the analysis can watch the recording as many times as necessary. If possible, it is a good idea to review the recording before the subject leaves in case the process needs to be repeated for any reason. In addition, this is an opportunity to show the subject a video recording of their gait, which can be very helpful in many cases. Also, when a therapist is working with a subject to correct a gait abnormality, the subject may gain a clearer idea of exactly what the therapist is concerned about if they can observe their own gait from the 'outside'.

The analysis is performed by replaying the video recording, looking for specific gait abnormalities in the different views and interpreting what is seen in light of the subject's history and physical examination. It is particularly helpful if two or more people work together to perform the analysis. Although visual gait analysis using simple video recording is largely subjective, the use of two-dimensional analysis software has been shown to provide useful measures of sagittal plane joint movements and to have high inter-rater and intra-rater reliability (Reinking et al., 2018).

Temporal and Spatial Parameters of Gait

Temporal and spatial parameters of gait, sometimes referred to as the *general gait parameters*, include cycle time (or stride time), stride length and speed. These provide the simplest form of objective gait evaluation (Robinson and Smidt, 1981) and may be made using only a stopwatch and a tape measure. Other temporal and spatial parameters of gait include step time, double support time, single support time, step length, base width and foot angle. These measurements require the use of specialised equipment which will be described in the next section.

Cycle time, stride length and speed tend to change together in most locomotor disabilities. This means a subject with a long cycle time will usually also have a short stride length and a low speed (speed being stride length divided by cycle time). The general gait parameters give a guide to the walking ability of a subject, but little specific information. They should always be interpreted in terms of the expected values for the subject's age and gender, such as those covered in Chapter 2, Normal Gait. Fig. 4.4 shows one way in which these data may be presented; the diamonds represent the 95% confidence limits for a healthy control subject of the same age and gender

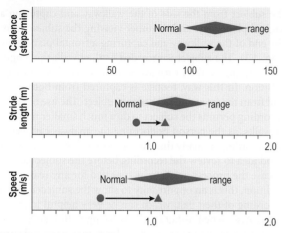

Fig. 4.4 Display of the general gait parameters, with normal ranges appropriate for a patient's age and gender. Pre- and postoperative values for a 70-year-old female patient undergoing knee replacement surgery.

as the subject under investigation. Although cycle time is gradually replacing cadence in the gait analysis community, it is more convenient to use cadence on plots of this type, since abnormally slow gait will give values on the left-hand side of the graph for all three of the general gait parameters.

Cycle Time or Cadence

Cycle time or cadence may be measured with the aid of a stopwatch, by counting the number of individual steps taken during a known period of time. It is seldom practical to count for a full minute, so a period of 10 or 15 seconds is usually chosen. The loss of accuracy incurred by counting for such short periods of time is unlikely to be of any practical significance. The subject should be told to walk naturally and should be allowed to reach their full walking speed before the observer starts to count the steps. The cycle time is calculated using the formula:

$$\text{cycle time (s)} = \text{time (s)} \times 2\,/\,\text{steps counted}$$

The 2 allows for the fact that there are two steps per stride. The cadence is calculated using the formula:

$$\text{cadence (steps/min)} = \text{steps counted} \times 60\,/\,\text{time (s)}$$

The 60 allows for the fact that there are 60 seconds in a minute.

Stride Length

Stride length can be determined in two ways: by direct measurement, or indirectly from the speed and cycle time. The simplest direct method of measurement is to count the strides taken whilst the subject covers a known distance. More useful methods include putting ink pads on the soles of the subject's shoes (Rafferty and Bell, 1995) or attaching markers to the subject's shoes (Gerny, 1983), and then having them walk on paper. A messier option is to have the subject step with both feet in a shallow tray of talcum powder and then walk along a strip of brown wrapping paper or coloured construction paper, leaving a trail of footprints. The resultant prints may be measured, as shown in Fig. 2.3, to derive left and right step lengths, stride length, walking base, toe-out angle and some idea of the foot contact pattern. This can provide a great deal of useful and surprisingly accurate information, for the sake of a few minutes of mopping up the floor afterwards! If both the cycle time and the speed have been measured, stride length may be calculated using the formula:

$$\text{stride length (m)} = \text{speed (m/s)} \times \text{cycle time (s)}$$

The equivalent calculation using cadence is:

$$\text{stride length (m)} = \frac{\text{speed (m/s)} \times 2 \times 60}{\text{cadence (steps/min)}}$$

The multiplication by 2 converts steps to strides and by 60 converts minutes to seconds. For accurate results, the cycle time and speed should be measured during the same walk. However, simultaneous counting, measuring and timing may prove too difficult, and the errors introduced by using data from different walks are not likely to be important unless the subject's gait varies markedly from one walk to another.

Speed

Speed may be measured by timing the subject whilst they walk a known distance; for example, between two marks on the floor or between two pillars in a corridor. The distance walked is a matter of convenience, but somewhere in the region of 6 to 10 metres (20 to 33 feet) is probably adequate. Again, the subject should be told to walk at their natural speed, and they should be allowed to hit their stride before measurement starts. The speed is calculated as follows:

$$\text{speed (m/s)} = \text{distance (m)}\,/\,\text{time (s)}$$

General Gait Parameters from Video Recording

Determining the general gait parameters from a video recording of the subject as they walk is relatively easy, so long as the recording shows the subject passing two landmarks whose positions are known. One simple method is to have the subject walk across two lines on the floor which are a known distance apart, such as lines of adhesive tape. Space should be allowed for acceleration before the first line and for slowing down after the second line. When the recording is replayed, the time taken to cover the distance is measured and the steps taken are counted. It is easiest to take the first initial contact *beyond the start line* as the point to begin both timing and counting, and the first initial contact *beyond the finish line* as the point to end. The first step beyond the start line must be counted as zero, not one. This method of measurement is not strictly accurate, since the position of the foot at initial contact is an unknown distance beyond the start and finish lines, but the errors introduced are unlikely to be significant. As mentioned earlier, this method can also be employed without the use of video recording. Since the distance, time and number of steps are all known, the general gait parameters can be calculated using the formulae:

$$\text{cycle time (s)} = \text{time(s)} \times 2 / \text{steps counted}$$

$$\text{cadence (steps/min)} = \text{steps counted} \times 60 / \text{time (s)}$$

$$\text{stride length (m)} = \text{distance (m)} \times 2 / \text{steps counted}$$

$$\text{speed (m/s)} = \text{distance (m)} / \text{time (s)}$$

MEASUREMENT OF TEMPORAL AND SPATIAL PARAMETERS OF GAIT

A number of systems are capable of automatically measuring the timing of the gait cycle, sometimes called the *temporal gait parameters*. Such systems may be divided into two main classes: footswitches and instrumented walkways.

Footswitches

Footswitches are used to record the timing of gait and are usually connected to a small transmitter or a portable recording device. If one switch is fixed beneath the heel and one beneath the forefoot, it is possible to measure the timing of initial contact, foot flat, heel rise and toe off, as well as the duration of the stance phase. Data from two or more strides make it possible to calculate cycle time and swing phase duration. If switches are mounted on both feet, the single and double support times can also be measured. Footswitches are most conveniently used within shoes, although they may also be taped directly to the underside of the foot. In addition to

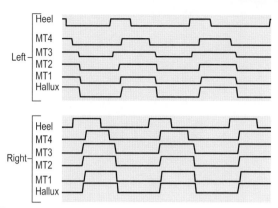

Fig. 4.5 Output from footswitches under the heel, four metatarsals (*MT1* to *MT4*) and hallux of both feet. The switch is 'on' (i.e., the area is in contact with the ground) when the line is high.

the basic heel and forefoot switches, further switches may be used in other areas of the foot to give greater detail regarding the temporal patterns of loading and unloading (Fig. 4.5).

Instrumented Walkways

Instrumented walkways can be used to measure the timing of foot contacts, the position of the foot on the ground, foot fall patterns with assistive devices, and many other temporal and spatial parameters. Conductive walkways are covered with an electrically conductive substance, such as a metal mesh or bars, or conductive rubber. Suitably positioned electrical contacts on the subject's shoes complete an electrical circuit, recording the position and timing of the foot contact. Timing information from the foot contacts is used to calculate the cycle time, and the combination of cycle time, step and stride length may be used to calculate speed.

An alternative arrangement is to have the walkway itself contain a large number of switch contacts. A number of commercial systems are available to perform these measurements, with some also providing some information on the magnitude of the forces between the foot and the ground. One such system in common use today is the GAITRite, which has been used to assess a wide variety of patient groups (Fig. 4.6) (Bilney et al., 2003).

CAMERA-BASED MOTION ANALYSIS

Kinematics refers to the measurement of movement or, more specifically, the geometrical description of motion. Kinematic systems are used in gait analysis to record the position and orientation of the body segments, the angles of the joints and the corresponding linear and angular velocities and accelerations.

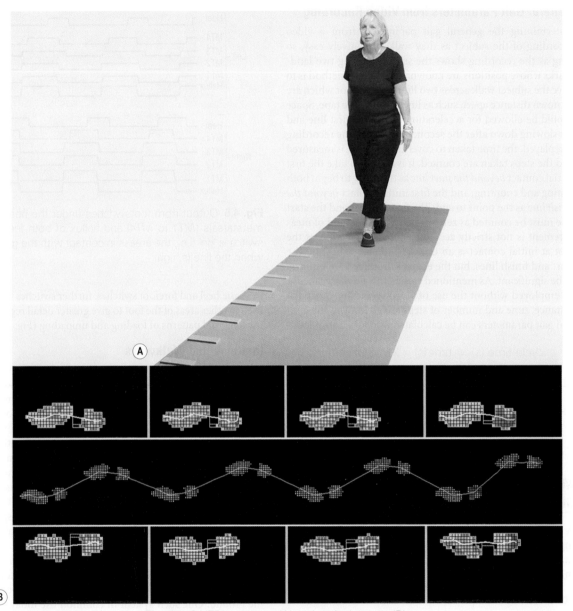

Fig. 4.6 GAITRite system (A) and typical output (B).

Following the pioneering work of Marey and Muybridge in the 1870s, photography remained the method of choice for measuring human movement for about 100 years, until it was replaced by electronic systems. Two basic photographic techniques were used: *cine photography* and *multiple-exposure photography*. In cine photography, a series of separate photographs are taken in quick succession. Multiple-exposure photography has existed in many different forms over the years, and is based on the use of either a single photograph or a strip of film on which a series of images are superimposed, sometimes with a horizontal displacement between each image. The 1960s and 1970s saw the development of gait analysis systems based on *opto-electronic techniques*, including camera-based systems, and these have now superseded the photographic methods. The general principles of kinematic measurement are common to all systems and will be discussed before considering particular systems in detail.

General Principles

Kinematic measurements may be made in either two or three dimensions. Three-dimensional measurements usually require the use of two or more cameras, although methods have been devised in which a single camera can be used to make limited three-dimensional measurements.

The simplest kinematic measurements are made using a single camera in an uncalibrated system. Such measurements are fairly inaccurate, but they may be useful for some purposes. Without calibration, it is impossible to measure distances accurately, so such a system is usually used only to estimate joint angles in the sagittal plane. The camera is positioned at right angles to the plane of motion and as far away from the subject as possible, to minimise the distortions introduced by perspective. To give an image of reasonable size and with a long camera-to-subject distance, a telephoto (long focal length) lens is often used. The angles measured from the image are projections of three-dimensional angles onto a two-dimensional plane, and any part of the angulation which occurs outside that plane is ignored. Although single-camera systems can be used to make approximate measurements of distance if some form of calibration object is used, measurement accuracy will be lost by any movement towards or away from the camera.

To achieve reasonable accuracy in kinematic measurements, it is necessary to use a calibrated three-dimensional system, which involves making measurements from more than one viewpoint. A detailed review of the technical aspects of the three-dimensional measurement of human movement was given in four companion papers by Cappozzo et al. (2005), Chiari et al. (2005), Leardini et al. (2005) and Della Croce et al. (2005). Although there are considerable differences in convenience and accuracy among cine film, video recording, camera systems and optoelectronic systems, the data processing for the different image capture techniques is similar.

Most commercial kinematic systems use either a three-dimensional calibration object, or a wand with markers at known points which is simultaneously viewed by all the cameras. Computer software is used to calculate the relationship between the known three-dimensional positions of the markers on the calibration object and the two-dimensional positions of the markers in the fields of view of the different cameras. An alternative method of calibration is used by the Codamotion system, whose optoelectronic sensors are in a fixed position in relation to each other, permitting the system to be calibrated in the factory.

When a subject walks in front of the cameras, the calibration process is reversed and three-dimensional positions are calculated for the markers fixed to the subject's limbs, so long as they are visible to at least two cameras.

Data are collected at a series of time intervals known as *frames*. Most systems have an interval between frames of either 20 ms, 16.7 ms or 5 ms, corresponding to data collection frequencies of 50 Hz, 60 Hz or 200 Hz, with some systems offering frame rates of up to 500 Hz and beyond.

Technical descriptions of kinematic systems use, and sometimes misuse, the terms *resolution*, *precision* and *accuracy*. In practical terms, resolution means the ability of the system to measure small changes in marker position. Precision is a measure of system noise based on the amount of variability between one frame of data and the next. For the majority of users, the most important parameter is accuracy, which describes the relationship between where the markers really are and where the system says they are.

Most commercial systems are sufficiently accurate to measure the positions of the limbs and the angles of the joints. However, calculation of linear or angular velocity requires mathematical differentiation of the position data, which magnifies any measurement errors. A second differentiation is required to determine acceleration, and a small amount of measurement noise in the original data can lead to unusable results for acceleration. The usual way of avoiding this problem is to use a low-pass filter to smooth the position data before differentiation. This achieves the desired objective but means that any genuinely high accelerations, such as heelstrike transients, may be lost. Thus, kinematic systems are good at measuring position but poorer at determining acceleration because of the problems of differentiating even slightly noisy data. Conversely, accelerometers are good at measuring acceleration but poor at estimating position. Highly accurate data could be obtained by combining the two methods, using each to correct the other and calculating the velocity from both. Some research studies have been conducted using this combined approach.

As well as the errors inherent in measuring the positions of the markers, further errors are introduced because considerable movement may take place between a skin marker and the underlying bone. The amount of error this causes in the final result depends on which parameter is being measured. For example, marker movement has little effect on the sagittal plane knee angle, because it causes only a small relative change in the length of fairly long segments, but it may cause considerable errors in transverse plane measurements or on measurements involving shorter segments, such as in the foot. Skin movement may also introduce errors in the calculation of joint moments and powers. For these reasons, the development of marker sets and anatomical models has been at the forefront of the evolution of gait analysis alongside the ability of new motion analysis systems capable of coping with larger numbers of markers.

Camera-Based Motion Analysis Systems

In addition to augmenting observational gait analysis, video recordings may also be used as the basis for a kinematic system. This has considerable advantages in terms of cost, convenience and speed, although it is not as accurate due to the poorer resolution of a video image and the sampling frequency compared with data collected from motion analysis cameras. Another considerable advantage, however, is that it is possible to automate the digitisation process using digital image processing, especially if skin markers are used, which show up clearly against the background. A number of commercial systems are available and can be used either as a two-dimensional system with a single camera, or as a three-dimensional system using two or more cameras. Most systems of this type use conventional video cameras which can now record at sufficiently high frame rates for the majority of movement tasks.

A number of different camera-based motion capture systems have been developed over the years. Although the systems differ in detail, the following description is typical. Reflective markers are fixed to the subject's limbs, either close to the joint centres or fixed to limb segments in such a way as to identify their positions and orientations. Close to the lens of each camera is an infrared or visible light source which causes the markers to show up as very bright spots (Fig. 4.7). The markers are usually covered in Scotchlite, the material that makes road signs show up brightly when illuminated by car headlights. To avoid smearing, which occurs if the marker is moving, only a short exposure time is used. This may be achieved by using:

- stroboscopic illumination,
- a mechanical shutter on the camera, and/or
- a charge-coupled device (CCD) camera which allows an image to be captured for a short interval within each frame.

For normal purposes, frame rates of between 50 Hz and 200 Hz are used, although most systems are now able to collect data at frame rates up to 500 Hz without loss of pixel resolution. Cameras either are connected via a special interface board (e.g., VICON), or are daisy-chained (e.g., Qualisys) (Fig. 4.8); both methods allow each frame to be synchronised. Most commercially available systems locate the *centroid* or *geometric centre* of each marker within the camera image, which is typically calculated using the edges of any bright spots in the field of view. Because a large number of edges are used to calculate the position of the centroid, its position can be determined to a greater accuracy than the horizontal and vertical resolutions of the image. This is known as making measurements with *subpixel accuracy*. Marker centroids may also be calculated using the optical density of all the pixels in the image rather than just the marker edges, again with an improvement in accuracy.

The computer stores the marker centroid positions from each frame of data for each camera. The process of identifying which marker image is which and following the markers from one frame of data to the next is known as *tracking* (Fig. 4.9). The speed and convenience of this process differ considerably among systems. In the past, this has been the least satisfactory aspect of motion capture systems, however many systems are now capable of real-time marker identification, allowing for much more straightforward and faster analysis. Whichever method is used, the end result of the tracking is a three-dimensional reconstruction of the position of each marker.

Common Marker Sets

In order to calculate accurate joint kinetics, it is essential to locate the centre of rotation of a joint in a repeatable manner through the definition of an anatomical frame. This issue was highlighted by Della Croce et al. (1999), who identified the errors associated with incorrect anatomical frame definitions. Therefore, the identification and modelling of joint centres has been key to the assessment of joint angles,

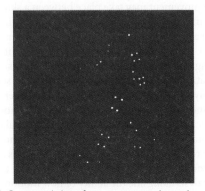

Fig. 4.7 Captured data from a camera-based system.

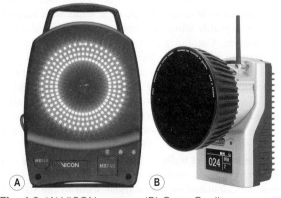

Fig. 4.8 (A) VICON camera; (B) Oqus Qualisys camera.

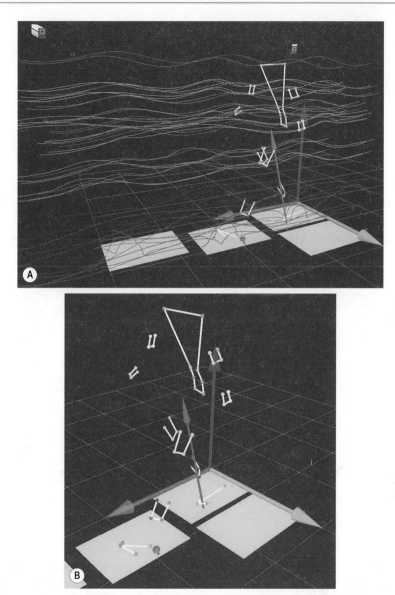

Fig. 4.9 (A, B) Automatic digitising of a full-body Calibrated Anatomical System Technique (CAST) marker set using Qualisys Track Manager.

moments and powers. Joint centres are generally found by using palpable anatomical landmarks to define the medial-lateral axis of the joint. From these anatomical landmarks, the centre of rotation is generally calculated in one of two ways: through the use of regression equations based on standard radiographic evidence or simply as a percentage offset from the anatomical marker based on some kind of anatomical landmark (Bell et al., 1990; Cappozzo et al., 1995; Davis et al., 1991; Kadaba et al., 1989).

Several different marker sets are commonly used today, which illustrates how improvements have continued to be made. The simplest marker set involves directly fixing markers on the skin over a bony anatomical landmark close to the centre of rotation of a joint. The position and orientation of the limb segment are then defined by a straight line between the two markers (Fig. 4.10A). This method requires fewer markers and so theoretically has less interference with movement, but it does not allow the calculation of axial

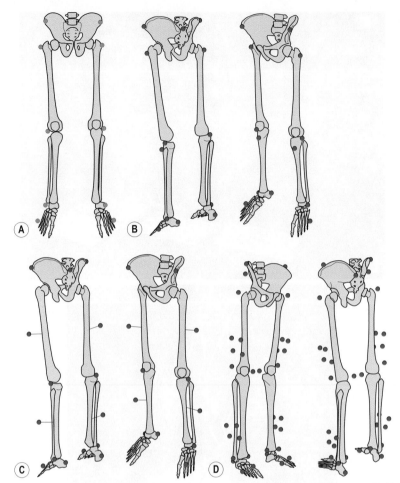

Fig. 4.10 Common marker sets. (A) Simple marker set; (B) Vaughan marker set; (C) Helen Hayes marker set; and (D) Calibrated Anatomical System Technique (CAST).

rotation of the body segments. The anatomical landmarks generally used are the head of the fifth metatarsal, the lateral malleolus, the lateral epicondyle of the femur, the greater trochanter and the anterior superior iliac spine.

The Vaughan marker set consists of 15 markers on the lower limb and pelvis (Fig. 4.10B). This allows for more detail on the location of the knee joint centre by including a marker in the coronal plane on the tibial tuberosity. The inclusion of the heel marker allows a more appropriate functional reference for the long axis of the foot to be determined between this and the metatarsal heads, with the point of rotation of the foot determined by the malleoli markers. The inclusion of the sacral marker also allows for a more functional reference for pelvis inclination in the sagittal plane and a meaningful measurement of pelvic tilt.

The anatomical landmarks used are the head of the fifth metatarsal, the lateral malleolus, the heel, the tibial tuberosity, the lateral femoral epicondyle, the greater trochanter, the anterior superior iliac spine and the sacrum.

The Conventional Gait Model (CGM), which is sometimes referred to as the Helen Hayes marker set (Fig. 4.10C), also includes a heel marker and the sacral marker for a more appropriate functional reference for the foot and pelvis. Additionally, it includes tibial and femoral wands, each comprising a single marker on a short stick which is attached to a pad fixed to the segment using tape or a bandage. These are not placed on any anatomical position as such, and variations on wand length and positioning, anterior versus lateral, have been used. Inclusion of these wands allows femoral and tibial rotations to be quantified. The joint markers are placed on anatomical landmarks including the head of the second metatarsal, the lateral malleolus, the heel, the lateral femoral epicondyle, the anterior superior iliac spines and either the sacrum or the posterior superior iliac spines.

The pelvis can be imagined as an equilateral triangle with its front edge formed by the line between the anterior superior iliac spine markers and the mid-point of the posterior superior iliac spine markers. The hip joint centre is assumed to be fixed in relation to this triangle at a position estimated using regression equations (Bell et al., 1990). The thigh segment can be imagined as another equilateral triangle with its apex between the hip joint centre and the centre of the base at the knee joint axis. This is assumed to pass through the knee in the plane defined by a lateral knee marker, a thigh marker and a hip joint centre. The knee joint centre is defined as lying half the knee width along this axis from the knee marker. The tibia segment is modelled in a similar way to the femur. The foot is defined on the basis of the line between the ankle joint centre and the toe marker. This method does not require the inclusion of joint markers on the medial side and therefore can be potentially susceptible to errors in the estimation of the rotational axis as it uses a medial projection of both the knee and the ankle markers.

The Calibrated Anatomical System Technique (CAST, Fig. 4.10D) was first proposed by Cappozzo et al. (1995) to contribute towards standardising descriptions of movement in research labs and clinical centres for the pelvis and lower limb segments. This method involves identifying an anatomical frame for each segment using anatomical landmarks and segment tracking markers, or marker clusters. Anatomical markers are placed on both the lateral and medial aspects of the joints to further improve estimation of the joint centres. Marker clusters are placed on each body segment. The exact placement of the clusters does not matter, although positioning them on the distal third of the body segment is typical. At least three markers are required to track each segment position and orientation in six degrees of freedom (Cappozzo et al., 2005); however, up to nine have been used. Usually, four or five markers are used per cluster, allowing for one or two markers to be lost. This is sometimes referred to as *marker redundancy*; if you lose a marker during tracking, the model will still work. This method determines the position and orientation of each body segment separately, which then allows each joint to be assessed in what is referred to as six degrees of freedom. Six degrees of freedom is best thought of as three orientations of rotation (i.e., flexion/extension, abduction/adduction and internal/external rotation) and three orientations of translation (i.e., anterior posterior and medial lateral translation, and compression and distraction), although the translational movements are more susceptible to soft tissue movement artifacts.

Active Marker Systems

Another type of kinematic system uses active markers, typically light-emitting diodes (LEDs), and an array of opto-electronic photo diodes. One such system is Codamotion (Fig. 4.11A). Codamotion performs a correlation between the shadow cast on the array by a shadow mask of lines when the LED flashes, and a software template of the shadow. This makes use of information from all photodiodes in the array to calculate the three-dimensional marker positions. Active markers produce infrared light at a given frequency, so these systems do not require illumination, and as such the markers are more easily identified and tracked (Chiari et al., 2005). The LEDs are attached to a body segment in the same way as passive markers, but with the addition of a power source and a control unit for each LED. Active markers can have their own specific frequency which allows them to be automatically detected. This leads to very stable real-time three-dimensional motion tracking, as no markers can be misidentified for adjacent markers.

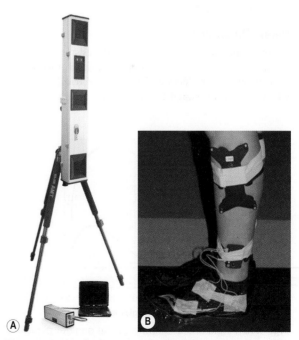

Fig. 4.11 (A) Codamotion opto-electronic movement analysis system (Charnwood Dynamics). (B) Codamotion Active LED marker clusters (Charnwood Dynamics).

An added advantage of active markers is that they can be used outdoors, whereas passive marker systems are usually confined to indoor use as they are sensitive to incandescent light and sunlight. The LEDs are arranged to flash on and off in sequence so that only one is illuminated at a time. The photo diodes are thus able to locate each marker in turn, without the need for a tracking procedure to determine which one is which. The penalty for this convenience is that the subject must carry a small power supply with wires running to each marker. These can be both single markers and clusters of markers (Fig. 4.11B), and therefore all the models considered in the previous section may be used.

ELECTROGONIOMETERS AND POTENTIOMETERS

Electrogoniometers and potentiometers are devices for making continuous measurements of joint angles. The outputs are usually plotted as a chart of joint angle against time, as shown in Fig. 2.5. However, if measurements have been made from two joints (typically the hip and knee), the data may be plotted as an *angle-angle diagram*, also known as a *cyclogram* (Fig. 4.12). This format allows the interaction between two joints to be plotted on one graph and makes it possible to identify characteristic patterns, although these can sometimes be difficult to interpret.

Rotary Potentiometers

A rotary potentiometer is a variable resistor similar to that used as a radio volume control, in which turning the central spindle produces a change in electrical resistance which can be measured by an external circuit. It can be used to measure the angle of a joint if it is fixed in such a way that the body of the potentiometer is attached to one limb segment and the spindle to the other. The electrical output thus depends on the joint position, and the device can be calibrated to measure the joint angle in degrees.

Although potentiometers could be used to measure the motion of any joint, they are most often used for the knee and less often for the ankle and hip. Fixation is achieved by cuffs, which wrap around the limb segment above and below the joint. The position of the potentiometer is adjusted to be as close to the joint axis as possible. A single potentiometer will only make measurements in one axis of the joint, but two or three may be mounted in different planes to make multiaxial measurements (Fig. 4.13). Concerns have been expressed about the accuracy of measurements provided by such devices and about the fact that they can be cumbersome, and because of these problems,

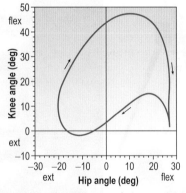

Fig. 4.12 Angle-angle diagram of the sagittal plane hip angle *(horizontal axis)* and knee angle *(vertical axis)*. Initial contact is at the lower right. Normal subject; same data as Fig. 2.5.

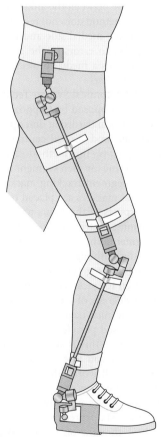

Fig. 4.13 Subject wearing triaxial goniometers on hip, knee and ankle (adapted from manufacturer's literature [Chattecx Corporation]).

flexible strain gauge electrogoniometers have become more popular in clinical and research settings.

Electrogoniometers

Flexible strain gauge electrogoniometers consist of a thin, flat strip of metal, one end of which is fixed to the limb on each side of the joint being studied (Fig. 4.14). The bending of the metal as the joint moves is measured by strain gauges and their associated electronics. Because of the way in which metal strips respond to bending, the output depends simply on the angle between the two ends, with linear motion being ignored. Electrogoniometers can be fixed simply and quickly across a joint using double-sided sticky tape; they usually measure in a single axis but can measure motion in more than one axis if twin or tri-axis electrogoniometers are used. Other designs which have been used in the past include mercury-in-rubber, in which the electrical resistance of a column of mercury in an elastic tube changes as the tube is stretched across a joint, and an optical system known as the polarised light goniometer.

Shamsi et al. (2019) demonstrated high intra-rater reliability when examining active knee flexion using a flexible strain gauge electrogoniometer, and showed an intraclass correlation coefficient (ICC) of 0.99, with a standard error of measurement of 2.16 degrees. Other studies have also demonstrated electrogoniometers to have high reliability when assessing ankle range of motion (ICC = 0.954) (Bronner et al., 2010a) and hip range of motion (ICC = 0.983) (Bronner et al., 2010b). Furthermore, electrogoniometers demonstrate high concurrent validity when compared to motion capture systems for the range of motion at the hip (ICC = 0.949), knee (ICC = 0.991) and ankle (ICC = 0.954) (Bronner et al., 2010b). Due to the increased use of camera-based systems, electrogoniometers are declining in popularity, however, they still serve as a viable mid-tier option for motion analysis if the cost of camera-based kinematic systems is prohibitive.

ACCELEROMETERS AND INERTIAL MEASUREMENT UNITS

Accelerometers, as their name suggests, measure acceleration. Historically, they contained a small mass connected to a stiff spring, with some electrical means of measuring the spring deflection when the mass is accelerated. Today, they usually consist of electronic microchip sensors with an onboard solid-state tri-axial accelerometer. They are usually very small, weighing only a few grams, and are of great value in gait analysis for providing feedback and assessments of motion in remote settings. Typically, accelerometers are used for gait analysis in one of two ways: either to measure transient events or to measure the motion of the limbs.

Measurement of Transients With Accelerometers

Accelerometers are suitable for measuring brief, high-acceleration events, such as the deceleration of the leg at heel strike, sometimes referred to as the *heel strike transient*. The main difficulty with this type of measurement is in obtaining an adequate mechanical linkage between the accelerometer and the skeleton, since movement occurs in both the skin and the subcutaneous tissues. On a few occasions, experiments have been performed with accelerometers mounted on pins screwed directly into the bones of volunteers, however, this is clearly not acceptable for common use.

Measurement of Motion With Accelerometers

The use of accelerometers for the kinematic analysis of limb motion has been explored countless times since Morris first explored this in 1973 (Morris, 1973). If the acceleration of a limb segment is known, a single mathematical integration will give its velocity and a second integration its position, provided both position and velocity are known at some point during the measurement period. However, these requirements, combined with the drift from which accelerometers often suffer, have prevented them from enjoying widespread use for this purpose. If the limb rotates as well as changing its position, which is usually the case, further sensors to measure the angular velocity are required to improve the accuracy of these estimations. However, the most common use of accelerometers is to measure step count, and with all smartphones now having onboard accelerometers combined with further developments of the algorithms, the assessment of the level of activity is now widely available.

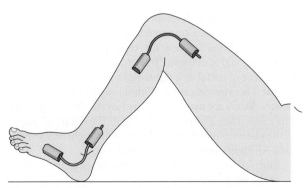

Fig. 4.14 Subject wearing flexible goniometers on knee and ankle (adapted from manufacturer's literature [Biometrics]).

Inertial Measurement Units

With the advent of newer technologies, researchers have been measuring gait kinematics and kinetics through the use of inertial measurement units (IMUs). IMUs integrate accelerometers, gyroscopes and magnetometers to track motion in three-dimensional space Seel et al. (2014). Costing less than three-dimensional motion capture camera systems, IMUs are becoming increasingly popular as a means of measuring joint angles. Due to their portable nature, they can be used to evaluate a variety of physical activities and even have the potential to assess movement in the community Fennema et al. (2019). Multiple studies have found the validity and reliability of IMUs in the assessment of lower extremity function to be satisfactory. For example, Leardini et al. (2014) examined the accuracy of an IMU system in measuring thoracic and knee angles during gait-specific rehabilitation exercises. They compared an IMU system against that of a three-dimensional motion capture system and found that the average difference in measurement was smaller than 5 degrees. In a separate study that compared IMUs against a three-dimensional motion capture system, Seel et al. (2014) found the average error in the sagittal plane to be around 3 degrees at the knee and only 1 degree at the ankle. In addition, Fennema et al. (2019) measured the reliability of IMUs by attaching them to a phantom leg that was moved by a robot controller. With fixed motion, they found that the maximum deviation between repeated measurements was ± 2.3 degrees. With IMUs having good reliability and validity, being less costly than three-dimensional motion capture systems and having greater potential for measuring patients in nonlaboratory settings, it is clear why they are becoming a more popular method for measuring joint angles.

Motion Capture Suits

In the past 10 years, considerable advances have been made in motion capture suits. Initially, the primary applications for motion capture suits were computer gaming and animation. Today they are now sensitive and reliable enough to be used in biomechanics and gait analysis. One such system is the XSENS MVN motion capture suit (Fig. 4.15). This suit uses small, three-dimensional gyroscopes, accelerometers and magnetometers. Because it does not require cameras or markers, it can be used indoors and outdoors, regardless of lighting conditions. The combination of the three sensor types allows the tracking of each segment in six degrees of freedom of up to 17 body segments. Although these systems sometimes suffer from drift, and it is often difficult to obtain a global reference which prevents them being linked with force platforms, the relative movement of one body segment about another has been shown to be accurate.

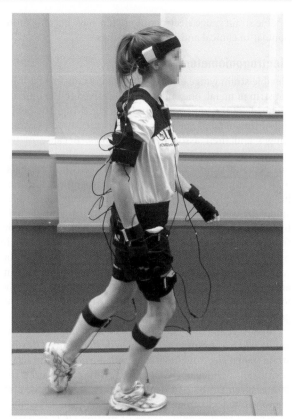

Fig. 4.15 XSENS MVN motion capture suit.

MEASURING FORCE AND PRESSURE

Force Platforms

The force platform, also known as a *force plate*, is used to measure the ground reaction force as a subject walks across it (Fig. 4.16). Although many specialised types of force platform have been developed over the years, most clinical laboratories use a commercial platform, typically about 100 mm high and with a flat rectangular upper surface measuring 400 × 600 mm. The upper surface is made of a large piece of metal or a lightweight honeycomb structure so that it is extremely rigid. Within the platform, a number of transducers are used to measure tiny displacements in all three axes when a force is applied to it. The electrical output of the platform may be provided as either eight or six channels. An eight-channel output consists of:

- four vertical signals from transducers near the corners of the platform;
- two fore–aft signals from the sides of the platform; and
- two side-to-side signals from the front and back of the platform.

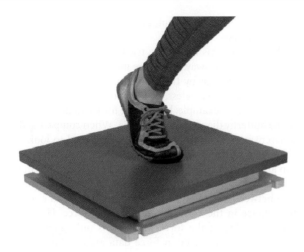

Fig. 4.16 AMTI multi-axis Optima force platform (Model: HPS464508, Advanced Mechanical Technology, Inc. [AMTI]).

A six-channel output generally consists of:
- three force vectors and
- three turning moments about the centre of the platform.

The output signals from force platforms are collected directly into a computer through an analogue-to-digital converter. The vertical, anterior-posterior and medial-lateral forces are calculated along with the position of the centre of pressure on the force plate, which can then be used for biomechanical calculations and integration with camera systems.

Ideally, a force platform should be mounted below floor level, with the upper surface flush with the floor. If this is not possible, a slightly raised walkway can be built to accommodate the thickness of the platform. It is highly undesirable to have the subject step up onto the platform and then down off it again, since such a step could never be regarded as normal walking. Force platforms are very sensitive to building vibrations, and many early gait laboratories were built in basements to reduce this form of interference. In the authors' opinion, this problem has been over emphasised, since although building vibrations can be seen in force platform data, they are negligible when compared with the magnitude of the signals recorded from subjects walking on the platform.

One problem which may be experienced when using force platforms is that of *aiming*. To obtain good data, the whole of the subject's foot must land on the platform. It is tempting to tell the subject where the platform is and to ask them to make sure their footstep lands squarely on it. However, this is likely to lead to an artificial gait pattern, as the subject aims for the platform. If at all possible, the

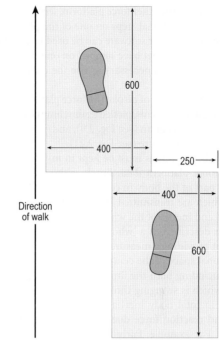

Fig. 4.17 Typical arrangement of two force platforms for use in studies of adults (dimensions in mm).

platform should be disguised so that it is not noticeably different from the rest of the floor, and the subject should not be informed of its presence. This may require that a number of walks be made before clean hits on the force plate are seen, and that slight adjustments in the starting position be made before acceptable data can be obtained.

Where it is required to record from both feet, the relative positioning of two force platforms can be a considerable problem. There is no single arrangement which is satisfactory for all subjects, and some laboratories have designed systems in which one or both platforms can be moved to suit the gait of individual subjects and to allow the examination of other activities such as running and jumping. Fig. 4.17 shows the arrangement used in a number of laboratories, which is a reasonable compromise for studies on adults but is unsatisfactory when the stride length is either very short or very long. For subjects who have a very short stride length, such as children or patients with disorders such as multiple sclerosis, better results may be obtained if the platforms are mounted with their shorter dimensions in the direction of the walk. For this reason, many laboratories use four or more force platforms with only a small gap between them. However, it is often impossible to get the whole of one foot on one force platform and the whole of the other foot on the other force platform, without also having unwanted additional steps on one of the platforms. To some extent, computer software can be used to unscramble the data when both feet have stepped on one platform, but more commonly it is necessary to use the data from only one foot at a time.

The usual methods of displaying force platform data are:
- individual components, plotted against time (see Fig. 2.20),
- the butterfly diagram (see Fig. 2.9), and
- the centre of pressure (see Fig. 2.21).

A number of things must be kept in mind when interpreting force platform data. Firstly, although the foot is the only part of the body in contact with the platform, the forces which are transmitted by the foot are derived from the mass and inertia of the whole body. The force platform has been described as a 'whole-body accelerometer', with its output providing a measure of the acceleration in three-dimensional space of the centre of gravity of the body as a whole, including both the limb that is on the ground and the leg which is swinging through the air. This means that changes in total body inertia may swamp small changes in ground reaction force due to events occurring within the foot. For example, fairly high moments are recorded about the vertical axis during the stance phase of gait (Fig. 4.18). Although these may be slightly modified by local events within the foot, they are mainly derived from the acceleration and retardation of the contralateral leg as it goes through the swing phase. The reactions to the forces responsible for this acceleration and retardation are transmitted to the floor through the stance phase leg and appear in the force platform output, principally as a torque about the vertical axis.

Force platforms have been used to test balance and to measure postural sway, which are important in some clinical assessments but by themselves are of limited value in gait analysis. Nevertheless, some laboratories use the data empirically; for example, by looking for particular patterns in the butterfly diagram (Rose, 1985). When comparing the different peaks and troughs they may be used to look for changes over time with an intervention. Some inferences can also be made from the shapes of the curves of the individual force components. For example, there is an association between stance phase flexion of the knee and a dip at mid-stance in the vertical component of force. However, the true value of the force platform is only appreciated when the ground reaction force data are combined with kinematic data. This combination provides a much more complete mechanical description of gait than either data set does by itself, and permits the calculation of joint moments and powers.

A number of devices have been developed which are not force platforms but have the same function. Typically, these consist of a number of force sensors which are fixed to the sole of a shoe. As the subject walks, electrical output gives a measure of the ground reaction force and the centre of pressure. Typically, only the vertical component of the ground reaction force is measured, although at least one tri-axial shoe-based force system has been described. The advantages claimed are:
- the ability to measure multiple steps,
- no problems with aiming,
- no risk of stepping on the platform with both feet, and
- no risk of missing the platform, either partly or completely.

The disadvantages are the presence of the force sensors beneath the feet, and the associated wiring. Also, the coordinate system for the force measurements moves with the foot, in contrast to the room-based coordinate system used for kinematic data. This makes it very difficult to combine force and kinematic data to perform a full biomechanical analysis.

Measuring Pressure Beneath the Foot

Measurement of the pressure beneath the foot is a specialised form of gait analysis which may be of particular value in conditions in which the pressure may be excessive, such as diabetic neuropathy and rheumatoid arthritis. Foot pressure measurement systems may be either floor mounted or in the form of an insole within the shoe. The SI unit for pressure is the pascal (Pa), which is a pressure of one newton per square metre. The pascal is inconveniently small, and practical measurements are generally made in kilopascals (kPa) or megapascals (MPa). For

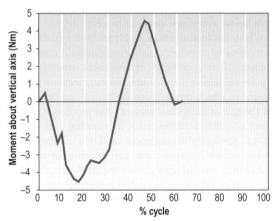

Fig. 4.18 Moments about the vertical axis at the instantaneous centre of pressure during the stance phase of gait. Normal subject, right leg. A positive moment occurs when the foot attempts to move clockwise relative to the floor.

conversions between different units of measurement, see Appendix 2.

Lord et al. (1986) highlighted that when making measurements beneath the feet, it is important to distinguish between force and pressure (force per unit area). Some measurement systems measure the force (or load) over a known area from which the mean pressure over that area can be calculated. However, the mean pressure may be much lower than the peak pressure within the area if high pressure gradients are present, which are often caused by subcutaneous bony prominences such as the metatarsal heads. A pitfall which must be kept in mind when making pressure measurements beneath the feet is that a subject will usually avoid walking on a painful area. Thus, an area of the foot which had previously experienced a high pressure and has become painful may show a low pressure when it is tested. However, this will not happen if the sole of the foot is anaesthetic, as commonly occurs in diabetic neuropathy. In this condition, very high pressures, leading to ulceration, may be recorded.

Typical pressures beneath the foot are 80 to 100 kPa in standing, 200 to 500 kPa in walking and up to 1500 kPa in some sports activities. In diabetic neuropathy, pressures as high as 3000 kPa have been recorded. To put these figures into perspective, the normal systolic blood pressure, measured at the feet in the standing position, is less than 33 kPa (250 mmHg); applied pressures higher than this will prevent blood from reaching the tissues.

Glass Plate Examination

Some useful semiquantitative information on the pressure beneath the foot can be obtained by having the subject stand on or walk across a glass plate, which is viewed from below with the aid of a mirror or video camera. It is easy to see which areas of the sole of the foot come into contact with the walking surface, and the blanching of the skin gives an idea of the applied pressure. Inspection of both the inside and outside of a subject's shoe will also provide useful information about the way the foot is used in walking; therefore, it is a good idea to ask patients to wear their oldest shoes when they come for an examination, not their newest ones!

Direct Pressure Mapping Systems

A number of low-technology methods of estimating pressure beneath the foot have been described over the years. The Harris or Harris–Beath mat is made of thin rubber, the upper surface of which consists of a pattern of ridges of different heights. Before use, it is coated with printing ink and covered by a sheet of paper, after which the subject is asked to walk across it. The highest ridges compress under relatively light pressures, with the lower ones requiring progressively greater pressures, making the transfer of ink to the paper greater in the areas of highest pressure. This gives a semiquantitative map of the pressure distribution beneath the foot. Other systems have also been described in which the subject walks on a pressure-sensitive film, a sheet of aluminium foil or carbon paper.

Pedobarograph

The pedobarograph uses an elastic mat laid on top of an edge-lit glass plate. When the subject walks on the mat it is compressed onto the glass, which loses its reflectivity, becoming progressively darker with increasing pressure. This darkening provides the means for quantitative measurement. The underside of the glass plate is usually viewed by a video camera, the monochrome image being processed to give a false-colour display in which different colours correspond to different levels of pressure.

Force Sensor Systems

A number of systems have been described in which the subject walks across an array of force sensors, each of which measures the vertical force beneath a particular area of the foot. Dividing the force by the area of the cell gives the mean pressure beneath the foot in that area. Many different types of force sensor have been used, including resistive and capacitive strain gauges, conductive rubber, piezoelectric materials and photoelastic optical systems. A number of different methods have been used to display the output of such systems, including the presentation shown in Fig. 4.19.

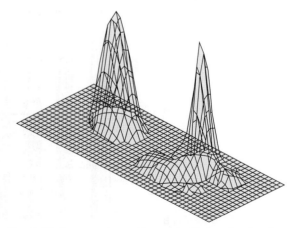

Fig. 4.19 Pressure beneath a cavus foot on landing from a jump (EM Hennig, 5th Biennial Conference, Canadian Society for Biomechanics/Société Canadienne de Bioméchanique, 1988.).

In-Shoe Devices

Many research groups have tackled the problem of measuring the pressure inside the shoe, and many commercial systems are available which can give clinically and scientifically useful data. The main challenges such systems try to overcome are the curvature of the surface, a lack of space for the transducers and the need to run large numbers of wires from inside the shoe to the measuring equipment.

MEASURING MUSCLE ACTIVITY

Electromyography

Electromyography (EMG) is the measurement of the electrical activity of muscles, which is often referred to as the motor unit action potential (MUAP). Since it is a measure of electrical and not mechanical activity, the EMG cannot be used to distinguish between concentric, isometric and eccentric contractions. In addition, the relationship between EMG activity and the force of contraction is far from straightforward. The most comprehensive textbook on EMG is *Muscles Alive: Their Functions Revealed by Electromyography* (Basmajian and De Luca, 1985), although a more recent textbook, *The Comprehensive Textbook of Clinical Biomechanics* (Richards, 2018), contains a useful summary chapter by De Luca and colleagues.

EMG can offer valuable insights within gait analysis, including information on the firing sequences of different muscles by considering the onset and offset of the activation of specific muscles (Fig. 4.20). EMG signals have both magnitude and a frequency. The frequency range of the usable EMG signal is between 1 Hz and 500 Hz and the amplitude of the EMG signal varies between 1 µV and 1 mV. The concept of magnitude and frequency can be applied to any signal, but the best way to think about this is the parallel with sound waves. The magnitude of a sound wave is how loud the signal is, and the frequency is the pitch. So, with EMG, the magnitude of the signal relates to the amount of electrical activity during muscle activation and the frequency relates to the average firing rate of all the motor units recorded. There are three common methods of recording EMG data: surface electrodes, fine wire electrodes and needle electrodes. In gait analysis, surface EMG electrodes are usually used unless deeper dwelling muscles are of interest, in which case fine wire electrodes may be required.

Surface Electrodes

Surface EMG is by far the most widely used method for gait analysis. Surface electrodes are fixed to the skin over the muscle, and the EMG is recorded as the voltage difference between two electrodes. It is usually necessary also to have a grounding electrode, either nearby or elsewhere on the body. Since the muscle action potential reaches the electrodes through the intervening layers of fascia, fat and skin, the voltage of the signal is relatively small and it is usually amplified close to, or onboard, the electrodes. The EMG signal picked up by surface electrodes is the sum of the muscle action potentials from many motor units within the most superficial muscle or muscles. Most of the signal comes from within 25 mm of the skin surface, so this type of recording is not suitable for deep muscles such as the

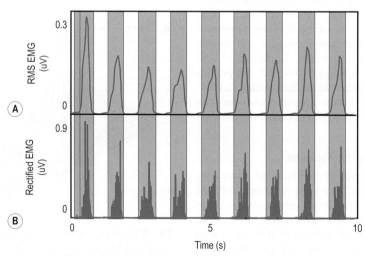

Fig. 4.20 Onsets and offsets of EMG signals from the gastrocnemius muscle during walking using (A) enveloped signals and (B) rectified signals.

iliopsoas. When targeting the EMG of a particular muscle we sometimes pick up activity from adjacent muscles; this is referred to as *cross talk*. Therefore, it is sometimes safest to regard the signal from surface electrodes as being derived from muscle groups rather than from individual muscles, although Õunpuu et al. (1997) showed that surface electrodes could satisfactorily distinguish between the three superficial muscle bellies of the quadriceps in children. There is often a change in the electrical baseline as the subject moves (*movement artifact*), and there may also be electromagnetic interference; for example, from nearby electrical equipment. The authors would recommend studying the wealth of information available in the SENIAM guidelines (www.seniam.org) and on the Delsys website (www.delsys.com).

Fine Wire Electrodes

Fine wire electrodes are introduced directly into a muscle using a hypodermic needle which is then withdrawn, leaving the wires in place. They can be quite uncomfortable or even painful. The wire is insulated, except for a few millimetres at the tip. The EMG signal may be recorded in three different ways:
- Between a pair of wires inserted using a single needle
- Between two fine wires inserted separately
- Between a single fine wire and a ground electrode

The voltage recorded within the muscle is generally higher than that from surface electrodes, particularly if separate wires are used, and there is less interference from movement and from electromagnetic fields. The signal is derived from a fairly small region of a single muscle, generally from a few motor units only, a fact which must be taken into account when interpreting the data. Because it is an uncomfortable and invasive technique, fine-wire EMG is usually only performed on selected muscles in patients in whom it is likely to be particularly useful.

Needle Electrodes

Needle electrodes are generally more appropriate to physiological research than to gait analysis. This technique uses a hypodermic needle which contains an insulated central conductor that records the EMG signal from a very localised area within the muscle into which it is inserted, and can only record a small number of motor units which may not represent the activation of the muscle bulk.

Signal Processing of EMG Signals
Raw EMG

EMG signals are low voltage and can be hidden by other electrical noise. Therefore, EMG signals have to be amplified to reduce the effect of this noise, typically between 1000 and 10,000 times to give a measurable signal. To decrease electrical interference the amplifiers can be positioned close to the electrodes, which reduces the length of wire that can pick up interference.

Often the EMG signal will oscillate on either side of a floating reference; this is referred to as *low voltage, direct current* (DC) *offset*, or *bias*. The way to remove the DC offset is to find the mean value of the entire signal and then subtract this from the original signal, therefore pulling the data to a 'zeroed' position. The threshold of the signal can then be set to give information as to whether or not the muscle is firing, which gives an on/off measurement of whether or not the muscle is active, known as muscle activity onset and offset.

If an individual is moving quickly, movement artifacts within the EMG signal can sometimes be seen. These artifacts can be minimised by filtering the signal at 20 Hz. This removes frequencies less than 20 Hz, which is where the majority of frequencies associated with limb movement are seen. At foot strike, higher-frequency movement artifacts can sometimes be seen which may require a higher-frequency high-pass filter. However, this may also remove some of the EMG signal as well, so care is needed to minimise the attenuation of the low-frequency components whilst minimising the effect on the EMG signal.

Rectified, Enveloped and Integrated EMG

Rectification is required as the DC offset–corrected EMG signal oscillates from positive to negative on either side of the zero line. Therefore, if we were to try to find the mean value, we would end up with zero. Rectification makes all the negative values in the signal positive. This can be achieved by first squaring the signal and then taking the square root (Fig. 4.21A). This is sometimes preferred when determining the threshold for the onset and offset of muscle contractions (Fig. 4.20B).

Enveloped EMG is a common method of showing the level of muscle activity which involves filtering or processing the EMG signal. A low-pass filter is used which lets the lower frequencies through whilst stopping the higher frequencies. The practical upshot of this is a smoothing effect similar to that used in kinematic analysis. There is much debate as to how much EMG signals should be filtered using low-pass filters, with typical amounts of cut-off frequency filtering used in the literature varying between 6 Hz and 25 Hz. Another method of filtering uses the root mean square, which is calculated using a moving average window. The calculation consists of three steps:
1. Square each data point in the signal.
2. Take the square root (Fig. 4.21A) which in essence rectifies the signal.
3. Perform a moving average over a specified window length (e.g., 0.125 seconds) (Fig. 4.21B).

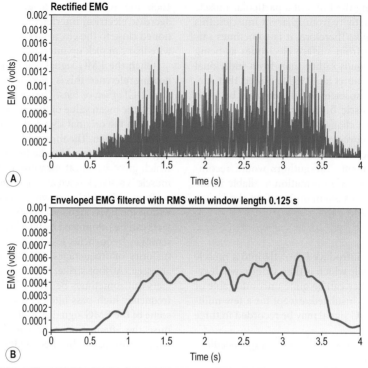

Fig. 4.21 (A) Rectified EMG. (B) Root mean square (RMS) EMG with a 0.125-second window length.

Integrated EMG (iEMG) refers to the area under the fully rectified EMG trace. iEMG has been used as an indicator of work done by the muscle. From this, the amount of relative work done by a muscle group during push off whilst walking could be found if the events at the start and end of the push off were identified. Therefore, iEMG would give us a single value for this period.

Limitations of EMG

EMG can give important information on the magnitude and timing of muscle activations, but it does not give a direct measure of the muscle force within individual muscles. Many attempts have been made over the years to estimate muscle forces, all with limited success. Within gait analysis, the EMG signal is generally processed to provide a visible indication of the onset and offset and the level of muscle activity. This information on muscle activation and level of activity can be of considerable value in gait assessment. For example, one form of treatment in cerebral palsy is to transfer the tendon of a muscle to a different position, thereby altering the action of the muscle. When contemplating this type of surgery, it is essential to use EMG first, to make sure the timing of the muscle contraction is

appropriate for its new role. It is also possible to determine any relative changes in activity due to immediate treatment (e.g., the use of orthoses, taping and bracing).

MEASURING ENERGY EXPENDITURE

The most accurate way to measure the total amount of energy used in performing an activity such as walking is *whole-body calorimetry*, in which the subject is kept in an insulated chamber from which the heat output of the body can be measured. This is, of course, quite impractical, except as a research technique. The most common way to estimate energy expenditure is based on measuring the body's oxygen consumption. There are also less direct methods, using either mechanical calculations or the measurement of heart rate.

Oxygen Consumption

The measurement of oxygen consumption requires an analysis of the subject's exhaled breath. If both the volume of exhaled air and its oxygen content are measured, the amount of oxygen consumed in a given time can be calculated. The amount of carbon dioxide produced can also be measured as the ratio of the carbon dioxide produced to the oxygen consumed, also known as the *respiratory quotient*, which provides information on the type of metabolism that is taking place, either aerobic or anaerobic. Except under abnormal environmental conditions, it is not necessary to measure either the oxygen or the carbon dioxide in the inspired air, since these are almost constant.

The classic method of measuring oxygen consumption and carbon dioxide production is to fit the subject with a noseclip and mouthpiece and to collect the whole of the expired air in a large plastic or rubberised canvas Douglas bag, or more commonly, by using a portable breath-by-breath gas analyser. After correcting for temperature, air pressure and humidity, a very accurate estimate of oxygen consumption can be obtained. The use of a portable system with a face mask is routine in some gait analysis centres; even children accept it well. Occasionally, studies of locomotion are made using a spirometer, an oxygen-filled, closed system into which the subject breathes and which absorbs the exhaled carbon dioxide. Since spirometers are not usually portable, they are practical only when the subject is walking on a treadmill. However, collecting the expirate can be uncomfortable for the subject, and consequently, spirometers can be unsuitable for some patients.

Oxygen consumption can be presented in one of two ways: energy expenditure per unit time and energy expenditure per unit distance. Energy expenditure per unit time (E_w) shows an increase in the energy consumed by an individual with the square of the walking speed, which is usually reported as calories per minute or joules per second (watt). This can be further developed by controlling for body mass, which allows comparison of the energy expenditure per kilogram among individuals of different mass (Fig. 4.22). The measurement of energy per unit distance walked (E_m) provides a quantitative measure of energy economy. Fig. 4.23 shows how the energy expenditure per metre walked varies

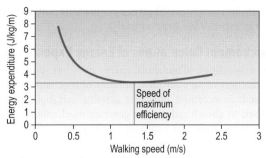

Fig. 4.23 Energy expenditure per metre (E_m) versus walking speed.

with walking speed. When this value is at a minimum the individual is walking at their most efficient speed. Therefore, we can determine that the most efficient walking speed is 1.33 metres per second, 80 metres per minute, 4.7 kilometres per hour or 2.9 miles per hour for healthy, able-bodied individuals. Any increase or decrease in walking speed will cause an increase in the energy expenditure per metre walked and a reduction in efficiency (Corcoran, 1970; Ralston, 1958). This method finds the most efficient walking speed for a particular individual and allows a useful comparison when studying pathological gait.

Heart Rate Monitoring

Rose (1983) stated that heart rate monitoring is a good substitute for the measurement of oxygen uptake, since a number of studies over the years have shown that there is a surprisingly close relationship between the two. One method of recording heart rate is to detect the heart's electrical activity using electrodes mounted on the chest. However, the development and commercialisation of wearable heart rate monitors has opened up this area for personal monitoring. As a general rule, energy consumption is related to the difference in heart rate between the resting condition and that measured during the exercise. Rather than attempting to relate the change in heart rate directly to energy consumption, some investigators use the *physiological cost index* (PCI), which is said to be less sensitive to differences among individuals (Steven et al., 1983). This can be calculated as follows:

PCI = (heart rate walking − heart rate resting)/speed

The calculation must be made using consistent units, with the heart rate in beats per minute and the speed in metres per minute, or the heart rate in beats per second and the speed in metres per second. The measurement unit for the PCI is net beats per metre. Since the heart rate tends to be somewhat variable, small changes in PCI may not be

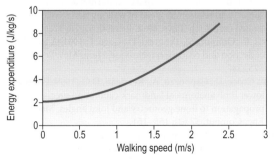

Fig. 4.22 Energy expenditure per second (E_w) versus walking speed.

significant; however, PCI gives a comparable pattern to the energy expenditure per metre (E_m).

Mechanical Calculations of Energy Expenditure

The expenditure of metabolic energy does not result in the production of an equivalent amount of mechanical work. Indeed, in eccentric muscular activity, metabolic energy is used to absorb rather than generate mechanical energy. Even when muscular contractions are used to do positive work, the efficiency of conversion is relatively low, is variable and is difficult to estimate. For these reasons, it is generally unsatisfactory to use mechanical calculations to estimate the total metabolic energy consumed in a complicated activity such as walking. Nonetheless, this method of estimating energy expenditure is used in some laboratories (Gage et al., 1984) and is known as the *estimated external work of walking* (EEWW). Calculations of this type are more reliable for activities in which the relationship between muscular contraction and mechanical output is extremely simple, such as in the concentric contraction of a single muscle. Even though mechanical calculations are generally unsatisfactory for estimating the total energy consumption of the body, measurement of energy generation and transfer at individual joints may be of great value in gait analysis using a combination of kinetic and kinematic measurements.

CONCLUSION

Clinical gait laboratories generally combine kinematic (movement) with kinetic (force) data. The capability of the combined data is greater than that of the sum of its component parts. The reason for this is that if the relationship is known between the limb segments and the ground reaction force vector, it is possible to perform inverse dynamics, which allows the calculation of joint moments and powers. Such calculations require knowledge of limb masses, moments of inertia and the location of their centres of gravity. Direct measurements of these are clearly impossible, but published data, modified to suit the subject's anthropometry, give an acceptable approximation. It is a common practice in such calculations to regard the foot as a single rigid object, although this simplification undoubtedly causes errors in calculating the ankle power, and multiple-segment foot inverse dynamic models have been suggested to answer specific hypotheses.

A fully equipped clinical gait laboratory can be expected to possess, at a minimum, a combined kinetic/kinematic system, with wireless EMG as well as video recording capabilities. Equipment may also be available for measuring oxygen uptake or pressure beneath the feet. If the laboratory is also used for research, further facilities and equipment may also be present. However, one of the challenges with fully equipped clinical gait laboratories is that they provide such a wealth of data that it may be very difficult to distinguish between those measurements which are important and those which are not. A number of mathematical, statistical and computational techniques have been used in an attempt to address this problem, some of which will be considered in more detail in Chapter 5.

REFERENCES

Basmajian, J.V., De Luca, C.J., 1985. Muscles Alive: Their Functions Revealed by Electromyography. Lippincott Williams & Wilkins, Baltimore, MD.

Bell, A., Pederson, D., Brand, R., 1990. A comparison of the accuracy of several hip centre location predication methods. J. Biomech. 23 (6), 617–621.

Bilney, B., Morris, M., Webster, K., 2003. Concurrent related validity of the GAITRite walkway system for quantification of the spatial and temporal parameters of gait. Gait Posture 17, 68–74.

Birch, I., Raymond, L., Christou, A., Fernando, M.A., Harrison, N., Paul, F., 2013. The identification of individuals by observational gait analysis using closed circuit television footage. Sci. Justice 53 (3), 339–342.

Bronner, S., Agraharasamakulam, S., Ojofeitimi, S., 2010a. Reliability and validity of a new ankle electrogoniometer. J. Med. Eng. Technol. 34 (5-6), 350–355.

Bronner, S., Agraharasamakulam, S., Ojofeitimi, S., 2010b. Reliability and validity of electrogoniometry measurement of lower extremity movement. J. Med. Eng. Technol. 34 (3), 232–242.

Cappozzo, A., Catani, F., Croce, U.D., Leardini, A., 1995. Position and orientation in space of bones during movement: anatomical frame definition and determination. Clin. Biomech. 10 (4), 171–178.

Cappozzo, A., Della Croce, U., Leardini, A., et al., 2005. Human movement analysis using stereophotogrammetry. Part 1: Theoretical background. Gait Posture 21, 186–196.

Chiari, L., Della Croce, U., Leardini, A., et al., 2005. Human movement analysis using stereophotogrammetry. Part 2: Instrumental errors. Gait Posture 21, 197–211.

Corcoran, B., 1970. Oxygen uptake in normal and handicapped subjects, in relation to speed of walking beside velocity controlled cart. Arch. Phys. Med. Rehabil. 51, 78–87.

Davis, R., Ounpuu, S., Tyburski, D., Gage, J., 1991. A gait data collection and reduction technique. Hum. Mov. Sci. 10, 575–587.

Della Croce, U., Cappozzo, A., Kerrigan, D.C., 1999. Pelvis and lower limb anatomical landmark calibration precision and its propagation to bone geometry and joint angles. Med. Biol. Eng. Comput. 37 (2), 155–161.

Della Croce, U., Leardini, A., Chiari, L., et al., 2005. Human movement analysis using stereophotogrammetry. Part 4: Assessment of anatomical landmark misplacement and its effects on joint kinematics. Gait Posture 21, 226–237.

Fennema, M.C., Bloomfield, R.A., Lanting, B.A., Birmingham, T.B., Teeter, M.G., 2019. Repeatability of measuring knee flexion angles with wearable inertial sensors. The Knee 26 (1), 97–105.

Gage, J.R., Fabian, D., Hicks, R., et al., 1984. Pre- and postoperative gait analysis in patients with spastic diplegia: a preliminary report. J. Pediatr. Orthop. 4, 715–725.

Gerny, K., 1983. A clinical method of quantitative gait analysis. Phys. Ther 63, 1125–1126.

Kadaba, M.P., Ramakrishnan, H.K., Wootten, M.E., Gainey, J., Gorton, G., Cochran, G.V., 1989. Repeatability of kinematic, kinetic, and electromyographic data in normal adult gait. J. Orthop. Res 7 (6), 849–860.

Larsen, P.K., Simonsen, E.B., Lynnerup, N., 2008. Gait analysis in forensic medicine. J. Forensic Sci 53 (5), 1149–1153.

Leardini, A., Chiari, L., Della Croce, U., et al., 2005. Human movement analysis using stereophotogrammetry. Part 3: Soft tissue artifact assessment and compensation. Gait Posture 21, 212–225.

Leardini, A., Lullini, G., Giannini, S., Berti, L., Ortolani, M., Caravaggi, P., 2014. Validation of the angular measurements of a new inertial-measurement-unit based rehabilitation system: comparison with state-of-the-art gait analysis. J. Neuroeng. Rehabil. 11, 136.

Lord, M., Reynolds, D.P., Hughes, J.R., 1986. Foot pressure measurement: a review of clinical findings. J. Biomed. Eng. 8, 283–294.

McGinley, J.L., Goldie, P.A., Greenwood, K.M., Olney, S.J., 2003. Accuracy and reliability of observational gait analysis data: judgments of push-off in gait after stroke. Phys. Ther 83 (2), 146–160.

Morris, J.R.W., 1973. Accelerometry – a technique for the measurement of human body movements. J. Biomech. 6, 729–736.

Õunpuu, S., DeLuca, P.A., Bell, K.J., et al., 1997. Using surface electrodes for the evaluation of the rectus femoris, vastus medialis and vastus lateralis in children with cerebral palsy. Gait Posture 5, 211–216.

Professional Staff Association of Rancho Los Amigos Medical Center, 1989. Observational Gait Analysis Handbook. Rancho Los Amigos Medical Center, Downey, CA.

Rafferty, D., Bell, F., 1995. Gait analysis – a semiautomated approach. Gait Posture 3 (3), 184.

Ralston, H.J., 1958. Energy speed relation and optimal speed during level walking. Int. Z. Angew. Physiol 17, 277.

Reinking, M.F., Dugan, L., Ripple, N., Schleper, K., Scholz, H., Spadino, J., et al., 2018. Reliability of two-dimensional video-based running gait analysis. Int. J. Sports Phys. Ther. 13 (3), 453–461.

Richards, J., 2018. The Comprehensive Textbook of Clinical Biomechanics. Churchill Livingstone, London.

Robinson, J.L., Smidt, G.L., 1981. Quantitative gait evaluation in the clinic. Phys. Ther 61, 351–353.

Rose, G.K., 1983. Clinical gait assessment: a personal view. J. Med. Eng. Technol. 7, 273–279.

Rose, G.K., 1985. Use of ORLAU-Pedotti diagrams in clinical gait assessment. In: Whittle, M., Harris, D. (Eds.), Biomechanical Measurement in Orthopaedic Practice. Clarendon Press, Oxford, UK, pp. 205–210.

Seel, T., Raisch, J., Schauer, T., 2014. IMU-based joint angle measurement for gait analysis. Sensors 14 (4), 6891–6909.

Shamsi, M., Mirzaei, M., Khabiri, S.S., 2019. Universal goniometer and electro-goniometer intra-examiner reliability in measuring the knee range of motion during active knee extension test in patients with chronic low back pain with short hamstring muscle. BMC Sports Sci. Med. Rehabil. 11, 4.

Steven, M.M., Capell, H.A., Sturrock, R.D., et al., 1983. The physiological cost of gait (PCG): a new technique for evaluating nonsteroidal antiinflammatory drugs in rheumatoid arthritis. Br. J. Rheumatol. 22, 141–145.

Toro, B., Nester, C.J., Farren, P.C., 2007. The development and validity of the Salford Gait Tool: an observation-based clinical gait assessment tool. Arch. Phys. Med. Rehabil. 88 (3), 321–327.

5

Applications of Gait Analysis

Michael Whittle, Hannah Shepherd,
Gabor Barton and Jim Richards

This chapter provides an overview of some of the ways in which gait analysis is currently used, and takes a look ahead at future possibilities. It is not intended to transform the reader into a gait analysis expert. To that end, we advise anyone planning to use gait analysis in clinical decision-making to attend courses and receive training on interpreting gait analysis data, and if possible, to spend some time studying or working in a clinical gait laboratory. Several national and international societies specialise in gait analysis courses and training, including the European Society for Movement Analysis in Adults and Children (ESMAC), the Gait and Clinical Movement Analysis Society (GCMAS) and the Clinical Movement Analysis Society (CMAS).

Applications of gait analysis may be divided into two main categories: *clinical gait assessment* and *gait research*. Clinical gait assessment aims to help individual patients directly, whereas gait research aims to improve our understanding of gait, either as an end in and of itself or to improve medical diagnoses or inform future treatments. There is obviously some overlap, in that many people performing clinical gait assessment use the results of their analyses as the basis for research studies. However, there are some differences that should be noted. Importantly, in gait research, it might be acceptable to spend several hours preparing the participant and taking measurements, with data processing happening at a later date, whereas in the clinical setting, patients often tire easily and the results are usually needed as quickly as possible.

CLINICAL GAIT ASSESSMENT

Clinical gait assessment seeks to describe the way in which a person walks. This may be all that is required, if the aim is simply to document their current status. Alternatively, it may be just one step in a continuing process, such as the planning of treatment or the monitoring of progress over time. Rose (1983) made a distinction between gait analysis and gait assessment. He regarded gait analysis as 'data gathering' and gait assessment as 'the integration of this information with that from other sources for the purposes of clinical decision making'. Gait assessment in the clinical setting is based on three components: the patient's history, the patient's physical examination and special investigations. In this context, gait analysis may be regarded as a special investigation, with the results augmenting other investigations such as X-ray reports and magnetic resonance imaging (MRI) scans.

The simplest form of gait assessment is practised every day in physicians' offices, rehabilitation clinics, orthotic and prosthetic clinics, sports centres and many other settings throughout the world. Every time a clinician watches an individual walk across a room, they are performing an assessment of the patient's gait. However, such an assessment is often non-systematic, and the most that can be hoped for is to obtain a general impression of how well the patient walks and perhaps some idea of one or two of the main problems relating to their gait. This could be termed an *informal* gait assessment.

A *formal* gait assessment requires careful examination using a systematic approach augmented by objective measurements where possible, usually resulting in a written report. The techniques used in clinical gait assessment vary enormously and are dictated by the nature of the patient's clinical condition and the skills and facilities available. In general, however, a clinical gait assessment is performed for one of three possible reasons: it may form the basis of clinical decision-making, it may help with the detailed characterisation of an abnormal gait or it may be used to document a patient's condition at a particular point in time.

CLINICAL DECISION-MAKING

Both Rose (1983) and Gage (1983; 2009) suggested that clinical decision-making in cases of gait abnormality should involve three clear stages: gait assessment, hypothesis formation and hypothesis testing.

Gait Assessment

The gait assessment starts with a full clinical history from the patient and from any others involved, such as doctors and other health professionals or family members. If the patient previously had surgery, details of the procedure should be obtained, if possible, from the operative notes. This is followed by a physical examination, with a particular emphasis on the patient's neuromusculoskeletal system. In many laboratories, physical examinations are performed by both a medical doctor and a physiotherapist. Finally, a formal gait analysis is carried out.

Hypothesis Formation

The development of hypotheses regarding the cause or causes of the observed abnormalities should be informed by specific questions raised by the referring clinician. It is very important that these hypotheses are reviewed along with the gait assessment data in a consultation involving a multidisciplinary team of colleagues. This is highlighted by Rose (1983), who emphasised that the patient's gait pattern is not entirely the direct result of the pathology, but is the net result of the original problem and the patient's ability to compensate for it. Therefore, the involvement of medical

doctors and allied health professionals in clinical decision-making to consider these aspects is key.

Hypothesis Testing

This stage is sometimes omitted when there is little doubt as to the cause of the abnormalities observed. However, where some doubt does exist, the hypothesis can be tested in two different ways: either by using a different method of measurement, or by attempting in some way to modify the patient's gait. Some laboratories routinely use a fairly complete standard protocol, including video recording, kinematic measurements, force platform measurements and surface electromyography (EMG). They will then add other measurements, such as fine wire EMG, when it is necessary to test a specific hypothesis. Others start the gait analysis using a simple method, such as video recording, and only add techniques such as EMG or the use of a force platform if they would clearly be helpful. Rose (1983) opposed the use of a standard protocol for all patients, since some of the procedures turn out to be unnecessary and there is a risk of ending up with 'an exhausted subject in pain'.

The other method of testing a hypothesis is to reexamine the gait after attempting some form of modification, typically through application of an orthotic to limit joint motion or a medication such as botulinum toxin to decrease spasticity; by anaesthetising a muscle; or through gait modification as a result of surgery and physical therapy.

Different gait analysis systems provide different amounts of technical data on the patient's gait, and examination of the data can be a long and painstaking process. One of the most important parts of the assessment is to identify deviations from normal, and details such as foot timing, joint angles, moments and powers and EMG are frequently included. Information on foot timing may be useful to identify asymmetries and may indicate problems with balance, stability and pain, whereas joint angles provide measures of the amount of movement in the different planes, and joint moments indicate which structures are coming under load and offer an estimation on the amount of load. Joint powers may help discriminate between concentric and eccentric muscle contractions, or whether soft tissues are under passive or active load. EMG analysis can also contribute to this process by identifying which muscles are active and are thus candidates for providing force at different times during the gait cycle, and can provide important information on functional deficits, motor patterns and motor control.

Once the preliminary gait analysis reports have been prepared, the team meets to discuss the case. The composition of the team varies considerably among facilities, but it commonly consists of a medical doctor, a physiotherapist and a kinesiologist or bioengineer, with the optional addition of other health professionals including prosthetists, orthotists and podiatrists. Indeed, anyone with an interest in providing the best possible care for the patient may be invited to join the team.

Having made a detailed assessment of the patient's functional problems, the team decides on an appropriate form of intervention which could involve physiotherapy, orthotics, surgery, drug treatment or a combination of these. At the end of the intervention, or after a suitable recovery period if surgery has been performed, the patient is often reassessed to determine the efficacy and effectiveness of the intervention and to decide whether further interventions may be required. This also gives the clinical team the opportunity to perform a critical review of the original diagnosis and treatment plan so that they can decide whether the correct decisions were made.

Another use of multiple assessments is to convince the patient and/or their relatives that progress has been made when they think it has not. An objective form of monitoring progress is particularly important for use in the evaluation of novel and controversial methods of treatment, where the enthusiasm of the investigators has been known to lead to errors in judgment.

Gait assessment may form part of the overall documentation of a number of medical conditions that involve the locomotor system. A deterioration in gait with the passage of time may be detected early, allowing remedial action to be taken. It may also identify clinical signs which should be looked for in other cases of the same condition, particularly if it is very uncommon.

Although clinical decision-making is the most direct way in which gait assessment may be used to help an individual patient, there are also instances when simply documenting the current state of a patient's gait may be of value. As part of the overall assessment of a patient with a disability, a clinician may require more detail about how well they walk. This type of gait assessment may be directly intended for use in clinical decision-making, but it is sometimes performed speculatively in case it should reveal a treatable cause for the patient's walking disorder.

DIAGNOSIS OF ABNORMAL GAIT

Most patients undergoing gait assessment have already been diagnosed with the principal disease or condition affecting their gait. In such cases, the assessment is carried out to make a more detailed exploration of functional problems relating to the exact state of particular joints and muscles. One method of charting gait abnormalities within common gait disorders, their possible causes and the type of evidence which would confirm or refute them is shown in Table 5.1. On occasion, however, a patient is seen in whom the cause of an abnormal gait is not clear.

A number of apparently abnormal gait patterns are, in fact, habits rather than the result of underlying pathology, and gait analysis techniques may be useful to identify them.

Since any pathology affecting the locomotor system generally reduces a person's ability to alter their gait pattern, a variable gait may be suggestive of a habit pattern and a highly reproducible gait may suggest a pathological process. Therefore, the assessment must take many other factors into account, including the possibility of a pathological process which includes an element of variability, such as ataxia or athetosis. One unusual application of gait analysis is to distinguish between a gait abnormality due to a genuine neuromuscular cause and one due to a psychogenic cause, such as may be seen in cases of malingering (Wesdock et al., 2003).

An example of the use of gait assessment to differentiate between pathological gaits and habit patterns is in the diagnosis of toe walking. Some children prefer to walk on their toes rather than on the whole foot, in a pattern known as *idiopathic toe walking*. It is important, but also quite difficult, to be able to differentiate between this relatively harmless and self-limiting condition and more serious conditions such as cerebral palsy. Hicks et al. (1988) stated that earlier attempts to establish the diagnosis using EMG alone had not been successful. In their study, they compared the gait kinematics of seven idiopathic toe walkers and seven children with mild spastic diplegia. There was a clear difference between the two groups in the pattern of sagittal plane knee and ankle motion. Both groups had initial contact by either flat foot or toe strike, but in the toe walkers this was due to ankle plantarflexion whereas in the children with cerebral palsy it was due to knee flexion. There were also other differences between the two groups, suggesting that gait assessment can add value in making a differential diagnosis.

CONDITIONS BENEFITING FROM GAIT ASSESSMENT

A large number of diseases affect the neuromuscular and musculoskeletal systems and may thus lead to gait disorders. Among the most important are:

- cerebral palsy,
- parkinsonism,
- muscular dystrophy,
- osteoarthritis,
- rheumatoid arthritis,
- lower limb amputation,
- stroke,
- traumatic brain injury,
- spinal cord injury,
- myelodysplastic syndromes and
- multiple sclerosis.

While it is possible that gait assessment may benefit a person affected by one of these conditions, it is clear that greater benefits are possible in some pathologies than in

TABLE 5.1 Common gait abnormalities, their possible causes and evidence required for confirmation.

Foot slap at heel contact	Below normal dorsiflexor activity at heel contact	Below normal tibialis anterior EMG or dorsiflexor moment at heel contact
Forefoot or flatfoot initial contact	(a) Hyperactive plantarflexor activity in late swing (b) Structural limitation in ankle range (c) Short step length	(a) Above normal plantarflexor EMG in late swing (b) Decreased dorsiflexor range of motion (c) See a–d immediately below
Short step	(a) Weak push off prior to swing (b) Weak hip flexors at toe off and early swing (c) Excessive deceleration of leg in late swing (d) Above normal contralateral hip extensor activity during contralateral stance	(a) Below normal plantarflexor moment or power generation or EMG during push off (b) Below normal hip flexor moment or power or EMG during late push off and early swing (c) Above normal hamstring EMG or knee flexor moment or power absorption late in swing (d) Hyperactivity in EMG of contralateral hip extensors
Stiff-legged weightbearing	Above normal extensor activity at the ankle, knee or hip early in stance[a]	Above normal EMG activity or moments in hip extensors, knee extensors or plantarflexors early in stance
Stance phase with flexed but rigid knee	Above normal extensor activity in early and mid-stance at the ankle and hip, but with reduced knee extensor activity	Above normal EMG activity or moments in hip extensors and plantarflexors in early and mid-stance
Weak push off accompanied by observable pull off	Weak plantarflexor activity at push off; normal, or above normal, hip flexor activity during late push off and early swing	Below normal plantarflexor EMG, moment or power during push off; normal or above normal hip flexor EMG or moment or power during late push off and early swing
Hip hiking in swing (with or without circumduction of lower limb)	(a) Weak hip, knee or ankle dorsiflexor activity during swing (b) Overactive extensor synergy during swing	(a) Below normal tibialis anterior EMG or hip or knee flexors during swing (b) Above normal hip or knee extensor EMG or moment during swing
Trendelenburg gait	(a) Weak hip abductors (b) Overactive hip adductors	(a) Below normal EMG in hip abductors: gluteus medius and minimus, tensor fascia lata (b) Above normal EMG in hip adductors, adductor longus, magnus and brevis, and gracilis

[a]Note: there may be below normal extensor forces at one joint but only in the presence of abnormally high extensor forces at one or both of the other joints.

Reproduced with permission from Winter, D.A.,1985. Concerning the scientific basis for the diagnosis of pathological gait and for rehabilitation protocols. Physiotherapy, Canada 37: 245–252.

EMG, Electromyography.

others. Many working in the field of clinical gait assessment have noted the difficulty of deducing an underlying cause from observed gait abnormalities due to the movement compensations which take place. Since gait patterns are seldom clear-cut, expert systems cannot generally use a fixed set of rules, but rather need to learn to recognise patterns within complex sets of data. We cover some of the latest techniques in the next section.

NEW DEVELOPMENTS IN GAIT ANALYSIS

Advanced Techniques Applied to Under Researched Pathologies

Gait analysis is a vital tool in clinical settings and for research purposes. The study of gait has been used to aid in identifying mechanisms, characterising classifications and making clinical decisions in a variety of well-known pathologies including cerebral palsy, stroke and osteoarthritis. However, there are several other, lesser-known diseases that have severe effects on gait and mobility but are often overlooked. A disease or disorder is considered rare if it has a prevalence of less than 1 per 2,000 (European Commission, 2022), and there are an estimated 7,000 known rare diseases (Wakap et al., 2020). Rare diseases that affect mobility could be musculoskeletal, such as alkaptonuria, osteogenesis imperfecta and achondroplasia; or neuromuscular, such as functional neurological disorders, Duchenne muscular dystrophy, and Huntington's disease. Sadly, due to the rarity of such diseases, there is often a lack of awareness and knowledge of them among clinicians. Additionally, funding is often limited, and access to specialised assessments and services means the lesser-known diseases are often neglected in the research community. With limited research on rare diseases and their effect on gait and mobility, it becomes a matter of starting from scratch. Therefore, when considering under-researched pathologies, research should be approached using advanced techniques and new technologies to help solve previously unidentified problems, as well as to improve gait and function and, ultimately, quality of life for patients with rare diseases. This section will walk through the process of understanding gait in an under researched pathology named alkaptonuria (AKU). A hereditary disease, AKU results in a process called *ochronosis*, which leads to a dark discolouration in fibrous connective tissues and changes the structural integrity of the joint, causing it to become brittle. The joints most affected by this process are those which are anatomically associated with greatest mechanical load, including the knees, hips and spine. The symptoms of AKU include joint decline, pain and premature osteoarthritis; by just 50 years of age, more than 50% of AKU patients have undergone at least one total joint arthroplasty (Ranganath et al., 2013). To understand gait in this population, there are innovative techniques and tools which can help us monitor disease progression across the life span; characterise and describe gait mechanisms for the first time and most importantly, inform treatment planning and interventions.

Self-Organising Maps and Single Summary Measures

A three-dimensional gait analysis provides a wealth of highly complex and interdependent data collated from multiple joints, in three planes of motion, across a full gait cycle. Data reduction techniques help manage the high dimensionality of gait data sets which enable us to identify gait patterns, monitor progression of gait over time, or quantify the effect of the disease on gait. One method is to cluster techniques which use self-organising maps (SOMs) (Kohonen, 2001). SOMs utilise a neural network which classifies inputs such as marker positions according to how they are grouped within an input space, identifying any clusters within the data set presented to it based on similarities. The results can be presented on an *n*-dimensional map, but for ease of interpretation they are typically presented in a one-, two- or three-dimensional topological map. If clear clustering appears within the results, this suggests that gait data in the patient group differs from unimpaired gait data and indicates whether there are common and similar gait patterns within the patient gait data.

Another way to reduce the complexity and dimensions of gait data is to produce a single summary gait measure. Well-known methods include the Gillette Gait Index (GGI) (Schutte et al., 2000), the Gait Deviation Index (GDI) (Schwartz and Rozumalski, 2008), Gait Profile Score (GPS) (Baker et al. 2009) and the Movement Deviation Profile (MDP) (Barton et al., 2012) (Fig. 5.1). Now used regularly in clinical practice, single summary gait measures enable us to easily identify when gait abnormalities appear during the life span and quantify the severity indicated by a single score.

In AKU, it was originally thought that ochronosis and other symptoms began around 30 years of age (Ranganath and Cox, 2011). However, when the MDP was used to map the natural progression of gait deviations in AKU in patients between the ages of 16 and 70, it was found that gait deviations began at the age of 16 (Barton et al., 2015; Cox et al., 2019) (Fig. 5.2). This coincided with other subclinical measures such as increased pain and pigmentation within the joint. These results suggested that gait problems began in younger adults with AKU, leading to treatment considerations at an earlier age than previously thought. When using clever data reduction techniques such as self-organising maps and summary gait measures, it is possible to simplify the interpretation of gait data, monitor the progression of disease and its effects on gait over time and measure the effectiveness of interventions which can be determined by a move of the MDP curve towards that of healthy control subjects.

Identifying Joint-Specific Mechanisms

For clinicians to identify and understand gait mechanisms and prescribe clinical interventions or treatments, they must be able to interpret gait at the joint level. Traditional approaches tend to extract predetermined, discrete scalar gait parameters such as peaks, troughs or ranges of motion. These discrete parameters are then tested for statistically significant differences between a pathological gait and a healthy reference. However, discrete parameters extracted in this way are extremely susceptible to regional focus bias, are limited to specific events during the gait cycle

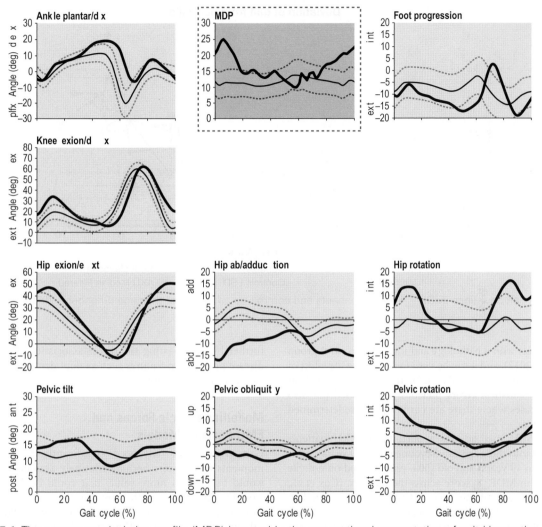

Fig. 5.1 The movement deviation profile (MDP) inserted in the conventional presentation of gait kinematics. Note that the axes and the presentation of a patient's MDP curve over the mean and SD of controls is identical to the other curves. The MDP chart *(surrounded by a dotted line)* summarises the other nine angle curves *(bold curves)* and shows the timing and extent of deviations from normality *(thin curves)* during the gait cycle (Barton et al., 2012).

and overlook any continuous effects. When considering under researched pathologies, it is often unknown which gait parameters at which point during the gait cycle have a strong association with clinical presentations.

When considering our understanding of gait in AKU, a full description of gait must be analysed to find joint-specific differences compared to healthy age-matched control subjects, and gait mechanisms need to be identified for the first time in a way that is statistically robust. A method which overcomes many of these issues is Statistical Parametric Mapping (SPM) (Friston et al., 2007). SPM was originally used to analyse multidimensional MRI information, but has recently been introduced in the processing of biomechanical data due to its ability to analyse waveforms (Castro et al., 2015; Pataky, Vanrenterghem and Robinson, 2015). Instead of statistically comparing specific data points at fixed events of the gait cycle, SPM allows analysis of the entire gait cycle, indicating where in the cycle there is a significant difference between data sets. This has been shown to be effective in determining differences among

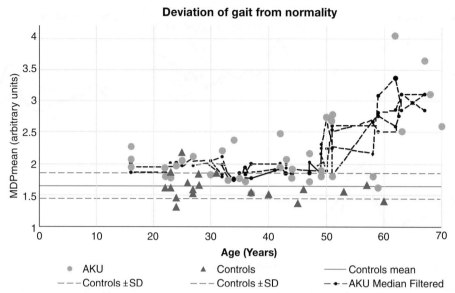

Fig. 5.2 Gait deviations (MDP$_{mean}$) of AKU patients and controls as a function of their age (Shepherd, 2020).

individuals with a pathology and those in a control group (Pataky, 2012), and it can be used to determine the effect of interventions (Klein et al., 2021). This method of analysis removes statistical errors previously mentioned but also aids in cases where there are currently no predetermined parameters.

The SPM method was applied to 36 AKU patients grouped into three age bands; young (16 to 29 years), middle (30 to 49 years) and old (50+ years); based on notable changes in MDP$_{mean}$ score across the life span (Cox et al., 2019). The gait of the AKU patients were compared to those in a speed-matched control group, and all lower-limb kinematics and kinetics were analysed. The results identified joint-specific mechanisms in the three age groups, with some interesting patterns. As age increased, there was an apparent shift from sagittal plane joint deviations to the frontal and transverse planes, demonstrating that AKU gait is affected in all three planes of motion throughout the gait cycle. In addition, there were potentially damaging, previously unidentified gait deviations in the younger group, and multiple gait mechanisms in the older group which contributed to a reduction in the frontal plane knee moment. Interestingly, the knee joint was affected in all three age groups, highlighting it as an important joint to focus on in future clinical interventions in the hope of delaying the progression of the disease (Shepherd et al., 2022). By using SPM to compare waveform gait data, joint mechanisms were identified and described for the first time in this patient group (Fig. 5.3). This can be expanded further by investigating the direct associations between disease progression features such as joint damage and the gait mechanisms identified.

Modelling Muscle Forces and EMG Assisted Models

Gait analysis has advanced significantly since joint moments and powers became routinely available. What would be of even more value, if it could be provided, would be knowledge of the forces in the different structures in and around the joints. The use of mathematical modelling permits estimates to be made of forces in tendons and ligaments and across articular surfaces. Unfortunately, a large number of unknown factors are involved, particularly the internal moments generated by different muscles and the extent of any co-contraction by antagonistic muscles. For this reason, such calculations can only be approximate, but they may nonetheless be extremely valuable, particularly in clinical and biomechanical research. One example is Motek's Human Body Model, which calculates multiple muscle forces in real-time from three-dimensional kinematic data and dual force plates (van den Bogert et al., 2013). The method uses inverse dynamics combined with optimisation performed by neural networks.

The output of mathematical models may be further refined using EMG. Most models offer a range of possible solutions based on different combinations of active

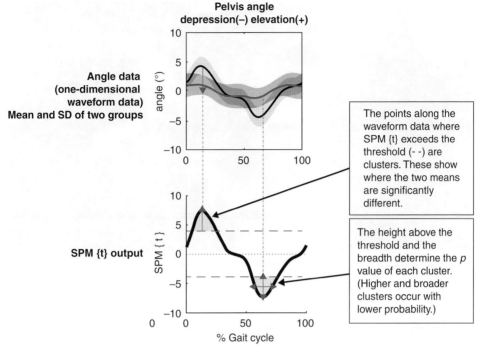

Fig. 5.3 An example of the SPM {t} output curve when comparing angle data (frontal plane pelvis angle) between two groups (alkaptonuria patients in blue and controls in black).

muscles. Even though it is not generally possible to convert EMG signals directly into muscle contraction forces, the knowledge that a muscle is either inactive, contracting a little or contracting strongly may make it possible to eliminate at least some of the possible model solutions and thereby to improve the reliability of the results. These models try to account for changes in musculotendinous length, velocity and the amount of electrical activity for both concentric and eccentric contractions from multiple muscles, and to correlate these with joint moments. Results have varied considerably from joint to joint, with the ankle showing the best correlations of up to 0.91 for normal walking (Lloyd and Besier, 2003; Bogey et al., 2005) and between 0.87 and 0.92 for stroke patients (Shao et al., 2009). However, as we consider the more proximal joints such as the knee and hip, the correlations are lower. Most authors support the use of this approach to estimate muscle forces during gait, yet research using such modelling techniques is still in the minority. This is mainly due to the fact that we do not always need to consider the internal forces in the tendinous and ligamentous structures, as these are rarely the primary outcome measures in gait assessment.

Moving Measurements Away From the Laboratory

Inertial Measurement Units

Full optoelectronic systems are considered the 'gold standard' for collecting accurate gait data in both clinical and research settings. However, these systems are often expensive, require trained specialists and have a limited measurement volume confined within a laboratory setting. The ability to collect accurate gait data outside the laboratory has been a goal for many years. Inertial measurement units such as gyroscopes, accelerometers and magnetometers have been developed to provide a solution to this problem. Comparisons between intertial measurement units (IMUs) and optoelectronic systems show a good match (Nüesch et al., 2017), but the main errors between the two measurements are associated with the differences between the underlying models used, protocols and calibrations (Robert-Lachaine et al., 2017).

One major downfall of IMUs is the lack of three-dimensional ground reaction forces and centre of pressure measurements, meaning vital gait information such as moments and powers using inverse dynamics cannot be calculated. The collection of GRF data is particularly important for pathologies such as AKU and osteoarthritis, where increased or abnormal loading can contribute

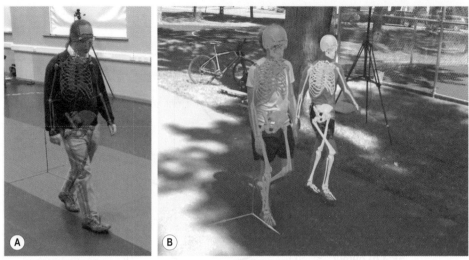

Fig. 5.4 Markerless tracking from standard video cameras using Theia3D (A) in the laboratory, and (B) outside (Theia Markerless, Inc., Canada).

to the progression of the disease, or when conducting load-reducing interventions. To overcome these problems, clever solutions utilising artificial neural networks have been developed to predict the kinetics from IMU kinematic data. Artificial neural networks require a large amount of data to train the network to produce valid results. However, continual development and validation of IMUs and GRF predictions, simple data collection of movement and its causes (moment) becomes feasible in real-world environments. Such systems would also have the potential to provide real-time biofeedback to allow gait modification interventions within home environments, reducing the need for laboratory visits.

Markerless Tracking Systems

It has recently become possible to estimate three-dimensional movements using an array of commercial video cameras, which record the movement and utilise deep neural network solutions to process the video images. This approach to motion capture does not rely on skin-based markers or sensors, hence the term *markerless tracking*. Instead, this uses a deep learning algorithm–based approach to markerless motion tracking utilises convolutional neural networks trained to recognize the joint centres of the human body (Mathis et al., 2020). The neural network approach requires the system to be trained to recognise human movement in a wide array of settings, including when subjects are wearing different types of clothing and performing various activities. Training the neural network using the anatomical features of the human body and its movements results in a probability

distribution for determining the most likely locations of joint centres. This produces a three-dimensional estimate of the position and orientation of every segment, thus producing a full-body model (Fig. 5.4). From the perspective of performing a movement analysis on a subject, this offers exciting new possibilities, as the use of markerless motion capture to measure joint kinematics removes the reliance on skin-mounted markers and the need for an experienced examiner to identify anatomical landmarks and the placement of markers, reducing data collection time, and allows subjects to wear the clothing of their choice. It also opens up the possibility of collecting data in settings outside the laboratory, in more ecologically valid environments which better match real-world contexts. One current issue is that the mean absolute errors are typically higher than standard motion capture systems.

CONCLUSION

Gait analysis has had a long history, and for much of this time it has remained an academic discipline with little practical application. This situation has now changed, and the value of this methodology has been unequivocally demonstrated in many musculoskeletal and neurological conditions. We are seeing decreases in cost and improvements in the ease of use of an ever-increasing variety of kinematic systems, along with increasing acceptance by clinicians of the results of gait analysis. This trend will hopefully continue so that the use of these techniques will increase, both in those conditions for which its value is already recognised and in other, lesser-known conditions.

REFERENCES

Baker, R., McGinley, J.L., Schwartz, M.H., et al., 2009. The gait profile score and movement analysis profile. Gait Posture 30, 265–269.

Barton, G.J., Hawken, M.B., Scott, M.A., Schwartz, M.H., 2012. Movement deviation profile: a measure of distance from normality using a self-organizing neural network. Hum. Mov. Sci. 31 (2), 284–294.

Barton, G.J., King, S.L., Robinson, M. A., Hawken, M.B., Ranganath, L.R., 2015. Age related deviation of gait from normality in alkaptonuria. JIMD 24, 39–44.

Bogey, R.A., Perry, J., Gitter, A.J., 2005. An EMG-to-force processing approach for determining ankle muscle forces during normal human gait. IEEE Trans Neural Syst Rehabil Eng 13 (3), 302–310.

Castro, M.P., Pataky, T.C., Sole, G., Vilas-Boas, J.P., 2015. Pooling sexes when assessing ground reaction forces during walking: statistical parametric mapping versus traditional approach. J. Biomech. 48 (10), 2162–2165.

Cox, T., Psarelli, E.E., Taylor, S., et al., 2019. Subclinical ochronosis features in alkaptonuria: a cross-sectional study. BMJ Innov 5, 82–91.

European Commission., 2022. Rare diseases. Available at: https://ec.europa.eu/info/research-and-innovation/research-area/health-research-and-innovation/rare-diseases_en#:~:text=In%20the%20European%20Union%2C%20a (Accessed 7 Jul. 2022).

Friston, K.J., Ashburner, J.T., Kiebel, S.J., Nichols, T.E., Penny, W.D. (Eds.), 2007. Statistical Parametric Mapping: The Analysis of Functional Brain Images. Elsevier, London.

Gage, J.R., 1983. Gait analysis for decision-making in cerebral palsy. Bull. Hosp. Jt. Dis. Orthop. Inst. 43, 147–163.

Gage, J.R., Schwartz, M.H., Koop, S.E., Novacheck, T.F., 2009. The Identification and Treatment of Gait Problems in Cerebral Palsy. John Wiley & Sons, United Kingdom.

Hicks, R., Durinick, N., Gage, J.R., 1988. Differentiation of idiopathic toe-walking and cerebral palsy. J. Pediatr. Orthop. 8, 160–163.

Klein, T., Lastovicka, O., Janura, M., Svoboda, Z., Chapman, G.J., Richards, J., 2021. The immediate effects of sensorimotor foot orthoses on foot kinematics in healthy adults. Gait Posture 84, 93–101.

Kohonen, T., 2001. Self-Organizing Maps. Springer, Berlin.

Lloyd, D.G., Besier, T.F., 2003. An EMG-driven musculoskeletal model to estimate muscle forces and knee joint moments in vivo. J. Biomech. 36, 765–776.

Mathis, A., Schneider, S., Lauer, J., Mathis, M.W., 2020. A primer on motion capture with deep learning: principles, pitfalls, and perspectives. Neuron 108, 44–65.

Nüesch, C., Roos, E., Pagenstert, G., Mündermann, A., 2017. Measuring joint kinematics of treadmill walking and running: comparison between an inertial sensor based system and a camera-based system. J. Biomech. 57, 32–38.

Pataky, T.C., 2012. One-dimensional statistical parametric mapping in Python. Computer Methods Biomech. Biomed. Engin. 15, 295–301.

Pataky, T.C., Vanrenterghem, J., Robinson, M.A., 2015. Zero- vs. one-dimensional, parametric vs. non-parametric, and confidence interval vs. hypothesis testing procedures in one-dimensional biomechanical trajectory analysis. J. Biomech. 48 (7), 1277–1285.

Ranganath, L.R., Cox, T.F., 2011. Natural history of alkaptonuria revisited: analyses based on scoring systems. J. Inherit. Metab. Dis. 34 (6), 1141–1151.

Ranganath, L.R., Jarvis, J.C., Gallagher, J.A., 2013. Recent advances in management of alkaptonuria (invited review; best practice article). J. Clin. Pathol. 66 (5), 367–373.

Robert-Lachaine, X., Mecheri, H., Larue, C., Plamondon, A., 2017. Validation of inertial measurement units with an opto-electronic system for whole-body motion analysis. Med. Biol. Eng. Comput. 55 (4), 609–619.

Rose, G.K., 1983. Clinical gait assessment: a personal view. J. Med. Eng. Technol. 7, 273–279.

Schutte, L.M., Narayanan, U., Stout, J.L., et al., 2000. An index for quantifying deviations from normal gait. Gait Posture 11, 25–31.

Schwartz, M.H., Rozumalski, A., 2008. The gait deviation index: a new comprehensive index of gait pathology. Gait Posture 28, 351–357.

Shao, Q., Bassett, D.N., Manal, K., et al., 2009. An EMG-driven model to estimate muscle forces and joint moments in stroke patients. Comput. Biol. Med. 39 (12), 1083–1088.

Shepherd, H., 2020. The development and evaluation of an individualised gait modification intervention to improve movement function in alkaptonuria patients. PhD thesis, John Moores University, Liverpool.

Shepherd, H.R., Robinson, M.A., Ranganath, L.R., Barton, G.J., 2022. Identifying joint specific gait mechanisms causing impaited gait in alkaptonuria patients. Gait Posture 91, 312–317.

van den Bogert, A.J., Geijtenbeek, T., Even-Zohar, O.E., Steenbrink, F., Hardin, E.C., 2013. A real-time system for biomechanical analysis of human movement and muscle function. Med Biol Eng Comput 51, 1069–1077.

Wakap, N.S., Lambert, D.M., Olry, A., Rodwell, C., Gueydan, C., Lanneau, V., et al., 2020. Estimating cumulative point prevalence of rare diseases: analysis of the Orphanet database. Eur. J. Hum. Genet. 28 (2), 165–173.

Wesdock, K., Blair, S., Masiello, G., et al., 2003. Psychogenic gait: when it is and when it isn't – correlating the physical exam with dynamic gait data. In: Gait and Clinical Movement Analysis Society, Eighth Annual Meeting, Wilmington, Delaware, USA, pp. 279–280.

6

Gait Assessment of Neurological Disorders

Michael Whittle, Richard Baker, Nancy Fell,
Derek Liuzzo, Jim Richards and Cathie Smith

OUTLINE

The aim of this chapter is to provide examples of how gait analysis can be used to determine the severity, progression and efficacy of non-surgical, surgical and pharmaceutical management of neurological disorders. This chapter will consider several common disorders and their management, including cerebral palsy, stroke, Parkinson's disease and muscular dystrophy.

GAIT ASSESSMENT IN CEREBRAL PALSY

Richard Baker

Definition, Causes and Prevalence

Cerebral palsy is defined as a group of permanent disorders of the development of movement and posture which can be attributed to brain damage to the foetus or infant (Rosenbaum et al., 2007). The condition is different from other forms of brain damage such as stroke or traumatic brain injury because it happens whilst the brain is still developing and this affects the subsequent neurological and musculoskeletal development of the child. The motor disorders of cerebral palsy are often accompanied by disturbances of sensation, perception, cognition, communication and behaviour. Cerebral palsy is the most common cause of physical disability affecting children in the developed world with a prevalence of around 2 cases for every 1000 live births (Stanley et al., 2000).

The brain damage is much more common in infants born prematurely, but the precise cause is unknown in the majority of cases. The ultimate effect is a failure of the oxygen supply to an area of the developing brain which may be a consequence of damage to the blood vessels, such as haemorrhage or embolism, or a more general drop in foetal blood pressure. The brain damage, once it has occurred, is static and will not get any better or any worse. The clinical manifestations, however, will continue to develop and change as the child grows and matures. This is particularly true of the musculoskeletal manifestations of cerebral palsy, which are very important in determining whether and how people with the condition will walk.

Classification

Gross Motor Function Classification System

The principal means of classifying children with cerebral palsy is with the Gross Motor Function Classification System (GMFCS) (Palisano et al., 1997, 2000), a five-point scale reflecting the severity of the condition as it affects motor function. There are different definitions for different age groups, but the definition for 6- to 12-year-olds is the most relevant to gait analysts (Table 6.1). It can be seen that most children who are suitable for gait analysis will be of levels I through III, and descriptors for 12- to 18-year-olds have also been produced (Palisano et al., 2008). These are similar to those in Table 6.1 but allow for some deterioration in motor ability that occurs in late childhood. While gait analysis is most often used for children with cerebral palsy, it is worth remembering that cerebral palsy is a lifelong condition, with between 25% and 50% of adults reporting further deterioration in walking ability in early adulthood (Day et al., 2007; Jahnsen et al., 2004; Murphy et al., 1995).

Classification by Motor Disorder and Topography

The brain damage that causes cerebral palsy can affect the nervous system in several different ways. In about 85% of people, the major limitation is spasticity, which leads to overactivity in specific muscles. A further 7% are dyskinetic (dystonic-athetoid), having mixed muscle tone (high or low), which leads to slow sinuous movements superimposed on the intended motor pattern. Another 5% have ataxia, which leads to rapid jerky movements and affects balance and depth perception. People with dyskinesia or ataxia tend to have very variable gait patterns, which can limit the usefulness of clinical gait analysis. Outcomes of orthopaedic surgery in people with dyskinesia can be unpredictable. Most children attending for clinical gait analysis are therefore those with a predominantly spastic motor type.

Before the advent of the GMFCS, the primary classification of children with cerebral palsy was with respect to the areas of the body that were most affected. *Hemiplegia* refers to one side of the body being affected, including an arm and leg on the same side. *Diplegia* refers to the involvement of both legs and *quadriplegia* to the involvement of all four limbs. Many children do not fall neatly into these categories and the distinction between quadriplegia and diplegia is rarely clear-cut; many diplegic individuals are affected much more on one side than the other. Such issues have led to recent advice that such terms be discontinued until they are defined more precisely. *Unilateral* and *bilateral motor involvements* are now the preferred terms for children who can walk with *total body involvement* being used for

TABLE 6.1 Gross Motor Function Classification System for children aged 6 to 12 years	
Level I	Children walk indoors and outdoors and climb stairs without limitation. Children perform gross motor skills including running and jumping, but speed, balance and coordination are impaired.
Level II	Children walk indoors and outdoors and climb stairs holding onto a railing but experience limitations walking on uneven surfaces and inclines and walking in crowds or confined spaces and with long distances.
Level III	Children walk indoors and outdoors on a level surface with an assistive mobility device and may climb stairs holding onto a railing. Children may use a wheelchair for mobility when travelling for long distances or outdoors over uneven terrain.
Level IV	Children use methods of mobility that usually require adult assistance. They may continue to walk for short distances with physical assistance at home but rely on wheeled mobility (pushed by adult or operate a powered chair) outdoors, at school and in the community.
Level V	Physical impairment restricts voluntary control of movement and the ability to maintain antigravity head and trunk posture. All areas of motor function are limited. Children have no means of independent mobility and are transported by adults.

non-walkers. Having said this, the original terms are still in widespread use.

Classification by Gait Pattern

There have been several attempts to classify cerebral palsy on the basis of gait pattern (Dobson et al., 2007). Some confusion has arisen because several authors have chosen to redefine terms used by previous authors and it is not always clear which classification system is being referred to. Two classifications for spastic hemiplegic gait have been proposed (Hullin et al., 1996; Winters et al., 1987) of which Winters et al., is more commonly used. This is described in Fig. 6.1 and Table 6.2, however, there is some confusion in how this

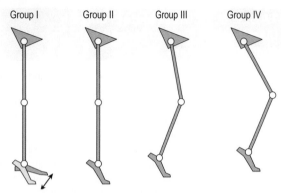

Fig. 6.1 Common gait patterns in hemiplegic cerebral palsy. (Reproduced with permission and copyright © of the British Editorial Society of Bone and Joint Surgery. [Rodda et al., 2004].)

TABLE 6.2 Classification of gait patterns in hemiplegia[a]	
Group I	Ankle equinus in the swing phase of gait due to underactivity of the ankle dorsiflexors in relation to the plantarflexors.
Group II	Plantarflexion throughout stance and swing from either static or dynamic contracture of the triceps surae. Knee is often forced into slight hyperextension in middle or late stance.
Group III	Findings of group II with reduced range of knee flexion/extension. Reference is now common to subgroups IIIa, reduced knee extension during stance; and IIIb, hyperextension in stance and reduced flexion in swing.
Group IV	Findings of group III with involvement of the hip musculature.[b]

[a]Summary by Thompson et al. (2002) of original by Winters et al. (1987).

[b]In the original paper, in which measurements were restricted to the sagittal plane, this was attributed to flexor and adductor involvement. A three-dimensional analysis would almost certainly have included increased internal rotation.

is applied clinically. The original paper refers exclusively to the sagittal plane and is based purely on the gait pattern. It is not at all uncommon to hear clinicians incorporating considerations of the transverse plane (particularly at the hip) and inferences about the nature of the underlying pathology (rather than just the gait pattern) in classifying children. Agreement among clinicians in applying this classification is substantial (Dobson et al., 2006). A more recent population-based study suggested that groups I, II and IV are far more common than group III.

Classifications of gait patterns in spastic diplegia are less clear-cut. One example is the classification by Rodda et al. (2004) in which the whole gait pattern is described (Fig. 6.2 and Table 6.3). There is particular confusion with regard to a number of terms that different people have chosen to define differently. Sutherland and Davids (1993), for example, defined *jump* as referring to a pattern in which the knee is flexed in early stance but extends rapidly in a pattern reminiscent of jumping. Rodda et al. (2004) used the same term to refer to a posture of flexed knee and plantarflexed ankle in late stance. *Crouch* gait is another term that has been defined differently by a range of authors. Many studies simply use the term to refer to a gait pattern exhibiting knee flexion of no less than a certain value (30 degrees is commonly used) throughout stance. Gage et al. (2009) used a kinetic definition for patterns in which an extensor internal knee moment is present throughout stance, whereas Rodda et al. (2004) required ankle dorsiflexion as well as knee flexion.

Classification by gait pattern does not give the whole picture. The two most commonly used schemes are based on sagittal plane data only (Rodda et al., 2004; Winters et al., 1987). Winters et al. proposed their classification system for people who had had no previous orthopaedic intervention and it is not clear how much value the scheme has for people who have had surgery. Rodda et al. did not discuss how surgery or other interventions would affect classification by gait pattern. There is considerable variability within grades and some people clearly have patterns on the boundary between one grade and the next. Indeed, two studies which include data that can be used to infer whether natural groupings exist (Dobson, 2007; Rozumalski and Schwartz, 2009) would suggest, on the contrary, that gait patterns vary continuously across a multidimensional spectrum and groupings will only ever be a rather gross guide to the general pattern of movement. They can, however, still be useful in giving an overall impression of the person's gait pattern, particularly if full instrumented gait analysis is not available. However, a full gait analysis is still essential if we want to be specific about how a person is walking and what is causing them to do so in a particular manner.

Impairments

An *impairment* is something that is wrong with a person's body structures or the way they function (World Health Organization [WHO], 2001). Primary impairments in people

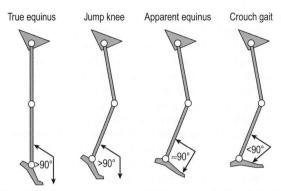

True equinus   Jump knee   Apparent equinus   Crouch gait

Fig. 6.2 Common gait patterns in spastic diplegic cerebral palsy (Rodda et al., 2004).

TABLE 6.3 Common gait patterns in spastic diplegic cerebral palsy (Rodda et al., 2004)	
Group I	The ankle is in equinus. The knee extends fully or goes into mild recurvatum. The hip extends fully and the pelvis is within the normal range or tilted anteriorly.
Group II	The ankle is in equinus, particularly in late stance. The knee and hip are excessively flexed in early stance and then extend to a variable degree in late stance, but never reach full extension. The pelvis is either within the normal range or tilted anteriorly.
Group III	The ankle has a normal range but the knee and hip are excessively flexed throughout stance. The pelvis is normal or tilted anteriorly.
Group IV	The ankle is excessively dorsiflexed throughout stance and the knee and hip are excessively flexed. The pelvis is in the normal range or tilted posteriorly.

with cerebral palsy are direct consequences of the brain damage, and thus affect neurological function, whereas secondary impairments are indirect consequences arising from the effects of altered neurology on other structures over a long period of time. Thus muscles may become contracted or bones misaligned. Impairments generally fall into four broad categories: spasticity, weakness, muscle contracture and bony malalignment.

Spasticity

The term *spasticity* means different things to different people. Most clinicians working with people with cerebral palsy tend to use it to refer to a very specific 'velocity-dependent increase in tonic stretch reflexes, with exaggerated tendon jerks resulting from hyperexcitability of the stretch reflex' (Lance, 1980). In other words, if a tendon is stretched rapidly then its muscle will become active. Depending on the severity of the spasticity, this might be for a short period and the muscle may thus show phasic but inappropriate activity, and may be active throughout the gait cycle. This stretch reflex is present in all of us, but in most people, it is suppressed by signals originating in the brain and passing down the spinal column (descending control). In people with cerebral palsy, the brain damage reduces the capacity to send such signals and the reflexes are effectively out of control. Thus, although it is common to hear reference to *spastic muscles*, spasticity is really a property of the nervous system.

In cerebral palsy, spasticity commonly affects some muscles more than others. In particular, the biarticular and multiarticular muscles appear to be most susceptible (Gage et al., 2009). Thus, spasticity is commonly found in the gastrocnemius, hamstrings, rectus femoris and psoas muscles. In more severely affected children, spasticity of the monoarticular hip adductors is a particular issue. Spasticity is not the only alteration to neurological function, and in some people with cerebral palsy, particularly those most severely affected, there can be inappropriate muscle activity in the absence of movement as well, and this is generally referred to as *resting tone*.

Muscle Contractures

Spasticity occurs in a wide range of conditions, and in most of these the muscles affected are susceptible to the development of *contractures*. In these, the passive length of the muscle and its tendon are reduced, and this leads to a restriction in the range of movement available at the joints. Most children with cerebral palsy are relatively free from contractures at birth and in infancy, and then develop them through childhood. They are commonly named by the position they are held in: for example, a flexion contracture of the knee means the knee is held in some degree of flexion and cannot fully extend, with the most commonly seen contractures including knee flexion, ankle plantarflexion and hip flexion.

The mechanisms by which contractures develop are not fully understood. In relation to children with cerebral palsy, it is quite common to hear contractures talked about as a failure of normal growth, where the bone keeps on growing but the muscle does not. This cannot be the full picture, as some children, particularly those with hemiplegia, can develop contractures over a short period of time which are too severe to be explained simply by failure of growth. Another common belief is that contractures are a result of immobilisation, which is supported by some early clinical and animal work suggesting that this reduces the length of the muscle fibres (Shortland et al., 2002). More recent work suggests that a reduction in muscle belly length through shortening of the aponeuroses is much more significant than any reduction in fibre length (Shortland et al., 2002), but no mechanism has been proposed for this. In summary, the development of contractures is probably related to failure of growth, immobilisation and the consequences of spasticity, but the relative contributions of these factors remain unknown.

Weakness

It is only relatively recently that the effect of muscle weakness on the gait of people with cerebral palsy has been fully acknowledged. Wiley and Damiano (1998) surveyed the strength of children with cerebral palsy and demonstrated that muscle weakness is also important with the gluteal muscles, with the plantarflexors also being particularly weak with respect to those of age-matched able-bodied children. Muscle weakness can arise either because of the anatomy and physiology of the muscles or through reduced neural activity to stimulate contraction. Despite cerebral palsy being an essentially neurological problem, there have been few investigations to establish the relative proportions of the muscular and neurological components of weakness.

The weakness has generally been attributed to a muscle's reduced physiological cross-sectional area and to short muscle belly length, and may therefore be strongly related to the development of contracture in both spastic hemiplegia and diplegia (Elder et al., 2003; Fry et al., 2007). However, the clinical picture does not always agree with this, with some muscles appearing to be quite weak without evidence of contracture. Recent evidence suggests that these changes are quite different from those that arise simply through either chronic stimulation or disuse (Foran et al., 2005) but, as with the development of contractures, the underlying mechanisms are not understood. During movement, there is a further factor in that contractures or specific walking patterns may result in muscle fibres functioning away from their optimal length to generate contractile force. The clinical picture appears to be that the muscles get weaker with age with respect to those of children without cerebral palsy. A particular issue arises in late childhood and early adolescent when weight increases rapidly and relative weakness becomes significant.

Bony Malalignment (and Capsular Contracture)

Children with cerebral palsy are also susceptible to developing malalignment of the bones. Anteversion of the femur is the most common example of this. It is essentially a twist somewhere along the shaft of the femur which results in the femoral neck pointing too far forwards in relation to the knee joint axis. Although it is commonly referred to as a developmental deformity, it is actually a result of persistence of the original bony alignment. At birth, most children have anteversion of about 40 degrees, but this reduces in normal growth to about 10 degrees at skeletal maturity. This reduction does not occur in many children with cerebral palsy. It is not uncommon for the tibia to be twisted externally along its shaft, a condition known as *tibial torsion*; malalignment of the bones of the foot, particularly the calcaneus, is also common. In more severely affected children, spinal, thoracic and upper limb deformities are also common.

As with the other impairments, the precise mechanisms are unclear, but at least three factors need to be considered. Bones grow in length at the *growth plates*. Most long bones have a growth plate proximally and distally. The rate at which the bones grow is determined by the stress exerted across the growth plate. In areas of the growth plate across which large compressive stresses are exerted, longitudinal growth will be suppressed and elsewhere growth may be stimulated. Thus, normal bone growth requires normal stress distributions. Walking is believed to be a major contributor to such stresses, and thus, if children do not walk normally the bones will not grow normally. *Remodelling* is another factor. Once bones have grown, the bone continues to be replaced on an ongoing basis and this can lead to a change in shape of the bone. Interestingly, the opposite law applies here. High compressive stresses tend to stimulate the production of more bone whereas lower stresses suppress this. The third factor is that cartilaginous bone can actually be deformed mechanically, and this may be particularly important in the feet where some bones are not fully calcified until around the age of 10 years.

A further common impairment is contracture of the joint capsule. This is particularly common at the knee but may also restrict extension and internal/external rotation of the hip. It results from contracture of the ligaments which form the joint capsule and is thus quite distinct from contracture of the muscle. It is included with bony deformities because the capsule is a deep structure and quite difficult to approach surgically. Management of joint contractures is thus often achieved through bony surgery similar to surgeries used to manage bony malalignment.

Clinical Management
Natural History

Children seen for gait analysis will typically have had delayed motor milestones such as the age at which they first sat, crawled or walked. Spasticity may be evident very early, and weakness (particularly around the hips) is also common in early childhood but contracture and bony malalignment are less evident. These tend to develop in middle and late childhood. Although weakness can be a significant issue from quite early on, it becomes much more significant as children increase their bodyweight rapidly through adolescence.

Spasticity Management

The focus of management in early childhood is generally on trying to reduce spasticity, and a range of options are available. Although there are some anecdotal reports of responses to stem cell implants, there is little scientific evidence so far that anything can be done to repair the original brain damage. *Botulinum toxin* is a chemical that disrupts the neuromuscular junction and thus prevents the neural input to a muscle activating it. If injected into the muscle, it is selectively absorbed by these junctions and suppresses activity. The direct effect of the toxin wears off over a period of between 3 and 9 months (Eames et al., 1999). This can be useful as it is possible to test the effects of injections without the risk of doing permanent harm but does mean that, if successful, injections need to be repeated. In children with cerebral palsy who can walk, the gastrocnemius muscles are the most commonly injected (Baker et al., 2002; Eames et al., 1999). However, in severe spasticity, it may be more effective simply to release specific muscles surgically rather than perform repeat injections.

If spasticity affects many muscles, a specific intervention such as botulinum toxin is less appropriate. *Selective dorsal rhizotomy* (SDR) is surgery to the spine which cuts a proportion of the nerves in the dorsal roots, typically in the lumbar and sacral spine. This reduces neural activity in the reflex arc and thus reduces spasticity in all muscles innervated from that level of the spine. The word *selective* in SDR refers to using electromyography (EMG) during the surgery to select which rootlets to cut and how many to cut. SDR is only suitable for a small number of children and requires highly specialised surgical teams. Another approach is to use baclofen, which is an analogue of a naturally occurring inhibitory neurotransmitter and thus suppresses spasticity generally. It can be taken orally but little of it crosses the blood–brain barrier into the cerebrospinal fluid; therefore large doses are required. Another option is intrathecal baclofen (ITB) therapy, in which a surgically inserted pump delivers the drug directly into the intrathecal space of the spine. ITB tends to be used only for more severely involved children, occasionally in GMFCS III but most commonly for GMFCS IV and V.

Muscle and Tendon Surgery

As children age, muscle contractures generally become more significant. As these are not a direct consequence of neural activity, they will not be affected by any of the spasticity reduction techniques. A variety of surgical procedures performed on either muscle or tendon are thus required. Perhaps the most common is the gastrocnemius recession in which the tendon linking the muscle to the Achilles tendon is cut. This is also referred to as Achilles tendon lengthening or heel cord lengthening. Partial releases of muscles such as the hamstrings, psoas and hip adductor muscles can also be performed to allow for more normal gait and posture. If the rectus femoris is contracted, it can be useful not just to release it but to transfer its insertion from the patella (where it acts as a knee extensor) to the posterior aspect of the proximal tibia (where it may act as a knee flexor). The longer tendons of the tibialis anterior and posterior can be divided longitudinally and part of the tendon can be transferred to the other side of the foot to provide a 'stirrup' that can stabilise the ankle and subtalar joint in the coronal plane.

Bony Surgery

Femoral anteversion and tibial torsion are rotational deformities of the bone and can be corrected by surgical procedures such as cutting the bone transversely, untwisting the bone and attaching a metal plate by screws to hold the bone in this new alignment whilst it heals. External fixation may also be used to correct rotational deformities. Bony malalignment of the feet can be corrected by performing various osteotomies to the bones of the foot. The most common of these is calcaneal lengthening in which the calcaneus is cut through and a bone graft placed in the gap to lengthen the bone and swing the foot internally.

Joint capsule contractures can also be improved by bony surgery. Thus, severe knee capsule contractures can be corrected by taking a wedge out of the anterior aspect of the distal femur. Milder contractures can be managed by *guided growth*. In this, staples or eight plates are inserted across the anterior aspect of the distal femoral growth plate. This prevents the bone from growing anteriorly, and the growth that does occur posteriorly negates the effect of the capsular contracture. Placing staples anteriorly and posteriorly can prevent any longitudinal growth and can be useful to correct any leg-length discrepancy.

In the past, surgeons tended to perform different surgical procedures on different occasions. More recently, and particularly as surgeons' confidence has grown, there has been a tendency towards performing a range of different procedures, to bone and muscle, within the same operation. This is often known as *single-event multilevel surgery (SEMLS)* acknowledging the intention that only one operation would be required.

Strengthening

Now that the importance of weakness in cerebral palsy has been acknowledged, there has been considerable research into physiotherapy programmes to actively strengthen muscles (Damiano and Abel, 1998; Damiano et al., 1995, 2002; Dodd and Taylor, 2005; Dodd et al., 2002, 2003). These generally used the principles of progressive resistive strength training, which have now been demonstrated to result in increases in muscle strength in children with cerebral palsy of up to 25%, which is consistent with their use in many other conditions. Such programmes are now being used more and more routinely.

Clinical Gait Analysis

The most obvious use of clinical gait analysis is for planning complex, multilevel orthopaedic surgery. In most cases the surgeon already knows that surgery is required, and the aim of the gait analysis is to determine exactly which combination of surgical procedures will be of most benefit to the individual child. Many centres will also perform follow-up analysis, often between 1 and 2 years after surgery, to assess outcomes as part of a clinical audit. This allows the clinical team to benefit from the experience in managing each child and is important to maintain and improve levels of service provision. Gait analysis can also be useful in planning botulinum toxin injections, physiotherapy, orthotic interventions and more general monitoring of progress. Unfortunately, the cost, availability and time required for the analysis often precludes its use for routine clinical purposes.

We will now focus on how clinical gait analysis is able to support surgical decision-making. Gait analysis is only part of this process, which also includes capturing gait data, performing a comprehensive physical examination and providing a biomechanical analysis of the results. The actual decision as to whether surgery is required and which procedures should be included requires consideration of a number of other issues, such as medical imaging, the patient's history and psychosocial background and the surgeon's competences and level of support, which are beyond the scope of this book. Clinical gait analysis works within a framework of clinical governance that ensures that the services delivered to patients are both safe and of the highest quality. This includes a commitment to evidence-based practice, which requires that all techniques used should be well established and have been the subject of rigorous research.

Data Capture

Most clinical services focus on obtaining good-quality kinematic and kinetic data based on the measured positions of retroreflective markers using techniques documented elsewhere in this book. The Conventional Gait Model (CGM) (Baker and Rodda, 2003; Davis et al., 1991; Kadaba et al., 1990; Ounpuu et al., 1996) is by far the best documented and most common approach (see Chapter 4, Methods of Gait Analysis). Other models are used, but it is questionable whether they have yet been sufficiently well validated in clinical practice to satisfy the strict demands of clinical governance. Many centres will also capture EMG data concurrently with kinematic data.

Children are generally asked to walk back and forth in bare feet first and with minimum walking aids to achieve a reasonable gait pattern. This information gives the best indication of what their body is capable of. They may then be asked to walk when wearing their ankle foot orthoses (AFO) and any other usual walking aids to give an indication of how they usually walk. As well as capturing full three-dimensional gait analysis data, it is important to capture good-quality standardised video recordings of the child walking.

Clinical Examination

In addition to the gait analysis, a full clinical examination is also completed. The range of movement of various joints is assessed which helps identify muscle and joint contractures. Muscle testing is generally carried out, grading muscles on the conventional five-point scale (Kendall and Kendall, 1949), and this is often accompanied by a simple assessment of the degree of selectivity with which the child can control muscle activation. The Tardieu test (Boyd and Graham, 1999) is used to measure spasticity and the modified Ashworth scale (Bohannon and Smith, 1987), while often referred to as a measure of spasticity, should probably be regarded as a measure of resting tone. Measures of bony malalignment, such as femoral anteversion and tibial torsion, are also recorded. An example of the results of such a clinical examination are included in Fig. 6.3. The results of the clinical examination give additional information which aids the process of interpreting the gait analysis data to elucidate exactly which impairments are most affecting the gait pattern. This process can be thought of as having four stages: orientation, mark-up, grouping and reporting.

Orientation

The first thing the clinician must do is obtain a general impression of the child and how they are walking. This will require a knowledge of the diagnosis (assumed here to be cerebral palsy), motor type, GMFCS classification and topographical distribution. Scales indicating the child's general level of functions, such as the Functional Assessment Questionnaire (Novacheck et al., 2000) or the Functional Mobility Scale (Harvey et al., 2007), may also

	Left	Right
Hip extension range (Thomas)	7° ext	8° ext
Hip flexor strength	5 (2)	5 (2)
Hip extensor strength (knee 0°)	5 (2)	5 (2)
Hip extensor strength (knee 90°)	5 (2)	5 (2)
Hip abduction range (hip 0°, knee 0°)	44° abd	53° abd
Hip abduction range (hip 0°, knee 90°)	NT	NT
Hip abductor strength	5 (2)	5 (2)
Hip internal rotation range	41° int	33° int
External rotation range	31° ext	42° ext

	Left	Right
Femoral anteversion	11° int	12° int

	Left	Right
Knee extension range (capsule)	5° hyp	10° hyp
Popliteal angle	27° flex	26° flex
True popliteal angle	20° flex	25° flex
Dynamic popliteal angle	43° flex	40° flex
Knee flexor strength	5 (2)	5 (2)
Knee extensor strength	5 (2)	5 (2)
Quadriceps lag	0° flex	0° flex
Duncan-Ely (slow)	none	none
Duncan-Ely (fast)	none	none

	Left	Right
Dorsiflexor strength	4 (2)	4 (2)
Confusion (+/−)	neg	neg
Dorsiflexion (knee 90°)	5° pf	4° df
Dorsiflexion (knee 0°)	5° pf	4° df
Plantarflexor spasticity (Tardieu)	10° pf	3° df
Plantarflexor tone (Ashworth)	0	0
Plantarflexor strength (knee 90°)	4 (2)	4 (2)
Invertor strength	5 (2)	5 (2)
Evertor strength	4+ (2)	4 (2)

	Left	Right
Tibial torsion	20° ext	13° ext

	Left	Right
Thigh-hindfoot angle	0°	2° ext
Hindfoot-forefoot angle	14° int	16° int
Ankle equinus/calcaneus	mild equinus	neutral
Hindfoot valgus/varus	neutral	mild varus
Planus/cavus	neutral	mild planus
Forefoot abd/add	mod add	mod add

Weight (kg)	31 kg	
Height (cm)	133 cm	
True leg length (cm)	69 cm	69 cm
Apparent leg length (cm)	75 cm	75 cm

Fig. 6.3 Typical physical examination for clinical gait analysis. Range of motions measures are in the ☐ boxes, muscle strength in the ☐, neurological signs in ☐ and bony or capsular deformities in ☐ boxes.

be useful. It is also important to have an overview of the child's medical and surgical history and the precise reason they have been referred for gait analysis. The final part of orientation is to look at the video to get an overall impression of the gait pattern. During the assessment, the child or family should be asked whether the walking pattern adopted during the analysis is representative of the way they usually walk.

Markup

The next stage is to look at the data and identify *gait features*. These are regions of the traces that are different from reference data from a population that has no neuromusculoskeletal impairments. Many gait analysts do this in their head, but it can be extremely useful to actually annotate the graphs to mark up these features using symbols (Fig. 6.4 and Table 6.4).

Grouping

Once the gait features have been identified, the next stage of the process is to group the features that are thought to indicate the presence of a specific impairment and to relate these to relevant aspects of the clinical examination. It can be useful to list the evidence for a particular impairment as illustrated in Table 6.5.

Reporting

The final stage requires a report of the findings to be written to the referring clinician. If the process outlined

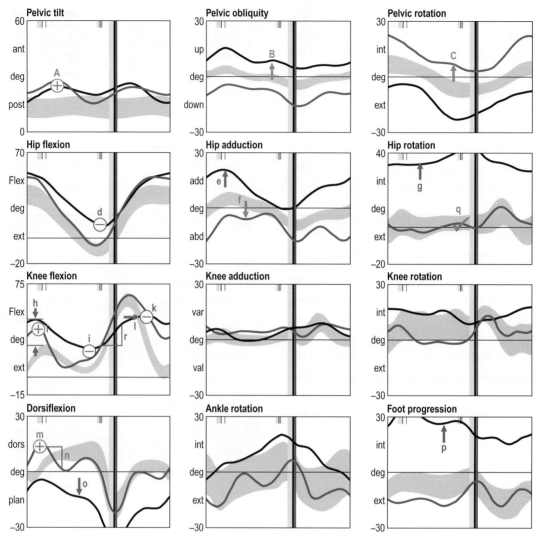

Fig. 6.4 Representative graph marked up to identify features of the gait pattern.

previously has been followed, this can be as simple as listing the impairments and including the evidence boxes and the marked-up gait traces in support of the analysis.

Key Points

- Cerebral palsy is caused by brain damage but this leads to a wide range of impairments including spasticity, weakness, muscle and joint contracture and bony malalignment.
- Common gait deviations during swing phase include equinus, excessive flexion of the knee and hip, and foot drop.
- Common gait deviations during stance include minimal to no heel contact and excessive hip and knee flexion.

- Each child with cerebral palsy has a distinct and unique gait pattern depending on their impairments and how they compensate for these.
- There are a wide range of options for improving walking ability and preventing deterioration, including botulinum toxin, selective dorsal rhizotomy, intrathecal baclofen, physiotherapy, orthotics, strengthening programmes and orthopaedic surgery.
- Gait analysis may be used to plan complex orthopaedic surgery. The goal is to identify which impairments are having the largest effect on walking from features in the gait data and the clinical examination.

TABLE 6.4 Symbols for markup

Symbol	Meaning
⊖	Too little (during particular phase in gait cycle)
⊕	Too much (during particular phase in gait cycle)
↓	Too little (throughout gait cycle)
↑	Too much (throughout gait cycle)
⤒	Increased range
⤓	Decreased range
▽ or △	Abnormal slope
→	Too late
←	Too early
↔	Increased duration
▶ ◀	Decreased duration
✓	Within normal limits
?	Possible artifact
⬭	Other feature (ring around feature)

Symbols are written on the charts in blue for the right side, and black for the left side. Capital letters indicate bilateral features (including those of the pelvis).

TABLE 6.5 Lists some of the features and supplementary data identified in Fig. 6.3 that suggest the child has femoral anteversion

Features	Comments
g.	Too much left int. hip rot^n throughout cycle
p.	Too much int. foot prog^n throughout cycle
c.	Too much ext. rot^n of left pelvis throughout cycle
	Partial compensation for hip int. rot^n

Supplementary data	Left	Right	Comments
Hip internal rotation range	50°	35°	
Hip external rotation range	0°	30°	
Femoral anteversion	30°	10°	From clinical exam

Impairment: **left femoral anteversion**
Evidence: **clear**
Effect on walking: **major**

GAIT ASSESSMENT IN STROKE

Nancy Fell

Definition, Causes and Prevalence

Stroke is a term which broadly refers to a collection of central nervous system vascular pathologies resulting in brain, spinal cord or retinal cell death. Common vascular pathologies include *ischemic stroke* due to thrombosis, and *nontraumatic hemorrhagic stroke* within the brain or spinal cord parenchyma, meninges or ventricular system (Sacco et al., 2013). Worldwide, 25% of adults over the age of 25 will have a stroke within their lifetime, with 13.7 million people experiencing a first stroke each year (World Stroke Organization, 2021). Of these, 5 million experience permanent disability (WHO, 2021). Disability from stroke affects millions of individuals in the United States, with over 795,000 cases annually. US statistics show that stroke is a leading cause of death and the leading cause of serious long-term disability. Stroke management is estimated to cost the United States $46 billion annually (Centers for Disease Control and Prevention, 2019).

Gait dysfunction post-stroke is common, arising from the primary impairments associated with the neurologic event as well as from secondary cardiovascular and musculoskeletal consequences from disuse and physical inactivity. Muscle weakness, tone dysfunction, impaired motor control, decreased soft tissue flexibility and reduced cardiovascular function are major contributors (Carr and Shepherd, 2003). Walking is considered important for return to independent living and full community access. So, whenever possible, rehabilitation professionals provide gait examination and rehabilitation as part of post-stroke management.

Temporal and Spatial Parameters

Post-stroke gait is frequently characterised as slow and asymmetrical (Hesse et al., 1997; Olney and Richards, 1996; Roth et al., 1997; Woolley, 2001) with reduced cadence (Woolley, 2001), and there is significant inter- and intra-subject variability (Olney and Richards, 1996; Woolley, 2001). Given the heterogeneity of post-stroke gait, a common set of performance measures is required. Gait speed using the 10-Meter Walk Test (Tyson and Connell, 2009; Lewek and Sykes, 2019) and distance walked/time using the 6-Minute Walk Test (Fulk and He, 2018) are essential post-stroke clinical gait assessments. These measures can be particularly important for prediction. Jarvis and colleagues (2019) documented young-adult stroke survivors' walking as significantly slower and less efficient than healthy age-matched control subjects, and found a low level (23%) of return to employment post-stroke, with walking speed as the strongest predictor for return to work. Individuals who were able to walk >0.93 m/s were significantly more likely to return to work post-stroke than those who walked slower (Jarvis et al., 2019). Awad and colleagues (2019) explored the clinical prediction of community walking ability in stroke survivors and found that a co-assessment of distance-induced changes in walking speed during the 6-Minute Walk Test (6MWT) and the total distance walked provided the best prediction. The total distance walked during the 6MWT explained 41% of the variance in stroke survivors' steps per day. Adding the change in distance walked within the first and last minutes of the test ($\Delta 6MWT_{min6-min1}$) expanded the prediction to 71% of variance. Further analyses showed that a decline in gait speed from the first to last minutes by ≥ 0.10 m/s positively correlated with significantly fewer steps per day.

Several authors suggest that hemiparetic gait deviations may be related to reduced gait speed (Carlsoo et al., 1974; Lehmann et al., 1987; Roth et al., 1997; Woolley, 2001). Roth and colleagues (1997) investigated the correlation between gait speed and 18 other temporal gait parameters for 25 people post-stroke. Since post-stroke gait speed was related to most, but not all, other temporal gait characteristics, the authors suggest that clinical gait examination must include gait speed with descriptions of asymmetry and paretic limb stance and swing phase durations and proportions. Many other spatiotemporal parameters frequently change post-stroke, including increased double support time, increased stance time by the nonparetic limb, shortened paretic limb step length, a moderately wider base of support, and slightly greater toe-out angles (Carr and Shepherd, 2003; Olney and Richards, 1996; Perry, 1969; Shumway-Cook and Woollacott, 2007; Woolley, 2001; Vistamehr et al., 2018).

Balasubramanian and colleagues (2009) explored temporal and spatial gait characteristics for an age-matched healthy control group and post-stroke groups of varying severity (severe, moderate, mild), step symmetry (longer, shorter, symmetrical) and fall risk (Dynamic Gait Index [DGI] ≤ 19 and DGI >19). The authors confirmed increased variability in step length, swing, pre-swing and stride times during hemiparetic walking as compared with healthy individuals. For subjects post-stroke, paretic leg swing time variability was increased compared with the nonparetic limb during gait. Between-leg differences in variability for other spatiotemporal characteristics were revealed in the participants with the most impaired performance. Slower walkers (speed <0.4 m/s) had significantly reduced step width variability as compared to age-matched controls. Patla et al. (2002) previously suggested that adaptation of step length, width and height is an important gait strategy

employed by persons post-stroke to avoid obstacles and maintain balance. Balasubramanian and colleagues (2009) went on to explore the impact of gait characteristics on function, by comparing gait characteristics across groups. They found that the post-stroke groups with increased step length variability and reduced step width variability also had poor performance outcomes (severe hemiparesis, asymmetric step and a DGI score of ≤ 19). The authors ultimately suggest that the presence of decreased step width variability as well as increases in the variability of other gait parameters correlate strongly with impaired walking performance.

Kinematics

Common post-stroke gait deviations have been described in the literature. For the paretic limb during stance phase, these include:
- decreased forward propulsion;
- forward flexion of the trunk with weak hip extension and/or hip flexion contracture notably contributing to a lack of hip extension in terminal stance;
- decreased or increased lateral pelvic displacement;
- poor hip position in hip adduction and/or flexion;
- Trendelenburg limp caused by weak hip abductors;
- leg scissoring caused by spastic hip adductors and/or muscle substitution for weak hip flexors;
- excessive knee flexion in early and/or late stance;
- knee hyperextension during forward progression in midstance;
- equinovarus foot position with absent or inadequate heelstrike;
- varus foot;
- decreased dorsiflexion with mid-stance forward progression;
- inadequate ankle plantarflexion at toe off; and
- unequal step lengths.

For the paretic limb during swing phase, these include:
- exaggerated trunk extension;
- inadequate forward pelvic rotation;
- vaulting on nonparetic stance limb;
- inadequate and/or delayed hip flexion with abnormal substitutions such as pelvic hike, hip circumduction, hip external rotation and/or adduction;
- exaggerated hip flexion;
- inadequate knee flexion in early swing;
- delayed swing knee flexion;
- poorly controlled knee extension, particularly prior to heelstrike;
- persistent ankle/foot equinus or equinovarus;
- foot drop/toe drag or exaggerated dorsiflexion; and
- excessive use of momentum resulting in an uncontrolled swing.

Van Criekinge et al. (2020) examined relationships between limb and trunk walking biomechanics after sub-acute stroke. They concluded that lower limb impairments may contribute to abnormal trunk motion but should not be assumed to be the sole or even primary contributor; and that there are likely intrinsic trunk deficits which require additional study. Moseley et al. (1993) and Moore et al. (1993) collectively hypothesise that both stance and swing phase gait deviations may be the result of an inability to selectively activate and coordinate muscle activity and/or maladaptive muscle shortening.

Olney and colleagues (1991) documented bilateral leg joint angles for individuals post-stroke walking at slow, medium and fast speeds. Joint angle amplitudes or joint ranges of motion differed from norms and were present at all gait speeds. Considered clinically important were the decreased amplitudes of knee flexion during swing and hip extension during stance for the paretic limb. A correlation between walking speed and maximum ankle plantarflexion on the nonparetic side was also documented. Hesse and colleagues (1997) first described significant differences in timing, step length mediolateral displacement of the centre of pressure and centre of mass movement velocity patterns when persons post-stroke initiated gait with the affected versus the nonaffected limb. Bensoussan et al. (2006) extended Hesse's work to assess the kinetic and kinematic gait initiation characteristics of three subjects post-stroke with spastic equinovarus foot and three control subjects. They observed that subjects post-stroke had asymmetrical movement strategies such as decreased support phase of the paretic limb when the nonparetic limb initiated gait; asymmetrical body weight distribution with the nonparetic limb accepting greater weight; more pronounced propulsive forces in the nonparetic versus the paretic limb; increased knee flexion during initial swing phase to accommodate for the equinovarus; and a foot flat position at initial contact on the paretic limb.

Lu et al. (2010) studied gait during an 8-metre walk and crossing obstacles of three different heights for both limbs for high-functioning individuals with chronic stroke (able to walk 100 metres without an assistive device and Berg Balance Score >50). High-functioning individuals post-stroke had significantly different joint kinematics compared with an age-matched healthy control group, including greater leading toe clearance for clearing an obstacle, trailing toe obstacle distance and posterior pelvic tilt regardless of leading limb. No significant differences were found for gait speed. The authors conclude that individuals post-stroke who are able to function at a high level develop a specific bilateral symmetrical strategy including increasing posterior pelvic tilt and elevating the swing toe. This strategy probably provides a more posterior placement of the trailing limb, increasing leading toe clearance during obstacle clearance and preventing tripping.

Kinetics

Similar to gait spatiotemporal characteristics, force patterns post-stroke are described as highly variable among individuals as well as between paretic and nonparetic limbs. Reduced vertical loading and significant variability of loading on initial contact have been documented for the paretic and nonparetic limbs post-stroke (Marks and Hirschberg, 1958; Wortis et al., 1951). Hesse and colleagues (1993) documented an increase in vertical loading after initial contact on the paretic limb when compared with the nonparetic limb, as well as delayed loading after initial contact, premature unloading and reduced vertical push-off forces during terminal stance. Iida and Yamamuro (1987) reported significantly greater post-stroke medial-lateral centre of gravity displacement widths as compared with healthy controls. They also described these differences to be more pronounced for individuals after a more severe stroke.

Gait muscle activation patterns have been extensively studied in persons post-stroke. Well established is the high variability post-stroke in muscle firing magnitudes and phasic patterns between limbs and among individuals. In a review of hemiplegic gait characteristics, Woolley (2001) concluded that the general muscular firing changes post-stroke include reduced magnitude for paretic limb muscles as well as premature onset and prolonged duration of firing across stance and swing phases for muscles in both limbs. Peat and colleagues (1976) reported a tendency for post-stroke paretic limb muscle activity to collectively peak at the same time after stance weight acceptance. A few studies have resulted in classification systems based on EMG patterns (Dimitrijevic et al., 1981; Knutsson and Richards, 1979; Waters et al., 1982), but none has gained broad translation into clinical practice.

Nasciutti-Prudente and colleagues (2009) examined the relationships between muscle moments and gait speed in individuals post chronic stroke. They only identified one muscle group, paretic knee flexors, to have significant impact for predicting gait speed post-stroke. The paretic knee flexors accounted for 61% of the variation in gait speed, consistent with a previous study which identified paretic knee muscle strength as a moderate to strong predictor of walking ability in individuals post chronic mild to moderate stroke (Flansbjer et al., 2006).

It has been suggested that for the typical person post-stroke, walking requires approximately 50% to 67% more metabolic energy expenditure than that of a healthy person walking at the same speed (Corcoran et al., 1970) and that the paretic leg performs approximately 40% of the mechanical work of walking (Olney et al., 1991). Bowden and colleagues (2006) examined the effect of leg paresis on anterior-posterior ground reaction forces for individuals with varying levels of hemiparetic severity post-stroke. They documented a percentage of total propulsion generated by the paretic leg at 16% for severe hemiparesis, 36% for moderate hemiparesis and 49% for mild hemiparesis. In a review of paretic propulsion post-stroke, Roelker and colleagues (2019) concluded that paretic propulsion is an important measure for both walking performance and functional motor recovery. They reported that paretic leg extension in terminal stance, including both hip extension and ankle plantarflexion, is strongly associated with paretic propulsion, both of which are related to spatiotemporal, kinematic and kinetic walking performance metrics. Vistamehr and colleagues (2018) gathered dynamic balance and walking adaptability data from 15 stroke survivors who were able to walk at least 10 metres independently or with supervision using a cane or an orthotic device and compared this with data from 10 healthy adults. The walking tasks, completed without assistive device(s), included forward and backward walking, obstacle negotiation and step-up tasks. The stroke survivors had deficits in the frontal plane compared to healthy controls, particularly with paretic limb stance, including significantly lower soleus motor activity.

One clinical point of concern is the possible effect of gait compensation, such as hip hiking, vaulting or knee hyperextension, on the nonparetic limb post-stroke. Kerrigan and colleagues (1999) estimated the nonparetic limb joint moments in all three planes about the hip, knee and ankle for individuals with spastic paresis and stiff-legged gait post-stroke. They compared average stresses of the nonparetic leg with healthy controls. In general, average peak nonparetic limb joint moments were not significantly different from that of controls, suggesting that the risk for biomechanical injury over time was minimal. More recently, Marrocco et al. (2016) explored knee joint loading with nine individuals post-stroke and 17 healthy adults, documenting external knee adduction and flexion moments using three-dimensional gait analysis. One objective of the study was to demonstrate feasibility of measuring proxies for dynamic medial knee joint loading with external knee adduction and flexion moments. Coronal and sagittal plane knee moments for each lower limb across the gait cycle were plotted. The first peak of knee adduction and flexion moments was identified from each trial and then averaged over five trials. The authors found greater variability and excessive knee loading on the paretic and nonparetic sides for the stroke survivors compared to healthy adults, which were unrelated to trunk lean or toe-out angles. Therefore, more research is needed before clinicians can accurately anticipate the effects of long-term gait compensation such as joint degeneration and/or pain.

Clinical Management

Already established in the rehabilitation community is the criterion of 1.1 to 1.5 m/s gait speed for safe pedestrian walking across different environmental and social contexts. Unfortunately, only approximately 7% of stroke survivors are discharged from rehabilitation able to walk 500 metres continuously at a speed necessary for safe street crossing (Hill et al., 1997). Much more research is needed to establish best practices for regaining safe community-level gait. That said, Hornby and colleagues (2020) published a clinical practice guideline to improve walking performance following chronic stroke (>6 months following acute onset), incomplete spinal cord injury and brain injury. They focused on how to best improve walking speed or distance and concluded that there is strong evidence for moderate- to high-intensity locomotor training to improve walking speed or distance while weak evidence exists that strength, circuit or cycling training or virtual reality–based balance training will support functional gains. The authors further concluded that strong evidence suggests that body weight–supported treadmill training, robotic-assisted training or balance training without virtual reality should not be prescribed to improve walking speed or distance in these ambulatory populations. From a spatiotemporal gait asymmetry management perspective, Ryan and colleagues (2020) studied individuals post chronic stroke comparing interventions focused on remediating step length asymmetry with interventions focused on remediating stance time asymmetry. They documented that step length–focused intervention resulted in improved walking distance while stance time–focused intervention resulted in improved metabolic cost of walking. Their conclusion was that targeted training, while focused on spatiotemporal gait asymmetries, did not result in more symmetrical gait. An additional observation was that improvements documented in the lab did not appear to translate to increased community mobility.

Many persons post-stroke are either directed to or independently elect to use a unilateral assistive walking device. Kuan and colleagues (1999) studied the temporal and spatial gait characteristics of 15 subjects post acute stroke and nine age-matched healthy control subjects walking with and without a cane. They found that cane use had more of an effect on gait spatial variables than on temporal variables for subjects post-stroke, and that gait phases remained similar regardless of cane use. For subjects post-stroke using a cane, the paretic side had increased pelvic obliquity, hip abduction and ankle eversion during terminal stance; increased hip extension, knee extension and ankle plantarflexion during pre-swing; and increased hip adduction, knee flexion and ankle dorsiflexion during swing when compared with walking without a cane. The authors concluded that persons post-stroke may have improved spatial gait characteristics, including enhanced centre of mass translation and push off in stance and decreased circumduction in swing, when using a cane.

Orthoses and functional electrical stimulation are also commonly considered prescriptions post-stroke. A recent clinical practice guideline (Johnston et al., 2021) presents strong evidence that AFOs and functional electrical stimulation (FES) can each increase gait speed, mobility and balance and moderate evidence that AFO and FES increase quality of life, walking endurance and muscle activation. One approach was not found superior to the other, however the AFO may lead to more compensatory effects while FES may lead to more therapeutic effects. Also, there is weak evidence for these strategies in the improvement of gait kinematics. The authors warn that the evidence shows that AFOs or FES should not be used to decrease plantarflexor spasticity.

Lewallen and colleagues (2010) documented gait characteristics for 13 individuals using an orthosis post-stroke; specifically, solid, articulated and posterior leaf spring ankle foot orthoses. They found that gait was most impaired for those individuals wearing the solid ankle foot orthosis with a significant decrease in step length and gait speed. Use of the solid orthosis also resulted in slower decline walking compared with incline and walking over a level surface. Lehmann and colleagues (1987) reported a correlation between improved gait speed and ankle foot orthosis–related stance phase duration. A 5-degree dorsiflexed orthotic ankle angle contributed to increased walking speed and increase in heelstrike as compared with walking with no orthotic or when the orthotic was set in 5 degrees of plantarflexion. The effect of a neutral ankle orthotic setting was not explored.

Also of interest to clinicians is the potential relevance of footwear choice to gait and balance for individuals post-stroke. Inadequate footwear has been identified as a fall risk factor for the elderly (Menz and Lord, 1999; Menz et al., 2006; Sherrington and Menz, 2003). While much more research is needed, footwear choice is probably important. Ng et al., 2010 documented that the majority of their study participants preferred loose-fitting slippers for indoor walking over close-fitting shoes and bare feet. Only 23% of participants reported they had received advice about wearing appropriate footwear. The authors concluded that for proper ground contact, stability and proprioceptive input, it is reasonable to recommend shoes with broad, flat heels; firm heel counter; thin firm midsole; laces or other fixation; and adequate slip resistance.

Key Points

- Clinicians should expect high gait variability within and among patients post-stroke.
- Gait speed, using a standardised protocol such as the 10-Meter Walk Test, and distance, using a protocol such as the 6-Minute Walk Test, are essential clinical measurements.
- To improve walking speed and/or distance for individuals >6 months post-stroke, moderate- to high-intensity locomotor training should be employed.
- To improve gait speed, knee flexion strength may be an important post-stroke measure as well as an intervention target.
- Interventions focused on improving spatiotemporal gait asymmetry do not necessarily translate to more symmetrical gait or improved function.
- Intervention methods should address flexibility, strength and task-specific dynamic ambulation activities.
- AFO and FES should be considered for paretic ankle management, but should not be used to manage plantarflexion spasticity.
- Other devices, including canes and footwear, are likely to impact gait characteristics on an individual basis. Exactly which gait characteristics change and to what extent are yet to be determined. Gait analysis can be helpful to determine optimal use of these devices.
- Environmental constraints must be considered when establishing goals for persons post-stroke.

GAIT ASSESSMENT IN PARKINSON'S DISEASE

Derek Liuzzo and Jim Richards

Parkinsonism, a disorder of the extrapyramidal system, is caused by degeneration of the basal ganglia of the brain and is a common condition that affects motor function and gait. Parkinson's disease is a significant cause of morbidity with an estimated prevalence of 1.8% in those over age 65 in Europe (de Rijk et al., 2000), with disease progression linked with a significant decline in quality of life (de Boer et al., 1996). The exact causal mechanism is not yet fully understood, however, it is associated with a significant decrease in the number of dopaminergic neurons and an increase in the presence of *Lewy bodies*, tiny spherical protein deposits found in nerve cells whose presence in the brain disrupts the action of important chemical messengers. Diagnosis of Parkinson's disease is based on the presence of two or more of the following symptoms: tremor, rigidity, postural instability and akinesia. *Akinesia* is defined as a lack or poverty of movement which can be subdivided into slowness and unskilful movement secondary to rigidity, a lack or poverty of movement and difficulty in initiation of movement known as *freezing*.

Early analysis of gait in Parkinson's disease focused on temporal and spatial characteristics such as speed and step length, with Knutsson (1972) being one of the first to use gait analysis techniques to report the temporal and spatial parameters of gait in Parkinson's disease. Murray et al. (1978) conducted the first kinematic assessment of the gait of 44 males with parkinsonism using interrupted-light photography to record the displacement patterns of multiple body segments during free-speed and fast walking to quantitatively characterise their gait patterns. They identified the following abnormalities:

- Stride length and speed were very much reduced, although cycle time and cadence were usually normal.
- The walking base was slightly increased.
- The range of motion at the hip, knee and ankle was decreased, mainly by a reduction in joint extension.
- The swinging of the arms was much reduced.
- The majority of patients rotated the trunk in phase with the pelvis, instead of twisting it in the opposite direction.
- The vertical trajectories of the head, heel and toe were all reduced, although others have commented on a distinct bobbing motion of the head.

Parkinsonian gait is now widely recognised by a characteristic stooped and shuffling appearance (Samii et al., 2004). This includes a reduction in extension during late stance phase and a reduction in flexion during mid-swing coupled with a forward inclination of the trunk (Fig. 6.5). The shuffling gait occurs because the foot is still moving forwards at the time of initial contact. In some patients initial contact is made with the foot flat; in others, there is a heelstrike but with the foot being much more horizontal than usual. Some patients also show scuffing of the foot in mid-swing. Unlike most gait patterns, which stabilise within the first two or three steps, the gait of patients with parkinsonism often evolves over the course of several strides. Fig. 6.5 shows steady-state walking in an individual with Parkinson's disease compared with an age- and gender-matched healthy subject.

Clinical Management

One of the most well-validated treatments for parkinsonism is L-DOPA, which is a dietary precursor to dopamine. L-DOPA is converted to dopamine, which improves the motor symptoms of rigidity and the ability to start and continue movements (bradykinesia) (Durrieu, 1998; Stowe et al., 2008; van Hilten et al., 2007). L-DOPA is recognised to have a short response (several hours) and a long response (several days or weeks) which both contribute to symptom relief. Newly treated patients typically experience a honeymoon period where the effects of L-DOPA help

significantly, typically for several years. As time progresses, this honeymoon period ends and the patient becomes more globally affected. As Parkinson's disease progresses, patients experience motor fluctuations and other autonomic symptoms, typically in distinct *on* and *off* phases, as the short response comes to an end (Morris et al., 2001).

Morris et al. (1996) found that both gait speed and step length increased for patients whilst they were on L-DOPA, and although the gait parameters were repeatable when *on* medication they fluctuated greatly in the *off* phase. O'Sullivan et al. (1998) found L-DOPA produced a significant increase in walking speed but not cadence, which again indicates that L-DOPA increases stride length, which was further confirmed by Defebvre et al. (2002). Ferrarin et al. (2004) used gait analysis to describe the inclination of the trunk and found a significantly reduced forwards inclination or stooped gait pattern in Parkinson's disease patients on L-DOPA.

In addition to gait analysis, clinical assessments are used. The Unified Parkinson's Disease Rating Scale (UPDRS), which is a validated scale for severity of Parkinson's disease, is commonly used (Box 6.1). The UPDRS has four components which have been largely derived from preexisting scales. Parts II and III have the greatest relevance to gait analysis. Part II evaluates activities of daily living in both the on and off phases, which include falling, freezing when walking and walking. Part III is an assessment of motor capabilities and includes arising from a chair, posture, gait, postural stability and body bradykinesia and hypokinesia.

Gait Initiation Problems in People with Parkinson's Disease

Difficulties in initiation of movement, known as *freezing* or *motor blocks*, remain one of the most debilitating aspects of Parkinson's disease (Halliday et al., 1998). Giladi et al. (1992) studied 990 people with Parkinson's disease and found 318 had motor blocks: 86% of these had blocks in initiation of gait, 45% had blocks in turning, 25% had blocks in doorways and 23% had blocks in open runways. Therefore, gait initiation affected the largest number of subjects with motor blocks, which accounted for 27% of the people with Parkinson's disease investigated.

Hass et al. (2005) investigated gait initiation and dynamic balance control in people with different severities of Parkinson's disease. They found that the peak magnitude of the centre of pressure (COP) to centre of mass (COM) distance was significantly greater during the end of the single-support phase in the less-disabled patients than in more balance-disabled patients. The differences in COP–COM distances between the groups suggest that people with Parkinson's disease who

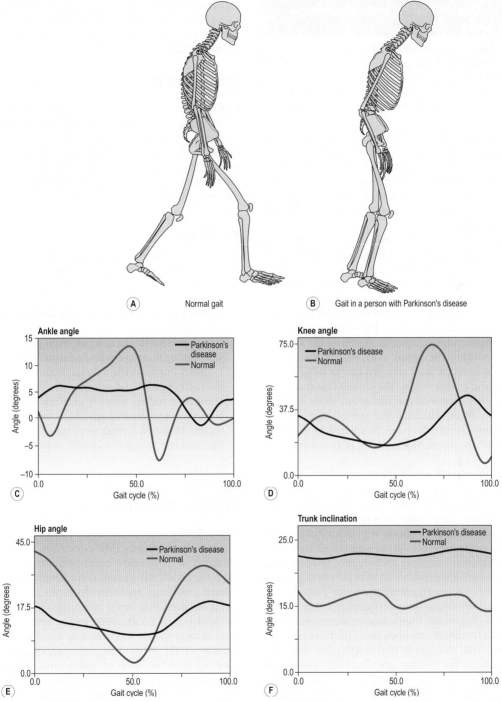

Fig. 6.5 (A, B) Representation of gait in a healthy subject and an individual with Parkinson's disease. (C) Ankle, (D) knee, (E) hip, and (F) trunk sagittal plane angles during gait in an individual with Parkinson's disease and an age-matched healthy individual.

Box 6.1   The Unified Parkinson's Disease Rating Scale

- Part I: Mentation, behaviour and mood
- Part II: Activities of daily living
- Part III: Motor examination
- Part IV: Complications of therapy (in the past week)

have impaired postural control produce shorter COM–COP distances than people without a clinically detectable balance impairment, which is an adaptation to prevent falls. Hass et al. (2005) concluded that this method of evaluation could prove a useful quantitative index to examine the impact of interventions designed to improve ambulation and balance in Parkinson's disease.

Jiang and Norman (2006) investigated the effects of visual and auditory cues on gait initiation in people with Parkinson's disease. They found a mean difference in the maximum forward propulsive force between people with Parkinson's disease who freeze and do not freeze. They also found a difference in the maximum horizontal force between the different cues. The auditory cues were rhythmic sounds with an interval matching the subject's average step time. The visual cues were high-contrast transverse lines on the floor adjusted for the subject's first step length and overall height. They found that transverse line visual cues improved gait initiation, while auditory cues had no effect. Although the use of high-contrast transverse lines on the floor can be applied to the home setting, these are not readily available in the community setting.

Portable cueing aids aimed at helping people overcome difficulties in initiating walking or freezing are becoming more common. McCandless et al. (2016) studied the effectiveness and acceptability of several of these devices on people with Parkinson's disease with gait initiation difficulties. Five randomised conditions were tested: laser cane, sound metronome, vibrating metronome, walking stick and uncued. Significant differences were seen in step length and COM and COP movement in the anterior-posterior and medial-lateral directions between freezing and nonfreezing episodes. Significant improvements were seen in the COM and COP movements when using the laser cane and the walking stick, and greater step length when using the laser cane during the freezing episodes. Participants rated the perceived effectiveness of the devices, which showed a significant improvement in satisfaction when using the laser cane for both starting and maintaining walking. Fig. 6.6 shows the COM and COP patterns for uncued, cued using a laser cane and age- and gender-matched gait initiation. The cued condition improves the medial-lateral

movement of the COP and the anterior movement of the COM, however there is still substantially less movement forwards when compared to the age- and gender-matched healthy individual.

CONCLUSION

Gait analysis for both steady-state gait and gait initiation is becoming more widely accepted as a sensitive tool for assessing Parkinson's disease. While general gait patterns can be identified, there is considerable variability of patients, particularly when in the *off* treatment phase. However, the use of clinically based gait analysis for this patient group is restricted to a small number of specialist clinics.

Key Points

- Trunk inclination and hip flexion/extension are useful clinical outcome measures, however temporal and spatial parameters are also good clinical markers.
- Clinicians should expect considerable gait variability among patients and between the *on* and *off* phases of the same patient.
- It is important to assess steady-state gait, gait initiation and turning in people with Parkinson's disease.
- L-DOPA improves the motor symptoms of rigidity and the ability to start and continue movements.
- Devices including walking aids and visual cues have been shown to improve gait characteristics and gait initiation. However, further work is required to determine the most effective devices in the community setting.

GAIT ASSESSMENT IN MUSCULAR DYSTROPHY

Cathie Smith

Muscular dystrophy (MD) describes a diagnostic subgrouping of progressive neuromuscular diseases resulting from genetically linked, noninflammatory, myopathic disease. Duchenne muscular dystrophy (DMD), the most common paediatric-onset neuromuscular disease with an incidence of 1:3500–6000 males, leads to progressive deterioration of gait mechanics as the disease progresses (Bushby et al., 2010). The combined effect of weakness resulting from the death of healthy muscle tissue and the hypoextensibility caused by deposition of fatty and fibrous tissue within the muscle produces relatively predictable changes in posture and movement patterns in children with DMD (Rahbek et al., 2005).

Considerable variance has been documented in timing of onset and speed of progression of DMD, however,

Paths of COM and COP during gait initiation

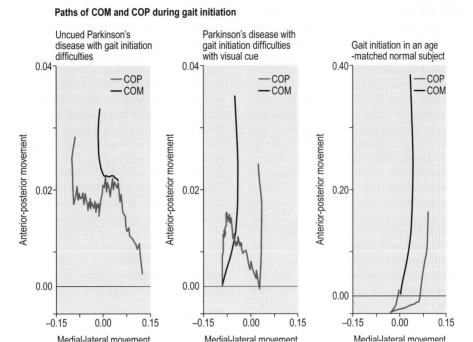

Fig. 6.6 Centre of mass (COM) and centre of pressure (COP) movement.

the typical clinical presentation is a functional deterioration of movement capacity in the lower extremities usually presenting 2 to 3 years before weakness in the upper extremities. This contributes significantly to the early compensatory patterns observed in children with DMD as they learn to accommodate for weaker muscle groups by modifying joint alignment and muscle activations. Early in the disease progression, children with DMD will reduce their walking speed as a subtle means of altering gait kinematics to more easily advance the leg during swing phase and to reduce the energy expenditure of walking (Campbell et al., 2012; Perry and Burnfield, 2010). A classic motor adaptation strategy demonstrated by children with DMD is the Gower's sign, where the arms are used to push against the thigh to assist with hip extension upon rising from sitting (Campbell et al., 2012).

The insidious nature of onset of this disorder between 2 and 5 years of age combined with these compensatory movement patterns may contribute to delayed identification of the early impairments associated with DMD. Monitoring changes in muscle strength and range of motion over time are essential examination components to help distinguish age-related variances in typical development from the atypical developmental trajectory demonstrated by children with DMD. Goniometric measurements or analysis of functional movement patterns can provide relatively objective assessments of change in joint mobility across all ages. However, obtaining reliable objective strength measures in very young children can be challenging. In children older than 5 years of age, classic manual muscle testing (MMT) can generally be applied to obtain serial strength measures. In older children, an alternative method for measuring decline in strength of specific muscle groups over time to more precisely interpret altered gait mechanics is quantitative muscle testing (QMT). QMT measures isometric force production capacity by using a force gauge to directly assess contractile activity in a particular muscle group whilst ensuring a constant muscle length (Stuberg and Metcalf, 1988). In addition to the specialised equipment required, the child must also demonstrate qualities of cooperation, motivation, attention and understanding of instructions to support the reliable use of QMT.

The diagnosis of DMD is most often made between 2 and 5 years of age, with the lack of gait maturation being one of the early hallmark signs. Early gait pathomechanics coupled with reports of walking reluctance, increased clumsiness with frequent falls, laboured efforts required to come to stand compared with age-matched peers, and absence of heelstrike are common early clinical presentations (Campbell et al., 2012). Sutherland et al. (1981) categorised gait disturbances of children with DMD into three groups: early, transitional and late ambulators. When examining the gait variables of

21 youngsters with DMD across these groups, these researchers identified three gait characteristics as predictors of disease progression with a 91% accuracy: cadence, dorsiflexion in swing and anterior pelvic tilt. Apart from the positive Gower's sign, the most notable early gait changes include altered cadence, a slight increase in hip flexion during swing phase and a decreased ankle dorsiflexion with foot drop occurring as the cadence continues to decrease. Associated with these gait pattern changes, the ground reaction force passes anterior to the knee joint during early single limb support with muscle weakness, most notably in the quadriceps. When examining gait patterns of a relatively homogeneous group of 21 children with DMD with a mean age of 72 ± 8.2 months, D'Angelo et al. (2009) confirmed previously reported data demonstrating excessive anterior tilt of the pelvis and abnormal knee pattern loading response. Additionally, these researchers reported significantly lower stride length values, significantly higher step width values with higher flexion and abduction movement patterns used to advance the limb during swing phase as compared with age-matched peers. When examining the effects of gait velocity on gait patterns of a cohort of children with DMD between 7 and 15 years of age, Gaudreault et al. (2010) reported higher cadence, shorter step length, a lower hip extension moment, a minimal or absent knee extension moment and reduced or absent dorsiflexion moment at heel strike when compared with age- and gender-matched peers. Gaudreault et al. (2009) examined the contribution of plantar flexion contractures during the gait of 11 children with a confirmed diagnosis of DMD with a mean age of 9.2 ± 2.6 years and reported that increased net plantar flexion moments at the end of the lengthening phase of the plantar flexors and forward shift of the COP served to help the children ambulate independently despite a significant weakness in the extensors.

During the late stage of ambulation, children with DMD demonstrate a marked increase in work output associated with a marked exaggeration of gait pathomechanics. Functional compensation for the increasing weakness in the gluteus maximus muscle produces an exaggerated anterior pelvic tilt with associated restricted hip extension during stance phase. Inability to maintain pelvic alignment during stance phase due to gluteus medius muscle weakness results in a positive Trendelenburg's sign where the non–weight-bearing hip drops excessively during single leg stance, and emergence of Trendelenburg gait pattern characterised by lateral flexion of the trunk towards the weight-bearing side resulting in increased shoulder sway and widened base of support. These gait alterations make it possible for the child with DMD to maintain the force line behind the hip joint and in front of the knee joint throughout single limb support, thereby helping to rely on deep joint structures to assist in the maintenance of upright stance as a compensation for increasing weakness in the hip and knee extensor muscles.

Reliable prediction of cessation of independent ambulation is an important management consideration for individuals with DMD. Sienko-Thomas et al. (2010) suggested that the loss of knee flexion in loading response may be an indicator of impending loss of ambulation while Bakker et al. (2002) found that strength loss in hip extension and dorsiflexion is the primary predictors. Siegel (1986) found that when the combined lag angle of active antigravity hip extension in prone (starting with hip flexed to 90 degrees) and active knee extension in sitting (starting with the knee flexed to 90 degrees) exceeds 90 degrees, loss of independent ambulation is likely to occur within a few months. Other reported clinical methods to identify impending cessation of independent ambulation include a MMT of below grade 3 for hip extensors or below grade 4 for ankle dorsiflexors (McDonald et al., 1995), reduction in lower-extremity strength by greater than 50% and a prolonged time to ascend four standard steps (Brooke et al., 1989).

Clinical Management

Advances in medical and pharmaceutical management of children with DMD have resulted in a change of the natural history of the disease process with increasing numbers of the children diagnosed with DMD surviving into adulthood. Advances have included delayed cessation of ambulation; delayed development of contractures and reduced numbers of surgical corrections; reduced use of long leg orthotics; decreased incidence of scoliosis and corrective back alignment surgeries; delayed pulmonary function decline; and increased survival into early adulthood. Moxley et al. (2010) reported an increase in mean survival to 30 years of age during the decade of the 2000s, with the potential for that age to further increase in the present decade. This represented an increase of almost 5 years between 1990 and 1999 as compared with 2000 and 2009. As preventive management of children with DMD becomes more precise, and as the survival likelihood continues to increase, it is important for clinicians to monitor gait patterns carefully for signs of impending degeneration.

To better understand the management needs of children with DMD across the life span, the International Standard of Care Committee for Congenital Muscular Dystrophy convened a 3-day workshop in Brussels, Belgium, in November 2009, to develop a consensus statement based on input from experts in the field and from families directly impacted by DMD (Wang et al., 2010). Management recommendations to meet the emerging needs of individuals with DMD across the life span drawn from the consensus statement on standard care for congenital muscular dystrophies developed during that meeting include coordinating transition of care from paediatric to adult services; identifying and planning for post-secondary educational and vocational needs; preparing patients to manage their own healthcare needs; supporting patients and families in making decisions regarding advance care directives; and advocating for services to meet independent living needs, aid services and healthcare coverage (Wang et al., 2010).

DMD is a representative example of multiple progressive neuromuscular disorders that result in altered gait characteristics. Understanding the underlying factors impacting gait pathomechanics in people with muscular dystrophy provides essential information to support optimal quality of life and promote prolonged independent ambulation for these individuals.

Key Points

- Quadriceps insufficiency is the key factor influencing compensatory postural adaptations of increased anterior pelvic tilt, restricted hip extension in stance and an equinus posture.
- Displacement of the weight-bearing force line anterior to the knee joint and posterior to the hip joint coupled with plantarflexion muscle tightness helps support independent ambulation despite significantly reduced extensor force generation capacity.
- Timing of cessation of independent ambulation may be reliably predicted.
- Advances in medical management leading to increasing life expectancy warrants inclusion of transition services as children with DMD transition from paediatric to adult services.

REFERENCES

Awad, L., Reisman, D., Binder-Macleod, S., 2019. Distance-induced changes in walking speed after stroke: relationship to community walking ability. J. Neurol. Phys. Ther. 43, 220–223.

Baker, R., Jasinski, M., Maciag-Tymecka, I., et al., 2002. Botulinum toxin treatment of spasticity in diplegic cerebral palsy: a randomized, double-blind, placebo-controlled, dose-ranging study. Dev. Med. Child Neurol. 44 (10), 666–675.

Baker, R., Rodda, J., 2003. All you Ever Wanted to Know about the Conventional Gait Model but Were Afraid to Ask (CD-ROM). Women and Children's Health, Melbourne.

Bakker, J.P., de Groot, I.J., Beelen, A., et al., 2002. Predictive factors of cessation of ambulation in patients with Duchenne muscular dystrophy. Am. J. Phys. Med. Rehabil. 81, 906–912.

Balasubramanian, C.K., Neptune, R.R., Kautz, S.A., 2009. Variability in spatiotemporal step characteristics and its relationship to walking performance post-stroke. Gait Posture 29, 408–414.

Bensoussan, L., Mesure, S., Viton, J., et al., 2006. Kinematic and kinetic asymmetries in hemiplegic patients' gait initiation patterns. J. Rehabil. Med. 38, 281–294.

Bohannon, R.W., Smith, M.B., 1987. Interrater reliability of a modified Ashworth scale of muscle spasticity. Phys. Ther. 67 (2), 206–207.

Bowden, M.G., Balasbramanian, C.K., Neptune, R.R., et al., 2006. Anterior-posterior ground reaction forces as a measure of paretic leg contribution in hemiparetic walking. Stroke 37, 872–876.

Boyd, R.N., Graham, H.K., 1999. Objective measurement of clinical findings in the use of botulinum toxin type A for the management of children with cerebral palsy. Eur. J. Neurol. 45 (Suppl. 96), 10–14.

Brooke, M.H., Fenichel, G.M., Grigs, R.C., et al., 1989. Duchenne muscular dystrophy: patterns of clinical progression and clinical effects of supportive therapy. Neurology 39, 475–481.

Bushby, K., Finkel, R., Birnkrant, D.J., et al., 2010. Diagnosis and management of Duchenne muscular dystrophy Part 1. Lancet Neurol. 9, 177–189.

Campbell, S.K., Palisano, R.J., Orlin, M.N., 2012. Physical Therapy for Children, fourth ed. WB Saunders/ Elsevier, St. Louis, MO.

Carlsoo, S., Dahllof, A., Holm, J., 1974. Kinetic analysis of the gait in patients with hemiparesis and in patients with intermittent claudication. Scand. J. Rehabil. Med. 6, 166–179.

Carr, J.H., Shepherd, R.B., 2003. Stroke Rehabilitation: Guidelines for Exercise and Training to Optimize Motor Skill. Elsevier, London.

Centers for Disease Control and Prevention. National Center on Health Statistics. Online: www.cdc.gov/nchs/fastats/stroke (accessed 1.3.22).

Corcoran, P.J., Jebsen, R.H., Brengelman, G.L., et al., 1970. Effects of plastic and metal leg braces in speed and energy cost of hemiparetic ambulations. Arch. Phys. Med. Rehabil. 51, 69–77.

Damiano, D.L., Abel, M.F., 1998. Functional outcomes of strength training in spastic cerebral palsy. Arch. Phys. Med. Rehabil. 79 (2), 119–125.

Damiano, D.L., Dodd, K., Taylor, N.F., 2002. Should we be testing and training muscle strength in cerebral palsy? Dev. Med. Child Neurol. 44 (1), 68–72.

Damiano, D.L., Vaughan, C.L., Abel, M.F., 1995. Muscle response to heavy resistance exercise in children with spastic cerebral palsy. Dev. Med. Child Neurol. 37 (8), 731–739.

D'Angelo, M.G., Berti, M., Piccinini, L., et al., 2009. Gait pattern in muscular dystrophy. Gait Posture 29, 36–41.

Davis, R., Jameson, E.G., Davids, J.R., et al., 1991. A gait analysis data collection and reduction technique. Hum. Mov. Sci. 10, 575–587.

Day, S.M., Wu, Y.W., Strauss, D.J., et al., 2007. Change in ambulatory ability of adolescents and young adults with cerebral palsy. Dev. Med. Child Neurol. 49 (9), 647–653.

de Boer, A.G., Wijker, W., Speelman, J.D., et al., 1996. Quality of life in patients with Parkinson's disease: development of a questionnaire. J. Neurol. Neurosurg. Psychiatry 61 (1), 70–74.

de Rijk, M.C., Launer, L.I., Berger, K., et al., 2000. Prevalence of Parkinson's disease in Europe: a collaborative study of population-based cohorts. Neurology 54 (11), S21–S23.

Defebvre, L.J.P., Krystkowiak, P., Blatt, J.L., et al., 2002. Influence of pallidal stimulation and levodopa on gait and preparatory postural adjustments in Parkinson's disease. Mov. Disord. 17 (1), 76–83.

Dimitrijevic, M.R., Faganel, J., Sherwood, A.M., et al., 1981. Activation of paralysed leg flexors and extensors during gait in patients after stroke. Scand. J. Rehabil. Med. 13, 109–115.

Dobson, F., 2007. Classification of Gait Patterns in Children with Hemiplegic Cerebral Palsy. School of Physiotherapy, University of Melbourne, Melbourne.

Dobson, F., Morris, M.E., Baker, R., et al., 2006. Clinician agreement on gait pattern ratings in children with spastic hemiplegia. Dev. Med. Child Neurol. 48 (6), 429–435.

Dobson, F., Morris, M.E., Baker, R., et al., 2007. Gait classification in children with cerebral palsy: a systematic review. Gait Posture 25 (1), 140–152.

Dodd, K., Taylor, N., 2005. Strength Training for Young People with Cerebral Palsy. La Trobe University, Melbourne.

Dodd, K., Taylor, N., Damiano, D., 2002. A systematic review on the effectiveness of strength training programs for people with cerebral palsy. Arch. Phys. Med. Rehabil. 83, 1157–1164.

Dodd, K., Taylor, N., Graham, H., 2003. A randomized clinical trial of strength training in young people with cerebral palsy. Dev. Med. Child Neurol. 45, 652–657.

Durrieu, G., 1998. Early combination therapy with levodopa and dopamine agonist for preventing motor fluctuations in Parkinson's disease. Cochrane Database Syst. Rev. 2, CD001311.

Eames, N.W.A., Baker, R., Hill, N., et al., 1999. The effect of botulinum toxin A on gastrocnemius length: magnitude and duration of response. Dev. Med. Child Neurol. 41 (4), 226–232.

Elder, G.C., Kirk, J., Stewart, G., et al., 2003. Contributing factors to muscle weakness in children with cerebral palsy. Dev. Med. Child Neurol. 45 (8), 542–550.

Ferrarin, M., Rizzone, M., Lopiano, L., et al., 2004. Effects of subthalamic nucleus stimulation and -dopa in trunk kinematics of patients with Parkinson's disease. Gait Posture 19 (2), 164–171.

Flansbjer, U., Downham, D., Lexell, J., 2006. Knee muscle strength, gait performance, and perceived participation after stroke. Arch. Phys. Med. Rehabil. 87, 974–980.

Foran, J.R., Steinman, S., Barash, I., et al., 2005. Structural and mechanical alterations in spastic skeletal muscle. Dev. Med. Child Neurol. 47 (10), 713–717.

Fry, N.R., Gough, M., McNee, A.E., et al., 2007. Changes in the volume and length of the medial gastrocnemius after surgical recession in children with spastic diplegic cerebral palsy. J. Pediatr. Orthop. 27 (7), 769–774.

Fulk, G.D., He, Y., 2018. Minimal clinically important difference of the 6-Minute Walk Test in people with stroke. J. Neurol. Phys. Ther. 42, 235–240.

Gage, J.R., Schwartz, M.H., Koop, S.E., et al., 2009. The Identification and Treatment of Gait Problems in Cerebral Palsy Clinics in Developmental Medicine. Mac Keith Press, London.

Gaudreault, N., Gravel, D., Nadeau, S., 2009. Evaluation of plantar flexion contracture contribution during the gait of children with Duchenne muscular dystrophy. J. Electromyogr. Kinesiol. 19, 180–186.

Gaudreault, N., Gravel, D., Nadeau, S., et al., 2010. Gait patterns comparison of children with Duchenne muscular dystrophy to those of control subjects considering the effect of gait velocity. Gait Posture 32, 342–347.

Giladi, N., McMahon, D., Przedborski, S., et al., 1992. Motor blocks in Parkinson's disease. Neurology 42, 333–339.

Halliday, S.E., Winter, D.A., Frank, J.S., et al., 1998. The initiation of gait in young, elderly, and Parkinson's disease subjects. Gait Posture 8, 8–14.

Harvey, A., Graham, H.K., Morris, M.E., et al., 2007. The Functional Mobility Scale: ability to detect change following single event multilevel surgery. Dev. Med. Child Neurol. 49 (8), 603–607.

Hass, C., Waddell, D., Fleming, R., et al., 2005. Gait initiation and dynamic balance control in Parkinson's disease. Arch. Phys. Med. Rehabil. 86 (11), 2172–2176.

Hesse, S., Reiter, F., Jhanke, M., et al., 1997. Asymmetry of gait initiation in hemiparetic stroke subjects. Arch. Phys. Med. Rehabil. 78, 719–724.

Hesse, S.A., Jahnke, M.T., Schreiner, C., et al., 1993. Gait symmetry and functional walking performance in hemiparetic patient prior to and after a 4-week rehabilitation programme. Gait Posture 1, 166–171.

Hill, K., Ellis, P., Bernhardt, J., et al., 1997. Balance and mobility outcomes for stroke patients: a comprehensive audit. Aust. J. Physiother 43, 173–180.

Hornby, T.G., Reisman, D.S., Ward, I.G., et al., 2020. Clinical practice guideline to improve locomotor function following chronic stroke, incomplete spinal cord injury, and brain injury. J. Neurol. Phys. Ther. 44, 49–100.

Hullin, M., Robb, J., Loudon, I., 1996. Gait patterns in children with hemiplegic spastic cerebral palsy. J. Pediatr. Orthop. 5, 247–251.

Iida, H., Yamamuro, T., 1987. Kinetic analysis of the center of gravity of the human body in normal and pathological gait. J. Biomech. 20, 987–995.

Jahnsen, R., Villien, L., Aamodt, G., et al., 2004. Locomotion skills in adults with cerebral palsy. Clin. Rehabil. 18, 309–316.

Jarvis, H.L., Brown, S.J., Price, M., et al., 2019. Return to employment after stroke in young adults: how important is the speed and energy cost of walking? Stroke 50, 3198–3204.

Jiang, Y., Norman, K.E., 2006. Effects of visual and auditory cues on gait initiation in people with Parkinson's disease. Clin. Rehabil. 20 (1), 36–45.

Johnston, T.E., Keller, S., Denzer-Weiler, C., Brown, L., 2021. A clinical practice guideline for the use of ankle-foot orthoses and functional electrical stimulation post-stroke. J. Neurol. Phys. Ther. 45, 112–196.

Kadaba, M.P., Ramakrishnan, H.K., Wootten, M.E., 1990. Measurement of lower extremity kinematics during level walking. J. Orthop. Res. 8 (3), 383–392.

Kendall, H., Kendall, F., 1949. Muscles Testing and Function. Lippincott Williams & Wilkins, Baltimore, MD.

Kerrigan, D.C., Frates, E.P., Rogan, S., et al., 1999. Spastic paretic stiff-legged gait: biomechanics of the unaffected limb. Am. J. Phys. Med. Rehabil. 78, 354–360.

Knutsson, E., 1972. An analysis of parkinsonian gait. Brain 95 (3), 475–486.

Knutsson, E., Richards, C., 1979. Different types of disturbed motor control in gait of hemiparetic patients. Brain 102, 405–430.

Kuan, T., Tsou, J., Fong-Chin, S., 1999. Hemiplegic gait of stroke patients: the effect of using a cane. Arch. Phys. Med. Rehabil. 80, 777–784.

Lance, J., 1980. Pathophysiology of spasticity and clinical experience with baclofen. In: Feldman, R., Young, R., Koella, W. (Eds.), Spasticity: Disordered Motor Control. Year Book Medical Publishers, Chicago, IL, pp. 485–495.

Lehmann, J.F., Condon, S.M., Price, R., et al., 1987. Gait abnormalities in hemiplegia: their correction by ankle-foot orthoses. Arch. Phys. Med. Rehabil. 68, 763–771.

Lewallen, J., Miedaner, J., Amyx, S., et al., 2010. Effect of three styles of custom ankle foot orthoses on the gait of stroke patients while walking on level and inclined surfaces. Am. Acad. Orthotists Prosthetists 22, 78–83.

Lewek, M.D., Sykes III, R., 2019. Minimal detectable change for gait speed depends on baseline speed in individuals with chronic stroke. J. Neurol. Phys. Ther. 43, 122–127.

Lu, T.W., Yen, H.C., Chen, H.L., et al., 2010. Symmetrical kinematic changes in higher function in older patients post-stroke during obstacle-crossing. Gait Posture 31, 511–516.

Marks, M., Hirschberg, G.G., 1958. Analysis of the hemiplegic gait. Ann. N. Y. Acad. Sci. 74, 59–77.

Marrocco, S., Crosby, L.D., Jones, I.C., et al., 2016. Knee loading patterns of the non-paretic and paretic legs during post-stroke gait. Gait Posture 49, 297–302.

McCandless, P.J., Evans, B.J., Janssen, J., Selfe, J., Churchill, A., Richards, J., 2016. Effect of three cueing devices for people with Parkinson's disease with gait initiation difficulties. Gait Posture 44, 7–11.

McDonald, C.M., Abresch, R.T., Carter, G.T., 1995. Profiles of neuromuscular diseases: Duchenne muscular dystrophy. Am. J. Phys. Med. Rehabil. 74 (Suppl), 570–592.

Menz, H.B., Lord, S.R., 1999. Footwear and postural stability in older people. J. Am. Podiatr. Med. Assoc. 89, 346–357.

Menz, H.B., Morris, M.E., Lord, S.R., 2006. Footwear characteristics and risk of indoor and outdoor falls in older people. Gerontology 52, 174–180.

Moore, S., Schurr, K., Wales, A., et al., 1993. Observation and analysis of hemiplegic gait: swing phase. Aust. J. Physiother 39, 271–278.

Morris, M.E., Huxham, F., McGinley, J., et al., 2001. The biomechanics and motor control of gait in Parkinson disease. Clin. Biomech. (Bristol, Avon) 16 (6), 459–470.

Morris, M.E., Matyas, T.A., Iansek, R., et al., 1996. Temporal stability of gait in Parkinson's disease. Phys. Ther. 76 (7), 763–777.

Moseley, A., Wales, A., Herbert, R., et al., 1993. Observation and analysis of hemiplegic gait: stance phase. Aust. J. Physiother 39, 259–267.

Moxley, R., Pandya, S., Ciafolnoi, E., et al., 2010. Change in natural history of Duchenne muscular dystrophy with long-term corticosteroid treatment: implications for management. J. Child Neurol. 25 (9), 1116–1129.

Murphy, K., Molnar, G., Lankasky, K., 1995. Medical and functional status of adults with cerebral palsy. Dev. Med. Child Neurol. 37, 1075–1084.

Murray, M.P., Sepic, S.B., Gardner, G.M., Downs, W.J., 1978. Walking patterns of men with parkinsonism. Am. J. Phys. Med. 57, 278–294.

Nasciutti-Prudente, C., Oliveira, F.G., Houri, S.F., et al., 2009. Relationships between muscular torque and gait speed in chronic hemiparetic subjects. Disabil. Rehabil. 31, 103–108.

Ng, H., McGinley, J.L., Jolley, D., Morris, M., Workman, B., Srikanth, V., 2010. Effects of footwear on gait and balance in people recovering from stroke. Age Ageing 39 (4), 507–510.

Novacheck, T.F., Stout, J.L., Tervo, R., 2000. Reliability and validity of the Gillette Functional Assessment Questionnaire as an outcome measure in children with walking disabilities. J. Pediatr. Orthop. 20 (1), 75–81.

Olney, S.J., Griffin, M.P., Monga, T.N., et al., 1991. Work and power in gait of stroke patients. Arch. Phys. Med. Rehabil. 72, 309–314.

Olney, S.J., Richards, C., 1996. Hemiparetic gait following stroke. Part 1: Characteristics. Gait Posture 4, 136–148.

O'Sullivan, J.D., Said, C.M., Dillon, L.C., et al., 1998. Gait analysis in patients with Parkinson's disease and motor fluctuations: influence of levodopa and comparison with other measures of motor function. Mov. Disord. 13 (6), 900–906.

Ounpuu, O., Davis, R., Deluca, P., 1996. Joint kinetics: methods, interpretation and treatment decision-making in children with cerebral palsy and myelomeningocele. Gait Posture 4, 62–78.

Palisano, R., Rosenbaum, P., Walter, S., 1997. Development and reliability of a system to classify gross motor function in children with cerebral palsy. Dev. Med. Child Neurol. 39 (4), 214–223.

Palisano, R.J., Hanna, S.E., Rosenbaum, P.L., et al., 2000. Validation of a model of gross motor function for children with cerebral palsy. Phys. Ther. 80 (10), 974–985.

Palisano, R.J., Rosenbaum, P., Bartlett, D., et al., 2008. Content validity of the expanded and revised Gross Motor Function Classification System. Dev. Med. Child Neurol. 50 (10), 744–750.

Patla, A.E., Niechwiej, E., Racco, V., et al., 2002. Understanding the roles of vision in the control of human locomotion. Exp. Brain Res. 142, 551–561.

Peat, M., Dubo, H.I.C., Winter, D.A., et al., 1976. Electromyographic analysis of gait: hemiplegic locomotion. Arch. Phys. Med. Rehabil. 57, 421–425.

Perry, J., 1969. The mechanics of walking in hemiplegia. Clin. Orthop. Relat. Res. 63, 23–31.

Perry, J., Burnfield, J.M., 2010. Gait Analysis: Normal and Pathological Function, second ed. Slack Inc., Thorofare, NJ.

Rahbek, J., Werge, B., Madsen, A., et al., 2005. Adult life with Duchenne muscular dystrophy: observations among an emerging and unforseen population. Pediatr. Rehabil. 8 (1), 17–28.

Rodda, J.M., Graham, H.K., Carson, L., et al., 2004. Sagittal gait patterns in spastic diplegia. J. Bone Joint Surg. Br. 86 (2), 251–258.

Roelker, S.A., Bowden, M.G., Kautz, S.A., Neptune, R.R., 2019. Paretic propulsion as a measure of walking performance and functional motor recovery post-stroke: a review. Gait Posture 68, 6–14.

Rosenbaum, P., Paneth, N., Leviton, A., et al., 2007. A report: the definition and classification of cerebral palsy, April 2006. Dev. Med. Child Neurol. 49 (Suppl. 2), 8–14.

Roth, E.J., Merbitz, C., Mroczek, K., et al., 1997. Hemiplegic gait relationships between walking speed and other temporal parameters. Am. J. Phys. Med. Rehabil. 76, 128–133.

Rozumalski, A., Schwartz, M.H., 2009. Crouch gait patterns defined using k-means cluster analysis are related to underlying clinical pathology. Gait Posture 30 (2), 155–160.

Ryan, H.P., Husted, C., Lewek, M.D., 2020. Improving spatiotemporal gait asymmetry has limited functional benefit for individuals poststroke. J. Neurol. Phys. Ther. 44, 197–204.

Sacco, R.L., Kasner, S.E., Broderick, J.P., et al., 2013. An updated definition of stroke for the 21st century. A statement for healthcare professionals from the American Heart Association/American Stroke Association. Stroke 44, 2064–2089.

Samii, A., Nutt, J.G., Ransom, B.R., 2004. Parkinson's disease. Lancet. 363 (9423), 1783–1793.

Sherrington, C., Menz, H.B., 2003. An evaluation of footwear worn at the time of fall-related hip fracture. Age Ageing 32, 310–314.

Shortland, A.P., Harris, C.A., Gough, M., et al., 2002. Architecture of the medial gastrocnemius in children with spastic diplegia. Dev. Med. Child Neurol. 44 (3), 158–163.

Shumway-Cook, A., Woollacott, M.H., 2007. Motor Control: Translating Research into Clinical Practice, third ed. Lippincott Williams & Wilkins, Philadelphia, PA.299–329.

Siegel, I.M., 1986. Muscle and Its Diseases: An Outline Primer of Basic Science and Clinical Method. Year Book Medical Publisher, Chicago, IL.

Sienko-Thomas, S., Buckon, C.E., Nicorici, A., et al., 2010. Classification of the gait patterns of boys with Duchenne muscular dystrophy and their relation to function. J. Child Neurol. 25 (9), 1103–1109.

Stanley, F.J., Blair, E., Alberman, E., 2000. Cerebral Palsies: Epidemiology and Causal Pathways. Mac Keith Press, Cambridge, UK.

Stowe, R., Ives, N., Clarke, C.E., et al., 2008. Dopamine agonist therapy in early Parkinson's disease. Cochrane Database Syst. Rev. 2, CD006564.

Stuberg, W.A., Metcalf, W.K., 1988. Reliability of quantitative muscle testing in health children and in children with Duchenne muscular dystrophy using a hand-held dynamometer. Phys. Ther. 68 (6), 977–982.

Sutherland, D.H., Davids, J.R., 1993. Common gait abnormalities of the knee in cerebral palsy. Clin. Orthop. Relat. Res. 288, 139–147.

Sutherland, D.H., Olshen, R.A., Cooper, L., et al., 1981. The pathomechanics of gait in Duchenne muscular dystrophy. Dev. Med. Child Neurol. 23 (1), 3–22.

Tyson, S., Connell, L., 2009. The psychometric properties and clinical utility of measures of walking and mobility in neurological conditions: a systematic review. Clin. Rehabil. 23 (11), 1018–1033.

Van Criekinge, T., Wim, S., Herssens, N., Van de Walle, P., De Hertogh, W., Truijen, S., et al., 2020. Trunk biomechanics during walking after sub-acute stroke and its relation to lower limb impairments. Clin. Biomech. 75, 105013.

van Hilten, J.J., Ramaker, C.C., Stowe, R., et al., 2007. Bromocriptine/levodopa combined versus levodopa alone for early Parkinson's disease. Cochrane Database Syst. Rev. 4, CD003634.

Vistamehr, A., Balasubramanian, C.K., Clark, D.J., et al., 2018. Dynamic balance during walking adaptability tasks in individuals post-stroke. J. Biomech. 74, 106–115.

Wang, C.H., Bonnemann, C.G., Rutkowski, A., et al., 2010. Consensus statement on standard of care for congenital muscular dystrophies. J. Child Neurol. 25 (12), 1559–1581.

Waters, R.L., Frazier, J., Garland, D.E., et al., 1982. Electromyographic analysis before and after operative treatment for hemiplegic equinus and equinovarus deformity. J. Bone Joint Surg. Am. 64, 284–288.

Wiley, M.E., Damiano, D.L., 1998. Lower-extremity strength profiles in spastic cerebral palsy. Dev. Med. Child Neurol. 40 (2), 100–107.

Winters Jr., T.F., Gage, J.R., Hicks, R., 1987. Gait patterns in spastic hemiplegia in children and young adults. J. Bone Joint Surg. Am. 69 (3), 437–441.

Woolley, S.M., 2001. Characteristics of gait in hemiplegia. Top. Stroke Rehabil. 7, 1–18.

World Health Organization, 2001. International Classification of Functioning, Disability and Health (ICF). https://www.who.int/classifications/international-classification-of-functioning-disability-and-health.

World Health Organization, 2021. The Atlas of Heart Disease and Stroke, Ch 15. Global Burden of Stroke., Online: www.WHO.int/cardiovascular_diseases/resources/atlas/en. (accessed 04.29.2021)

World Stroke Organization. 2021. Facts and Figures about Stroke. Online: www.world-stroke.org. (accessed 04.29.2021).

Wortis, B.S., Marks, M., Hirschberg, G.G., et al., 1951. Gait analysis in hemiplegia. Trans. Am. Neurol. Assoc. 76, 181–183.

7

Gait Analysis in Musculoskeletal Conditions, Prosthetics and Orthotics

Jim Richards, Frank Tudini, June Hanks, Hannah Shepherd, Gabor Barton, David Levine, Natalie Vanicek, Cleveland Barnett and Ashley Schilling

OUTLINE

This chapter discusses how gait analysis can improve our understanding of the treatment of musculoskeletal conditions, using examples of total hip arthroplasty, knee osteoarthritis, prosthetics and amputee gait and orthotic management.

TOTAL HIP ARTHROPLASTY

David Levine, Frank Tudini
and Jim Richards

Total hip arthroplasty (THA) is one of the most frequently performed and successful orthopedic surgeries for reducing pain and restoring function in individuals with osteoarthritis of the hip. The incidence of THA in the United States increased from 56.80 to 116.26 per 100,000 people between 2000 and 2014. The number of primary THA procedures increased from 159,856 to 370,770 during the same time frame. According to a linear progression model, this is projected to further increase by 71.2% to 635,000 by 2030 (Sloan et al., 2018).

Gait analysis is accepted as an objective measure of physical function and is one of the methods used to assess the success of THA. Most analyses concentrate on the spatiotemporal parameters, kinematics and kinetics of the lower extremities during gait. The majority of studies have compared THA status at 6 to 18 months postoperatively to preoperative levels or to healthy controls, and have concluded that gait improves but does not return to normal following THA.

Spatiotemporal Factors

Spatiotemporal factors include gait speed, cadence, step length and stride length (Foucher, 2016). After THA, there is moderate evidence for increased walking speed at 6 weeks, 3 months and 6 months (Bahl et al., 2018). Postoperatively, notable improvements in gait speed as well as several other gait performance parameters are typically seen by 12 months. Nevertheless, deficits often still exist for speed, step length, stride length and single limb support time (Bahl et al., 2018; Bolink et al., 2016; Mazzoli et al., 2017). Foucher et al. developed a postoperative gait speed goal of 1.34 m/s, which is well above the reported clinically important change of 0.32 m/s (Foucher, 2016). However, a recent meta-analysis observed improvements in gait velocity following surgery that did not meet these values (Bahl et al., 2018), indicating that recovery is multifactorial. This may be explained in part by an association between age and gait speed, with older adults performing at lower levels than younger patients with THA (Bahl et al., 2018; Mazzoli et al., 2017).

Kinematics

The most consistently reported kinematic gait deficit is reduced dynamic hip range of motion (ROM) in the sagittal plane (Foucher, 2016). This deficit is primarily observed as a decrease in peak hip extension prior to push off (Fig. 7.1) when compared with age-matched, healthy controls (Beaulieu et al., 2010; Bennett et al., 2008; Foucher et al., 2007; Perron et al., 2000). Bennett et al. (2008) and Perron et al. (2000) suggested that failure to fully extend the hip during late stance correlated to decreased gait speed. Several additional studies have suggested that this decrease in hip extension may be linked to passive resistance or contractures in the anterior hip structures (e.g., hip flexors) rather than hip extensor weakness (Miki et al., 2004; Nantel et al., 2009; Perron et al., 2000). There is moderate evidence

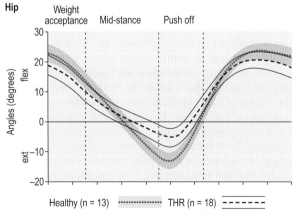

Fig. 7.1 Demonstrating decreased sagittal plane hip range of motion, mostly as a result of decreased hip extension during the late stages of stance. (From Perron et al., 2000.)

for small changes in postoperative sagittal plane hip motion at 6 weeks and moderate increases at 3 months, 6 months and 12 months (Bahl et al., 2018). However, asymmetrical side-to-side differences may still exist beyond 10 months after surgery (Tsai et al., 2015). Foucher suggested a postoperative benchmark increase of 30 degrees for sagittal plane dynamic hip motion, with a clinically important change of 13.3 degrees (Foucher, 2016).

A significant increase in ipsilateral lateral trunk bending has also been observed during single limb support on the operated limb (Nankaku et al., 2007; Perron et al., 2000) along with decreased peak hip adduction angle (Beaulieu et al., 2010; Perron et al., 2000) when compared with age-matched, healthy controls. Both deviations are considered strategies to decrease demand on the hip abductors and stabilise the pelvis in the frontal plane during single limb stance by moving the centre of mass closer to the axis of rotation (i.e., the hip). Beaulieu et al. (2010) suggested that lateral trunk bending may be an attempt to improve balance, however Nankaku et al. (2007) concluded that it may also lead to an increase in energy expenditure.

Kinetics

Preoperatively, people with hip osteoarthritis produce less power in the involved hip than in the uninvolved hip during level walking and stair negotiation. After THA, total power production increases, which may reduce the need for compensatory power production in other joints (Queen et al., 2019). Foucher suggested a postoperative strength goal of ≥4.2%, with an increase of 0.87% being necessary for a clinical improvement to be observed (Foucher, 2016). The most consistently reported kinetic gait deficit is reduced dynamic abductor strength and function when compared to a control group (Foucher, 2016; Beaulieu, et al., 2010). However, it has not yet been confirmed whether hip abductor weakness is due to disuse atrophy from pain avoidance strategies prior to surgery, or the effect of the surgery itself.

A direct anterior surgical approach spares the muscles surrounding the hip while an anterolateral approach detaches the gluteus medius and part of the minimus. A posterior surgical approach avoids the hip abductor muscles, and instead gaining access to the hip joint through the gluteus maximus and external rotators. Two recent systematic reviews compared these surgical techniques. The first review found that patients who underwent the direct anterior approach showed greater gait speed and peak hip flexion 3 months after surgery than patients who underwent the anterior lateral approach. The second review favoured the posterior approach for increased step length and greater frontal plane moments. However, the differences were few and the clinical meaningfulness of the results is unknown, which has led to the conclusion that there is little difference between these surgical approaches (Moyer et al., 2018; Yoo et al., 2019).

Perron et al. (2000) and Miki et al. (2004) observed a decreased internal hip extension moment during loading response, between 0% and 20% of the gait cycle, which correlated to decreases in walking speed. This is consistent with the kinematic findings of decreased hip extension ROM influencing gait speed and suggests that hip extensor strength is an important factor in the return to a normal gait pattern.

Additional Clinical Relevance

In addition to gait analysis, the success of THA surgeries is also measured by patient-reported outcome measures such as the Western Ontario and McMaster Universities Osteoarthritis Index (WOMAC) and the Harris Hip Score (HHS). Studies indicate that there are significant improvements in function in the first 3 months after surgery, with the majority of patients reaching near-maximum or maximum functional scores between 3 and 12 months postoperatively (Bolink et al., 2016; Foucher, 2016). However, up to 25% of patients may have moderate to severe limitations in walking and in other important activities of daily living 2 to 5 years after THA (Brunner and Foucher, 2018). Factors that may predict a less than optimal outcome include a lower preoperative HHS, a decreased peak external rotation moment and higher preoperative sagittal plane hip ROM (Foucher, 2017), with lower performance being expected in older subjects (Mazzoli et al., 2017).

Nantel et al. (2009) suggested that long-term follow-ups at 6 months and 1 year should be performed, with the goal of restoring normal gait patterns. Restoration of normal gait may help prevent falls and reduce the risk of injury in more challenging activities. Early and long-term intervention should focus on alleviating hip flexor tightness and strengthening the hip extensors and abductors.

Key Points

- A large increase in primary THA and THA revisions is expected over the next 10 years.
- The majority of studies indicate that gait improves but does not normalise following THA.
- Rehabilitation should focus on improving spatiotemporal variables such as gait speed and step length; kinematic variables, particularly hip extension ROM; and kinetic variables including hip abduction and extension strength.
- Researchers suggest that more long-term follow-ups are needed to address persistent hip ROM and strength deficits in efforts to normalise gait, decrease stresses on implants and restore overall function.

KNEE OSTEOARTHRITIS

Jim Richards, Frank Tudini, Hannah Shepherd and Gabor Barton

Gait Analysis in Knee Osteoarthritis

The global prevalence of knee osteoarthritis is 22.9% in individuals aged 40 and over, which corresponds to approximately 654 million individuals worldwide (Cui et al., 2020). Osteoarthritis most commonly affects the medial compartment of the knee (van Tunen et al., 2018). This is thought to be related to coronal plane biomechanics, which shows between 60% and 80% of the load acting on the medial compartment during normal gait (Andriacchi, 1994; Baliunas et al., 2002; Hurwitz et al., 2002) and up to 100% of the load acting on the medial compartment in subjects with medial compartment knee osteoarthritis (Schipplein and Andriacchi, 1991). A recent systematic review comparing the kinematics of osteoarthritic and healthy knees observed that the affected knee maintained a more adducted position, especially between 0 and 90 degrees of flexion (Scarvell et al., 2018) (Fig. 7.2). This finding is consistent with the observed association of osteoarthritis with a knee varus deformity, which gives rise to an external adduction moment at the knee throughout the stance phase (Telfer et al., 2017). The knee adduction moment is the product of the ground reaction force passing medial to the knee joint's centre of rotation in the coronal

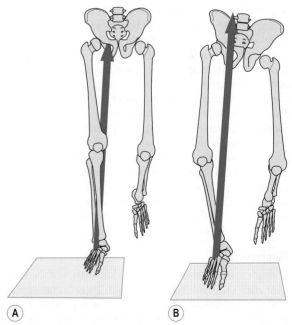

Fig. 7.2 Knee adduction moments in (A) a pain- and pathology-free individual, and (B) an individual with medial compartment knee osteoarthritis.

plane. It is unclear whether the knee starts in a varus position which leads to the adduction moment, which will then exacerbate the varus deformity, or whether the presence of an adduction moment causes the varus deformity. What is clear is the importance of the varus deformity and knee adduction moment in the mechanics of medial compartment knee osteoarthritis (Andriacchi, 1994; Crenshaw et al., 2000; Hurwitz et al., 1998).

Surgical Management

Several surgical approaches are available for managing knee osteoarthritis. These include total knee arthroplasty (TKA), unicompartmental knee arthroplasty (UKA) and high tibial osteotomy (HTO). The aim of these methods is to reduce excessive load on the medial compartment of the knee by correcting varus deformity, thereby reducing pain and improving function.

Total Knee Arthroplasty

The prevalence of TKA in the total US population was 1.52% in 2010. This corresponds to 4.7 million individuals: 3 million females and 1.7 million males (Maradit Kremers et al., 2015). TKA is the primary treatment for symptomatic late-stage osteoarthritis. In the traditional method, the knee prosthesis is aligned mechanically to create a neutral hip-knee-ankle axis, positioning the components perpendicular to the femoral and tibial mechanical axes and attempting to balance the load between the medial and lateral compartments. However, with dissatisfaction rates as high as 25%, other methods such as kinematic alignment are being explored. Kinematic alignment aims to restore the flexion-extension axis of the femoral component to the natural kinematic axis of the individual knee to match the anatomy. At present, kinematic and mechanical alignment have comparable clinical and radiological outcomes up to 96 months postoperatively (Luo et al., 2020; Sappey-Marinier et al., 2020). From a patient perspective, the most important outcomes after TKA are to decrease pain and improve function (Devasenapathy et al., 2019). In the weeks to months of rehabilitation following surgery, patients generally show decreased pain and improved function (Hatfield et al. 2011). Typical outcome measures after a TKA include WOMAC scores and objective measures such as walking velocity.

Kinematics

Multiple systematic reviews on the kinematics of the knee joint after TKA have been performed. There is consistency among the literature that the total (overall) knee ROM is decreased in comparison to controls, with a reduction in knee flexion during loading response (Milner, 2009) (Fig. 7.3). One systematic review found a range of 9.8 to

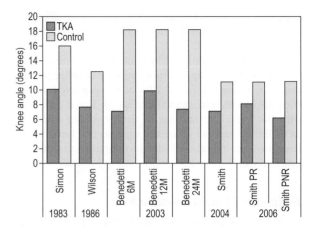

PR = With patellar resurfacing   PNR = Without patellar resurfacing

Fig. 7.3 Knee flexion excursion from footstrike to peak knee flexion during weight acceptance in total knee arthroplasty and control groups across studies. With kind permission from Springer Science and Business Media.

16.0 degrees of knee flexion during the loading response for TKA patients versus 16.0 to 19.7 degrees for controls (Milner, 2009). The same review found absolute differences of 3.0 to 11.2 degrees in ROM between loading response and peak knee flexion during stance. Additionally, TKA patients often demonstrate reduced knee flexion during swing and usually have a greater knee angle at heelstrike (McClelland et al., 2007; Milner, 2009).

Kinetics

Kinetic changes at the knee joint have been measured after TKA, particularly in the sagittal plane. In normal subjects, a biphasic moment pattern occurs during the stance phase of gait. An external moment across the knee, which causes extension, rapidly changes to a flexion moment, and then changes again to extend and then flex the knee towards the end of stance (McClelland et al., 2007). Internal moments are generated by the leg musculature to counteract these external moments. After TKA, this normal biphasic pattern is typically not present (McClelland et al., 2007). Depending on the alignment of the lower limb, a flexion moment or an extension moment may be present throughout the duration of stance. When an external flexion moment is present throughout stance, the quadriceps must generate the internal moment to a greater extent; this is termed a *quadriceps overuse pattern*. When an external extension moment is present throughout stance, there is an absence of quadriceps activity; this is termed a *quadriceps avoidance pattern* (Fig. 7.4). The quadriceps avoidance pattern is clinically important, as the hip or ankle must compensate for the

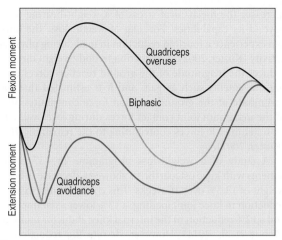

Fig. 7.4 Quadriceps avoidance and overuse patterns (McClellan et al., 2007).

reduced knee extensor moment, and studies have demonstrated that the hip extensor moment is typically increased in TKA patients compared with controls (Mandeville et al., 2007). In addition, the coronal plane often shows a decreased peak knee adduction moment and increased knee adduction angle (Sosdian et al., 2014).

Additional Clinical Relevance

Compared with healthy controls, people with knee osteoarthritis generally have lower muscle strength, longer sit-to-stand times, higher knee adduction moments, proprioception deficits and a higher fall risk (Sonoo et al., 2019; van Tunen et al., 2018). Poor preoperative function and decreased quadriceps strength are also common and may result in suboptimal outcomes (Devasenapathy et al., 2019). This has caused some clinicians to advocate for prehabilitation before surgery, which has been reported to result in increased motion, improved quadriceps strength and decreased length of stay after surgery (Moyer et al., 2017). Quadriceps strength has been correlated with functional performance at both 3 and 12 months postoperatively. Yoshida et al. (2008) found that improved quadriceps strength resulted in significantly faster times in the timed up and go test, stair-climbing test and 6-minute walk test.

Exercise interventions after surgery should focus on improving pain, physical function, stiffness, knee extension strength, active knee flexion ROM, gait speed, balance, proprioception and fall risk (Bragonzoni et al., 2019; di Laura Frattura et al., 2018; Umehara and Tanaka, 2018). However, another aim of exercise interventions should be to improve knee extension ROM which has been shown to improve knee extensor performance and function (Pua et al., 2013). The available extension ROM is a determinant of limb dominance during stance and walking. Harato et al. (2010) compared weight-bearing strategies of individuals with a diagnosis of bilateral arthritis who had undergone unilateral TKA. Their findings suggest that patients who have sufficient extension ROM during the stance phase utilise the operated lower extremity as the dominant side, and that patients with decreased extension ROM bear more weight on the contralateral limb, which could increase its rate of degeneration (Harato et al., 2010).

High Tibial Osteotomy and Unicompartmental Knee Arthroplasty

Uncertainty exists with regards to surgery versus non-surgical management for patients with moderate knee osteoarthritis (Palmer et al., 2019). In symptomatic knees, especially those that have failed nonsurgical management, surgical options include high tibial osteotomy (HTO) and unicompartmental knee arthroplasty (UKA). HTO is a surgical procedure used to alter the bony alignment and reduce the varus angle of the knee joint while causing minimal damage to the soft tissue and minimally affecting knee stability. The aim of an HTO is to evenly distribute the load between the medial and lateral compartments of the knee. There are two main types of osteotomy for knee osteoarthritis: an opening wedge and a closing wedge. In an opening wedge, a cut is made in the tibia and the two sides are separated; the wedge-shaped space is then filled with a bone graft. In a closing wedge, two cuts are made and a wedge-shaped piece of bone is removed; the two edges are then brought together, creating the desired change in angle. Both types of operation require the bone to be fixed, usually with a plate and screws. Fig. 7.5 shows an example of how an HTO was successful in reducing the external adduction moment and changing the varus alignment at the knee from 11 degrees to 1.5 degrees.

One systematic review and meta-analysis found that patients undergoing HTO had high rates of return to sport (75.7%) and work (80.8%) with low complication rates regardless of the technique used. One drawback to HTO is that there is a higher risk of revision to TKA (Chen et al., 2020). If a revision is needed, the 10-year survival rates, outcome measure scores, extension angle and radiographic results are similar to those who undergo primary TKA. However, there is a longer operative time, higher infection rate and poorer flexion angle (Sun et al., 2020). Current consensus is that HTO can be considered an alternate to TKA for younger patients with knee osteoarthritis (He et al., 2021).

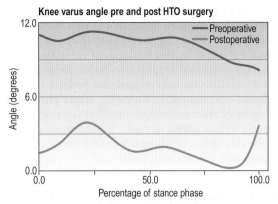

Fig. 7.5 Pre- and post-high tibial osteotomy.

A second option is the UKA or partial knee replacement, which resurfaces the cartilage of only the damaged compartment (usually medial). While there appear to be no significant differences in vertical ground reaction force or overall kinematics in the sagittal plane between UKA patients and healthy controls during level walking, the UKA group has a slower walking speed, slower cadence and shorter stride length (Kim et al., 2018). In comparing UKA outcomes to TKA outcomes, there are no significant differences in overall kinematics or walking speed during level walking, and UKA may result in a longer stride length (Nha et al., 2018). Additionally, with the UKA procedure, more bone mass is retained and cutting the cruciate ligament is not necessary. However, in UKA the joint may wear unevenly and there is an increased risk of revision (He et al., 2021).

In comparing UKA with HTO, a recent systematic review and meta-analysis found that both techniques showed satisfactory functional results. UKA has fewer complications and revisions compared with HTO. However, HTO achieved superior ROM and may be suitable for patients with high activity requirements (Cao et al., 2018). Another systematic review showed that those who underwent HTO were more physically active compared to those who underwent UKA, but that the UKA patients experienced a greater increase in physical activity levels overall compared to the HTO patients (Belsey et al., 2021).

Nonsurgical Management of Knee Osteoarthritis

Nonsurgical management of knee osteoarthritis includes weight loss, manual therapy, exercise and muscle strengthening, patient education, bracing (orthotics), gait retraining and pharmacological interventions.

Weight Loss

Obesity is widely acknowledged as one of the risk factors for the onset of knee osteoarthritis (Lau et al., 2000). Obesity increases the mechanical stress of a weight-bearing joint beyond its capabilities. For 1 kg of weight loss, the knee can experience a fourfold reduction in load during physical activity (Kuster, 2002). A reduction in body weight directly reduces the magnitude of the ground reaction forces during movements such as gait, and it is estimated that the magnitude of the ground reaction force contributes 30% of the maximum joint contact forces during level walking, with net muscle forces contributing to the remaining 70% (Kuster, 2002).

A study of a weight-loss programme in 157 obese patients with knee osteoarthritis showed a decrease in body weight of 13.5% over 16 weeks. This corresponded to a 7% reduction in knee joint loading, a 13% lower axial impulse, and a 12% reduction in the internal knee abductor moment (Aaboe et al., 2011). However, despite the reduction in loading, more recent studies have shown that weight loss causes only small to moderate improvements in pain and disability for those with osteoarthritis compared to minimal care (Robson et al., 2020).

Manual Therapy and Exercise Interventions

Manual therapy including soft tissue mobilisation, joint mobilisation and massage may be beneficial in reducing pain and stiffness, and can improve physical function in those with knee osteoarthritis (Xu et al., 2017). These techniques are commonly performed to reduce symptoms or improve mobility before exercising, which is the mainstay of rehabilitation. Participating in exercise programmes may improve physical function, decrease pain and impact psychosocial domains such as depression while improving self-efficacy and social function (Bartholdy et al., 2017). Providing advice and reassurance about how exercise can aide in controlling symptoms may improve patient adherence (Hurley et al., 2018). Despite the benefits of an overall exercise program, a systematic review that specifically analysed strengthening found that after training, strength was improved but there was not a significant impact on pain or disability.

Bracing and Foot Orthotics

Bracing and shoe inserts are also commonly used for patients with knee osteoarthritis and can influence the external forces applied to the knee, either by directly applying a system of forces or indirectly changing the line of action of the ground reaction force. The aims of knee valgus braces are to unload the painful compartment, through bending moments applied proximally and distally to the knee joint, and to reduce the varus deformity (Pollo, 1998). Bracing has been shown to reduce the degree of varus deformity by 3 degrees and reduce the knee adduction moment by 14.5%, providing significant pain relief (Jones et al., 2013). While valgus offloader bracing is an effective treatment for improving pain secondary to medial compartment knee osteoarthritis, effectiveness with regard to functional outcomes and stiffness is less clear (Gohal et al., 2018). Soft bracing does not have the biomechanical effects that valgus offloader bracing provides, but it has been shown to have moderate effects on pain and small to moderate effects on self-reported physical function in patients with knee osteoarthritis (Cudejko et al., 2018). Lateral wedge foot orthotics have also been used to impact the biomechanics of the knee by placing an insole with a thicker lateral border under the heel. This applies a valgus moment to the heel, attempting to move it into an everted position. Lateral wedge insoles have been shown to reduce knee adduction angles and external moments, however the impact on pain and function is less clear (Shaw et al., 2018; Zafar et al., 2020).

Gait Modification

Gait modification interventions are often considered a noninvasive solution which has the potential to reduce the risk of disease onset, delay the progression of disease and reduce pain. Gait modifications aim to retrain gait by subtly altering kinematics and optimising movement function in both neurological and musculoskeletal conditions. Gait modification interventions are not a new concept, and a systematic review identified and discussed 14 different gait modifications to reduce the frontal plane knee moment in knee osteoarthritis (Simic et al., 2011).

Gait modifications are a combination of complex but subtle kinematic changes, which may also have effects on the moments in the sagittal and transverse planes (Walter et al., 2010; Erhart-Hledik et al., 2015). Most importantly, a decrease in the frontal plane during a modified gait pattern may be at the expense of an increase in the sagittal and transverse planes, or even at adjacent joints. These considerations question the sole use of the frontal plane moment peaks and suggests that the net sum of all three knee-loading moments acting upon the joint during gait should be considered as a more robust outcome measure.

There are two ways to present feedback to train a gait modification. Indirect feedback provides information about the kinematic strategies that are understood to modify knee loading; that is, lateral trunk sway (implicit instructions). Direct feedback provides information on the specific parameter that is being modified, or the knee loading outcome measure (explicit instructions). Typically, in osteoarthritis research, indirect feedback is presented to the participants, but this have resulted in inconsistent findings. When presented with two modifications, lateral trunk sway and medial knee thrust, Gerbrands and colleagues (2017) found that optimal strategies differ among knee osteoarthritis patients. Not only does indirect feedback require prior knowledge and evidence of specific

kinematic movements that influence joint moment, but additionally prescribing a specific kinematic strategy may not be as well received by patients. Large variations in individual responses to multiple prescribed gait modifications have been shown in unimpaired adults who do not have any current movement constraints that would limit their ability to perform each modification (Lindsey et al., 2021). These large variations in response may be further amplified within patient populations when there are heterogeneous samples, current gait compensations, perceived effort and additional movement constraints due to pain, which may cause an inability to perform a particular avoidance strategy. To overcome these issues, direct feedback can be utilised, where patients are encouraged to create their own gait modification using direct feedback of the desired outcome measure. Not only has direct feedback tended to yield a higher reduction in knee moment parameters than indirect instructions (Barrios et al., 2010; Hunt et al., 2011; Shull et al., 2011), but it promotes a patient-specific individualised response with the potential to improve the desired outcome as well as patient adherence. Advancements in the technology of movement feedback devices which can aid home-based learning interventions are continuous. Monitoring gait interventions during daily living would provide a wealth of longitudinal data to understand the adherence to gait modification programs and the impact of these programmes on clinical measures and disease progression.

Key Points

- The prevalence of TKA surgery is expected to increase dramatically.
- TKA is an effective treatment for late-stage symptomatic knee osteoarthritis.
- HTO and UKA are both effective for moderate symptomatic unicompartmental knee osteoarthritis.
- Both nonsurgical and surgical procedures can affect anatomical realignment and cause a reduction in the knee adduction moment, leading to pain reduction.
- Participating in exercise programmes may improve physical function, decrease pain and impact psychosocial domains.
- Gait retraining using direct feedback may improve knee mechanics and clinical outcomes.

PROSTHETIC GAIT

Natalie Vanicek and Cleveland Barnett

Lower Limb Amputation and Prosthetic Components

An amputation is the surgical removal of a body extremity and results in the loss of part of a limb or the entire limb, its associated skeletal structures, muscle function and proprioception. Most amputations occur in the lower limbs, and at various levels: above the knee (transfemoral), through the knee, below the knee (transtibial), ankle disarticulation (Syme's disease) or partial foot (forefoot/toe) amputation. Most amputations are unilateral (one sided), with bilateral (two-sided) amputations being less common. In developed countries, diabetes mellitus and peripheral vascular disease are the main causes of lower limb amputation. Other, less common causes include trauma, infection and cancer. The level of discomfort and physical adaptation a person experiences following amputation varies, according to both internal factors (level of amputation, muscle strength) and external factors (prosthetic components, suspension type).

People with a lower limb amputation can often learn to walk safely and comfortably using a prosthesis. A prosthesis typically consists of a socket which is suspended securely from the residual limb, a 'knee' component (for through-knee amputations and above), a pylon component and a prosthetic ankle-foot component. Prosthetic knees and ankle-feet range from basic passive to bionic systems. Different commercially available prosthetic ankle-feet vary in the amount of energy that is stored and then returned during the stance phase of the gait cycle. Prosthetic knee components are designed to enhance stance phase stability and, in more advanced systems, aid in stumble recovery. Special prostheses also exist for specific activities; for example, running blades designed for sprinting. Pylon components are usually rigid cylinders but can also include longitudinal and rotational shock absorption. Typically, prosthetic suspension is achieved through belts, sleeves or suction/vacuum methods. Osseointegration is a suspension method where the prosthesis is directly anchored into weight-bearing bone eliminating socket-related and is more commonly used in people with a non-vascular-related amputation and upper extremity amputations.

Prosthetic Rehabilitation

Following lower limb amputation, a person will first practise walking and weight bearing using an early walking aid (EWA). An EWA can be used as early as 1 week postoperatively and has benefits such as reduced oedema, faster healing of the residual limb and less time between surgery and casting for the functional prosthesis (Redhead et al., 1978; Scott et al., 2000). EWAs differ according to the level of amputation and, for people with transtibial amputation, movement at the knee joint (articulated versus nonarticulated). Research has shown that, for people with a transtibial amputation, there are no clear, long-term benefits of walking with either an EWA that allows flexion and extension at the knee joint, such as Ortho Europe's Amputee Mobility Aid (AMA), or an EWA that maintains the biological knee joint in extension, such as Ortho Europe's Pneumatic Post Amputation Mobility (PPAM) aid. At discharge from rehabilitation, people using either the AMA or the PPAM had improved walking performance, with walking speeds of approximately 0.71 m/s, and did not show any differences in temporal-spatial or kinematic variables despite very different gait patterns with the EWAs during early rehabilitation (Barnett et al., 2009). A similar process is used for people following transfemoral amputation who use Ortho Europe's Femurett EWA.

Temporal-Spatial Parameters

Prosthesis users exhibit modified gait patterns and, in the case of unilateral amputation, often show asymmetrical profiles between the intact and affected limbs. Individuals with a lower limb amputation walk slower than age-matched, able-bodied people and expend more metabolic energy per unit distance walked (Waters and Mulroy, 1999). People with a transfemoral amputation often walk slower (0.78 to 0.96 m·s^{-1}) (Highsmith et al., 2010; Shirota et al., 2015) than people with a transtibial amputation (1.07 to 1.15 m·s^{-1}) (De Asha and Buckley, 2015; Vanicek et al., 2009; Wong et al., 2015). People who have a nontraumatic amputation tend to walk slower than those whose amputation was related to trauma, who are also often younger. The amount of energy expenditure differs according to the level of amputation, as well as the mass, alignment and inertial properties of the prosthesis. People with a unilateral amputation spend less time bearing weight on their prosthesis, causing a reduced stance phase compared with their intact limb. They also take longer steps with the affected limb than the intact limb.

Kinematics

People with a transtibial amputation have reduced joint ROM. The shape of the commonly used patellar tendon bearing (PTB) socket may limit joint mobility at the knee, particularly knee flexion, when performing more complex tasks such as stair ascent and descent. People with transtibial and transfemoral amputations do not typically exhibit ankle plantarflexion during the transition from terminal double support to swing. This is due to the prosthetic ankle-foot not allowing for active plantarflexion. Without the necessary energy generation for push off, muscles proximal to the site of the amputation must compensate for inadequate ankle joint function. These compensations are usually provided by the hip musculature. The muscles surrounding the knee joint are relatively unaffected in people with transtibial amputation, with the exception of gastrocnemius, however, kinematic adaptations still occur.

Some studies have shown that individuals with a transtibial amputation lack normal stance phase knee flexion (Powers et al., 1998; Sanderson and Martin, 1997). This could be due in part to weakness in the knee extensor muscles, which are required to contract eccentrically during this phase of the gait cycle, or to feelings of instability, which could result in a fall. The knee extensors often exhibit significant atrophy as a result of disuse and weakness. Maintaining the knee in a relatively extended position facilitates greater stability during the transition from initial double support to single support on the affected limb. The hip joint kinematics typically fall within normal ranges, although hip extension in pre-swing may be reduced. This adaptation could be related to slower walking speeds, reduced step length, greater anterior pelvic tilt, hip flexor contractures or a combination of these factors.

Kinetics

Examining the ground reaction force profiles, joint moments and powers of people with lower limb amputation could reveal internal adaptations that occur as a result of amputation. Propulsive forces and impulses for the affected limb are reduced, and this is related to the absence of the power-generating plantarflexor muscles, while the braking force and impulse are not too dissimilar to the intact limb during level walking. Vertical ground reaction force peaks on the affected side are flattened and reduced in magnitude, and may not show the typical 'double hump' profile seen in able-bodied participants. This could be due in part to slower walking speeds, but also an attempt to reduce loading on the residual limb/socket interface.

Internal joint moment and power profiles illustrate some compensatory adaptations related to the loss of musculature at either the transtibial or transfemoral level. Fig. 7.6 shows the sagittal plane hip, knee and ankle angles (A), joint moments (B) and joint powers (C) of the prosthetic limb of eight participants whilst walking. The participants had undergone a transfemoral amputation and were fitted with a prosthetic knee: either the C-Leg (a microprocessor-controlled knee) or the Mauch SNS (a non-microprocessor-controlled knee). The hip plays an important role during pre-swing when the hip flexor muscles contract concentrically to ensure adequate foot clearance in the absence of active ankle plantarflexion. This is seen by a larger hip flexor moment and power generation burst (labelled H3) on the prosthetic side compared with able-bodied subjects. The knee joint moments and powers during stance on the prosthetic side are typically very low or approach zero. By keeping the prosthetic knee in a more extended position, the moment arm between the knee joint and the ground reaction force vector is relatively short, resulting in small knee joint moments and hence joint powers. Ankle joint moment and power profiles are arguably the most affected joint kinetic parameters because of the mechanical limitations of the prosthetic ankle-foot. Without active

plantarflexion of the prosthetic ankle, and with inadequate power generation from the absent plantarflexor musculature, the ankle moment of the affected limb is substantially reduced. A small power absorption burst by the prosthesis (A1) is usually obvious, and this has been attributed to the prosthetic ankle-foot absorbing energy as it deforms in dorsiflexion in mid- to terminal stance. This may be a desired function of the prosthetic ankle-foot, providing energy storage and return. Depending on the mechanical energy return, the ankle power generation burst in pre-swing (A2) is minimal, but this will depend on the exact type of ankle-foot component.

Compared with able-bodied individuals, people with a lower limb amputation display modified gait profiles but can learn to walk proficiently and safely with their prosthesis. Technological advances are focused on developing and improving prosthetic components and fit to facilitate a more natural and comfortable walking pattern. Other recent research is aimed at improving gait biomechanics and balance and reducing the propensity to falling, with personalised exercise programmes demonstrating longer-term efficacy (Schafer and Vanicek, 2021; Schafer et al., 2018).

Movement Patterns During Activities of Daily Living

When encountering more challenging terrain, such as walking up and down inclined surfaces, as well as negotiating stairs, people with a lower limb amputation must make additional adaptations to their gait. When walking on an incline, there is greater instability in stance phase on the prosthetic side, as evidenced by shorter single support time and reduced ground reaction forces (Vickers et al., 2008). People with a transtibial amputation may demonstrate increased knee flexion on the affected limb: during uphill walking, this occurs following initial contact, but during downhill walking, it can be observed during late stance to early swing. However, people with a transfemoral amputation are often unable to flex the knee more during swing on the affected side, especially when using a non-microprocessor-controlled knee component, and compensations will likely occur at the ipsilateral hip. When walking downhill, it is common to see prosthesis users shorten their step length to facilitate positioning the foot and managing the height difference more comfortably. They also maintain the knee on the affected side in a more extended position during loading and stance (Vrieling et al., 2008).

Walking on stairs is more mechanically demanding than level walking, and stumbles and falls are more likely to occur on stairs; this is exacerbated for prosthesis users. People with a lower limb amputation tend to negotiate stairs at a significantly slower pace. They rely more

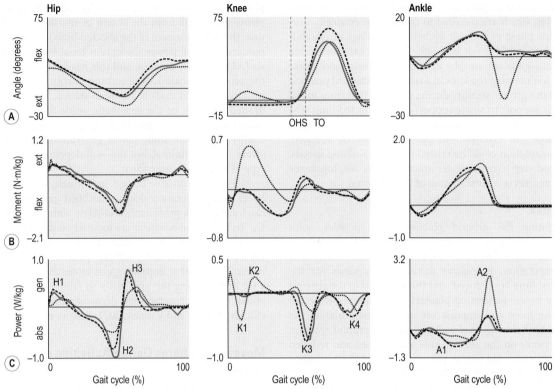

Fig. 7.6 Kinematics and kinetics of prosthetic limb for subjects wearing C-Leg *(solid line)* versus Mauch SNS *(dashed line)* versus control group *(dotted line)* (Adapted from Segal et al., 2006). For all subjects and trials, average (A) angle curves, (B) moment curves and (C) power curves are shown for hip, knee and ankle for a controlled walking speed (1.11 ± 0.1 m/s). H1 = peak sagittal-plane hip power in early stance (+) H2 = peak sagittal-plane hip power in mid-stance (–) H3 = peak sagittal-plane hip power in late stance (+) K1 = peak sagittal-plane knee power in early stance (–) K2 = peak sagittal-plane knee power in mid-stance (+) K3 = peak sagittal-plane knee power in late stance (–) K4 = peak sagittal-plane knee power in late swing (–) A1 = peak sagittal-plane ankle power in early stance (–) A2 = peak sagittal-plane ankle power in late stance (+) OHS = opposite heelstrike; TO = toe off. Positive (+) indicates power produced; negative (–) indicates power absorbed.

on handrails for support to unload the lower limbs, and they often present with alternate strategies such as using a 'step-to' rather than reciprocal 'step-over-step' pattern, especially during stair descent. During rehabilitation, prosthesis users are usually advised to lead with the stronger intact limb during stair ascent, but with the affected limb during descent. During the 'pull-up' phase of stair ascent, the knee normally generates energy to elevate the body (McFadyen and Winter, 1988). Weakness or absence of the knee extensors on the affected side means the task demands are usually met by the ipsilateral hip extensor muscles. During descent, the prosthetic ankle-foot cannot actively plantarflex to make initial contact with the forefoot. Therefore, prosthesis users will make contact with their heel or mid-foot, maintaining the knee on the affected limb in an extended position. The controlled lowering phase, a vulnerable time in the stance phase when the knee must flex to lower the body downwards, usually using eccentric activation of the knee extensors, can be avoided on the affected side by leading with the affected limb, maintaining knee extension and using a safer 'step-to' strategy (Vanicek et al., 2015).

Walking safety can be enhanced, even in more difficult environments, through targeted and ongoing strengthening of lower limb muscles in the intact and affected limbs, especially at the hip and knee. Improving the availability of functionally advanced prosthetic componentry, such as hydraulic and microprocessor-controlled components, could aid stability for many prosthesis users. Other strategies include the use of walking aids and/or hand or grab rails, adequate light for important visual feedback and adopting alternate safe movement strategies as required.

Measuring Prosthetic Gait

When performing gait analysis in people with lower limb amputation, some specific biomechanical considerations should be made. Principally, these considerations relate to the assumption of rigidity of segments. Violation of this assumption occurs at the suspension interface of the prosthetic device and residual limb, and in prosthetic components that are designed specifically to articulate and deform. This is problematic for more advanced biomechanical analyses, such as calculating joint moments and powers. However, methods have been developed to enable these analyses whilst accounting for the specific characteristics of prosthetic components (Takahashi et al., 2012). An increasing number of studies are incorporating activity monitoring to assess free-living behaviour in people with limb loss. For example, activity monitors have shown that the number of steps taken by people with a transfemoral amputation relates closely to their functional classification. Over 12 months, these authors found the average daily steps ranged from approximately 1150 to 2560 for the groups with the lowest and highest mobility classifications, respectively (Halsne et al., 2013). Another study found adults over 50 years of age with a transtibial, vascular-related amputation took on average, fewer than 1800 steps per day over 30 minutes throughout the day, describing the largely sedentary behaviour experienced by this group (Vanicek et al., 2021).

Key Points

- Compared with able-bodied individuals, people with a lower limb amputation display modified gait profiles but can learn to walk proficiently and safely with their prosthesis.
- Technological advances are focused on developing and improving prosthetic components and fit to facilitate a more natural and comfortable walking pattern.
- Recent research has focused on improving functional performance and reducing the propensity to falling, especially among older people with a vascular-related amputation.
- More challenging activities of daily living, such as incline and stair walking, require more complex compensatory gait patterns and possibly 'safer' strategies.

ORTHOTIC MANAGEMENT

Jim Richards, June Hanks and Ashley Schilling

Lower extremity orthoses include external braces and shoe inserts which are used to reduce the primary impairment, prevent secondary impairments and improve gait and performance of activities of daily living (Aboutorabi et al., 2017; Caliskan Uckun et al., 2014). These devices affect the biomechanics of the lower limb and foot by controlling alignment or providing support. While orthoses can be constructed of leather, metal and thermosetting materials, the majority of modern lower limb orthotics are made of lightweight thermoplastic or carbon fibre composite materials of varying designs, which are provided depending on the patient's biomechanical needs.

Foot Orthoses

Foot orthoses are shaped or moulded inserts for the shoe, which aim to:

- hold the foot in position,
- change the foot position,
- offload a part of the foot,
- change the ROM of either the whole foot or between the different segments of the foot, and
- change the line of action of the ground reaction force.

Foot orthoses and shock-absorbing insoles are commonly used for the prevention and management of many musculoskeletal disorders of the lower extremity. Foot orthoses can have direct effects on the segments of the foot, along with significant clinical effects indirectly much farther up the body to the pelvis and lower back, and arguably as far up as the shoulders and neck. Foot orthoses are available in many shapes and forms. Basic forms consist of simple ethyl vinyl acetate (EVA) wedges. Some are premade contoured devices which may or may not need modification to adequately address the patient's needs. Classification systems used to describe shoe inserts vary from a description of the properties of the materials used (i.e., soft, semirigid or rigid), to the type of procedure used to construct the appliance (i.e., moulded or non-moulded). The nature of each individual's muscle and joint function dictates which would be the most effective in achieving the desired outcomes.

Although the specific mechanisms are not completely clear, foot orthoses have been shown to alter plantar pressure distribution, sensory feedback, muscle activity and kinematics of the lower limb during standing, walking and running. Shock-absorbing insoles have a relatively flat profile. They are made from soft materials and are predominantly used to reduce impact forces. Full-length (Vanicek et al., 2015) foot orthoses are effective in relieving plantar fasciitis–related pain, especially when combined with tape and use of night stretching splints (Schuitema et al., 2019). Foot orthoses and AFOs may also help limit deformity progression in conditions such as posterior tibiailis insufficiency (Soliman et al., 2019).

The foot is an extremely complex system of articulating segments. Therefore, the movements of the foot and ankle cannot be completely explained by rotations about a single plane, but by a combination of movements in all three planes. This complexity makes biomechanical assessment of the foot and the action of foot orthoses exceptionally challenging. Advancements in technology allowing analysis beyond a single segment continue to inform our understanding of foot function and the effects of foot orthotic management.

Ankle Foot Orthoses

Ankle foot orthoses (AFOs) encompass much of the lower leg and foot and can be prefabricated (off-the-shelf) devices, custom devices to fit the patient with preshaped 'blanks' or component parts adapted as needed, or individually custom moulded to fit a patient's limb. Although no standardised description of AFOs exists, designs include rigid, posterior leaf spring, hinged, spiral, ground reaction and supramalleolar AFOs. Table 7.1 describes primary indications and special considerations regarding the different designs.

Rigid AFOs aim to block movement about the ankle joint and foot in all planes (Totah et al., 2018; Abe et al., 2009). These are usually made from moulded plastic and extend up the back of the leg and under the entire length of the foot or to the metatarsophalangeal joint. Rigid AFOs are designed to support a dorsiflexion moment produced by the ground reaction force about the ankle by providing a posteriorly directed force on the anterior tibial strap, which prevents or controls tibial movement over the foot. In this way, the stiffness of the rigid ankle foot orthosis produces a plantarflexion moment that opposes the moment about the ankle from the ground reaction force. Rigid AFOs can be used to resist knee flexion by setting the leg/foot angle into slight plantarflexion. However, excessive knee flexion may require a knee-ankle-foot orthosis (KAFO) to provide more direct control. A rocker sole may be added to the shoe to aid the progression of the body over the stance limb by assisting forward tibia movement over the foot. This design also reduces eccentric work required by the ankle plantarflexors.

TABLE 7.1	**Types of ankle-foot orthoses**	
Type	**Characteristic**	**Primary indication**
Rigid	Limits/blocks sagittal, coronal and transverse plane movement	• Weak/absent ankle dorsiflexors and plantarflexors • Severe spasticity causing foot equinovarus during swing and stance • Weak knee extensors • Proprioceptive sensory loss
Posterior leaf spring	Assists dorsiflexion in swing phase and provides inversion/eversion stability in stance phase	• Weak or absence of active dorsiflexion with good pronation/supination stability • Requires neutral dorsiflexion range of motion at midstance
Hinged	Allows free sagittal plane movement with restricted coronal and transverse plane movement; can limit sagittal plane movement with joint 'stops' as needed	• Weak medial/lateral ankle stabilisers
Spiral	Controls sagittal, coronal and transverse plane movement	• Motor weakness affecting all compartments of the ankle-foot complex which may be flaccid or mild to moderately spastic • Medial-lateral instability during stance or swing phase • Slightly diminished motor power at the knee in addition to motor weakness at the ankle • Loss of ankle proprioception
Ground reaction	Maintains ground reaction force in front of knee joint centre	• Weakness of quadriceps or plantarflexors
Supramalleolar	Provides stability and improves alignment of the foot	• Pronation; foot malalignment

Posterior leaf spring AFOs, also known as flexible plastic shell orthoses, provide dorsiflexion assistance during the swing phase, while giving some stability for inversion/eversion of the ankle joint during the stance phase. Posterior leaf spring AFOs are usually too flexible to give support in the transverse plane, although this will in part depend on the *trim lines*, or the width and thickness of the material of the leaf spring (Fig. 7.7). The thickness of the trim lines must be balanced between the need to provide dorsiflexion assistance during the swing phase to prevent foot drop, whilst supporting the weight of the foot and/or resisting spastic activity of the ankle plantarflexors. A wider trim line may be needed to resist eccentric action of the plantarflexors during the stance phase, providing greater resistance to dorsiflexion movement and therefore improving the control of the movement over the stance limb. Posterior leaf spring AFOs require good knee stability, dorsiflexion ROM to neutral at midstance and an absence of significant foot varus or valgus and spasticity.

The hinged ankle foot orthosis, which can be constructed with an unrestricted or an assisted joint, is designed to permit movement of the ankle in plantarflexion and dorsiflexion whilst aiming to block pronation/supination and inversion/eversion movement in the ankle. If sagittal plane movement control is needed, plantarflexion and/or dorsiflexion stops may be added to the joint, setting an available ROM which is matched to the degree of control needed. A dorsiflexion stop may be set to limit tibial progression over the foot, and consequently knee collapse into flexion, whilst still allowing a degree of movement of the tibia forwards over the foot (Balaban et al., 2007). Hinged ankle foot orthosis designs use either metal or plastic hinges, with metal hinges providing greater rigidity to prevent coronal and transverse plane movement, while plastic hinges allow a lower profile and better fit inside a shoe (Daryabor et al., 2018) (Fig. 7.8).

Spiral AFOs provide controlled motion in the sagittal, coronal and transverse planes. The strut can originate from either the medial or lateral side of the footplate, and then passes posteriorly around the leg and terminates at the level of the medial tibial condyle. The design of spiral AFOs avoids the need for metal hinges by unwinding during weight-bearing to permit plantarflexion and rewinding during unloading to dorsiflex the foot.

Additional types of orthoses commonly used in pediatric populations include ground reaction and supramalleolar AFOs. Ground reaction AFOs pass from the front of the knee to the ankle to maintain the ground reaction force anterior to the knee joint centre in weight-bearing. The extension moment at the knee and limitation of excessive dorsiflexion contribute to knee joint stability and maintain hamstring length, thereby limiting knee flexion (crouched gait) during stance. Supramalleolar AFOs support the arches of the foot while maintaining a neutral heel, thus preventing excessive pronation. These are typically smaller than other types of AFOs and are generally well tolerated by users.

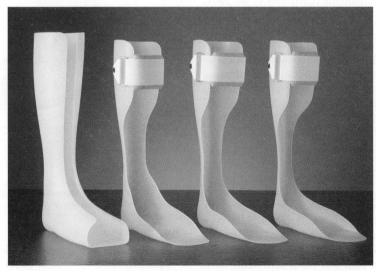

Fig. 7.7 Otto Bock moulded plastic ankle foot orthoses. Far left: rigid; middle: alternative trim lines; far right: posterior leaf spring.

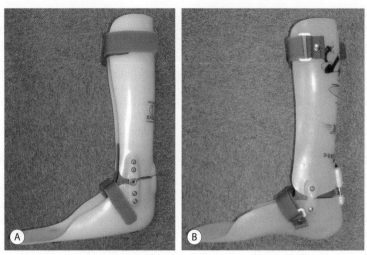

Fig. 7.8 (A) Metal-hinged ankle foot orthoses; (B) Plastic-hinged ankle foot orthoses.

Orthotic Walkers

Orthotic walkers, or walker boots, and total contact casts are frequently used in clinical practice to manage various pathologies and injuries including diabetes and ankle fractures. Orthotic walkers (Fig. 7.9) allow early weight-bearing while providing protection and immobilisation to the foot and ankle. The use of orthotic walkers has been shown to afford better clinical outcomes in terms of ankle function, bone strength and faster bone healing, with individuals showing improved quality of life. Several studies have explored the use of orthotic walkers and their effect on plantar pressure distributions (Crenshaw et al., 2004) and, more recently, on knee and hip function during gait (Richards et al., 2016). The effect of immobilising the ankle tends to slightly increase knee flexion and hip extension angles during midstance, but more notably increases knee extension moments and reductions in hip extension moments. Although the various designs of such devices look similar, differences in the knee and hip angles and moments exist among the different designs, which may be attributed to subtle differences in the rocker profile of the sole and tibial inclination angles.

Knee-Ankle-Foot Orthoses

Knee-ankle-foot orthoses (KAFOs) combine the benefits of ankle-foot orthoses and knee orthoses. They are generally used when larger moments are required to control the knee and when there is a substantial lack of control and stability of the ankle and knee joints. The KAFO may be constructed with leather straps and pads and metal side struts, or it could be plastic, with metal hinges forming the articulating sections (Fig 7.10). KAFOs are most often used in spinal

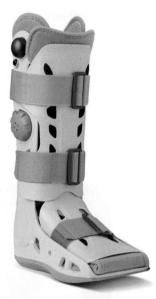

Fig. 7.9 Aircast AirSelect Elite Orthotic Walker (DJO, LLC).

cord injury, myelomeningocele, spinal muscle atrophy, muscular dystrophy, multiple sclerosis and poliomyelitis.

Key Points

- Different configurations of ankle-foot orthoses can be used to block movement about the ankle joint, assist with muscle function present or allow free movement within 'safe' limits.

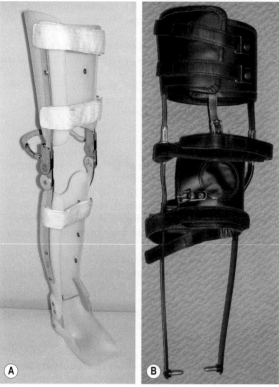

Fig. 7.10 Knee-ankle-foot orthoses (KAFO): (A) cosmetic KAFO; (B) conventional KAFO.

- The use of ankle-foot orthoses can have clinical effects at the ankle, knee, hip and pelvis.
- Foot orthoses can have a direct effect on foot and ankle movement and ground reaction forces, and a clinically significant effect on the control and function of the knee, hip and pelvis.
- The nature of each individual's muscle and joint function dictates which would be the most effective form of orthotic management.

REFERENCES

Aaboe, J., Bliddal, H., Messier, S.P., et al., 2011. Effects of an intensive weight loss program on knee joint loading in obese adults with knee osteoarthritis. Osteoarthritis Cartilage 19 (7), 822–828.

Abe, H., Michimata, A., Sugawara, K., et al., 2009. Improving gait stability in stroke hemiplegic patients with a plastic ankle-foot orthosis. Tohoku J. Exp. Med. 218 (3), 193–199.

Aboutorabi, A., Arazpour, M., Ahmadi Bani, M., et al., 2017. Efficacy of ankle foot orthoses types on walking in children with cerebral palsy: a systematic review. Ann. Phys. Rehabil. Med. 60 (6), 393–402.

Andriacchi, T.P., 1994. Dynamics of knee malalignment. Orthop. Clin. North Am. 25, 395–403.

Bahl, J.S., Nelson, M.J., Taylor, M., et al., 2018. Biomechanical changes and recovery of gait function after total hip arthroplasty for osteoarthritis: a systematic review and meta-analysis. Osteoarthritis and Cartilage 26 (7), 847–863.

Balaban, B.B., Yasar, E., Dal, U., et al., 2007. The effect of hinged ankle-foot orthosis on gait and energy expenditure in spastic hemiplegic cerebral palsy. Disabil. Rehabil. 29 (2), 139–144.

Baliunas, A.J., Hurwitz, D.E., Ryals, A.B., et al., 2002. Increased knee joint loads during walking are present in subjects with knee osteoarthritis. Osteoarthritis Cartilage 10, 573–579.

Barnett, C., Vanicek, N., Polman, R., et al., 2009. Kinematic gait adaptations in unilateral transtibial amputees during rehabilitation. Prosthet. Orthot. Int. 33, 141–153..

Barrios, J.A., Crossley, K.M., Davis, I.S., 2010. Gait retraining to reduce the knee adduction moment through real-time visual feedback of dynamic knee alignment. J. Biomech. 43 (11), 2208–2213.

Bartholdy, C., Juhl, C., Christensen, R., et al., 2017. The role of muscle strengthening in exercise therapy for knee osteoarthritis: a systematic review and meta-regression analysis of randomized trials. Semin. Arthritis Rheum. 47 (1), 9–21.

Beaulieu, M.L., Lamontagne, M., Beaule, P.E., 2010. Lower limb biomechanics during gait do not return to normal following total hip arthroplasty. Gait Posture 32, 269–273.

Belsey, J., Yasen, S.K., Jobson, S., et al., 2021. Return to physical activity after high tibial osteotomy or unicompartmental knee arthroplasty: a systematic review and pooling data analysis. Am. J. Sports Med. 49 (5), 1372–1380.

Bennett, D., Humphreys, L., O'Brien, S., et al., 2008. Gait kinematics of age-stratified hip replacement patients – a large scale, long-term follow-up study. Gait Posture 28, 194–200.

Bolink, S.A., Lenguerrand, E., Brunton, L.R., et al., 2016. Assessment of physical function following total hip arthroplasty: inertial sensor based gait analysis is supplementary to patient-reported outcome measures. Clin. Biomech (Bristol, Avon) 32, 171–179.

Bragonzoni, L., Rovini, E., Barone, G., et al., 2019. How proprioception changes before and after total knee arthroplasty: a systematic review. Gait Posture 72, 1–11.

Brunner, J.H., Foucher, K.C., 2018. Sex specific associations between biomechanical recovery and clinical recovery after total hip arthroplasty. Clin. Biomech. (Bristol) 59, 167–173.

Caliskan Uckun, A., Celik, C., Ucan, H., et al., 2014. Comparison of effects of lower extremity orthoses on energy expenditure in patients with cerebral palsy. Dev. Neurorehabil. 17 (6), 388–392.

Cao, Z., Mai, X., Wang, J., et al., 2018. Unicompartmental knee arthroplasty vs high tibial osteotomy for knee osteoarthritis: a systematic review and meta-analysis. J. Arthroplasty 33 (3), 952–959.

Chen, X., Yang, Z., Li, H., et al., 2020. Higher risk of revision in total knee arthroplasty after high tibial osteotomy: a systematic review and updated meta-analysis. BMC Musculoskelet. Disord. 21 (1), 153.

Crenshaw, S.J., Pollo, F.E., Brodsky, J.W., 2004. The effect of ankle position on plantar pressure in a short leg walking boot. Foot Ankle Int. 25, 69–72.

Crenshaw, S.J., Pollo, F.E., Calton, E.F., 2000. Effect of lateral-wedged insoles on kinetics of the knee. Clin. Orthop. Relat. Res. 375, 185–192.

Cudejko, T., van der Esch, M., van der Leeden, M., et al., 2018. Effect of soft braces on pain and physical function in patients with knee osteoarthritis: systematic review with meta-analyses. Arch. Phys. Med. Rehabil. 99 (1), 153–163.

Cui, A., Huizi, L., Wang, D., et al., 2020. Global, regional prevalence, incidence and risk factors of knee osteoarthritis in population based studies. EClinicalMedicine, 29–30..

Daryabor, A., Arazpour, M., Aminian, G., 2018. Effect of different designs of ankle-foot orthoses on gait in patients with stroke: a systematic review. Gait Posture 62, 268–279.

De Asha, A. R., Buckley, J. G., 2015. The effects of walking speed on minimum toe clearance and on the temporal relationship between minimum clearance and peak swing-foot velocity in unilateral trans-tibial amputees. Prosthet. Orthot. Int. 39 (2), 120–125.

Devasenapathy, N., Maddison, R., Malhotra, R., et al., 2019. Preoperative quadriceps muscle strength and functional ability predict performance-based outcomes 6 months after total knee arthroplasty: a systematic review. Phys. Ther. 99 (1), 46–61.

di Laura Frattura, G., Filardo, G., Giunchi, D., et al., 2018. Risk of falls in patients with knee osteoarthritis undergoing total knee arthroplasty: a systematic review and best evidence synthesis. J. Orthop. 15 (3), 903–908.

Erhart-Hledik, J.C., Asay, J.L., Clancy, C., et al., 2017. Effects of active feedback gait retraining to produce a medial weight transfer at the foot in subjects with symptomatic medial knee osteoarthritis. J. Orthop. Res. 35 (10), 2251–2259.

Foucher, K.C., 2016. Identifying clinically meaningful benchmarks for gait improvement after total hip arthroplasty. J. Orthop. Res. 34 (1), 88–96.

Foucher, K.C., 2017. Preoperative gait mechanics predict clinical response to total hip arthroplasty. J. Orthop. Res. 35 (2), 366–376.

Foucher, K.C., Hurwitz, D.E., Wimmer, M.A., 2007. Preoperative gait adaptations persist one year after surgery in clinically well-functioning total hip replacement patients. J. Biomech. 40, 3432–3437.

Gerbrands, T.A., Pisters, M.F., Theeven, P.J.R., et al., 2017. Lateral trunk lean and medializing the knee as gait strategies for knee osteoarthritis. Gait Posture 51, 247–253.

Gohal, C., Shanmugaraj, A., Tate, P., et al., 2018. Effectiveness of valgus offloading knee braces in the treatment of medial compartment knee osteoarthritis: a systematic review. Sports Health 10 (6), 500–514.

Halsne, E. G., Waddingham, M. G., Hafner, B. J., et al., 2013. Long-term activity in and among persons with transfemoral amputation. J. Rehabil. Res. Dev. 50 (4), 515-529.

Harato, K., Nagura, T., Matsumoto, H., et al., 2010. Extension limitation in standing affects weight-bearing asymmetry after unilateral total knee arthroplasty. J. Arthroplasty 25 (2), 225–229.

Hatfield, G.L., Hubley-Kozey, C.L., Astephen Wilson, J.L., et al., 2011. The effect of total knee arthroplasty on knee joint kinematics and kinetics during gait. J, Arthroplasty 26 (2), 309–318.

He, M., Zhong, X., Li, Z., et al., 2021. Progress in the treatment of knee osteoarthritis with high tibial osteotomy: a systematic review. Syst. Rev. 10 (1), 56.

Highsmith, M. J., Schulz, B. W., Hart-Hughes, S., et al.,. 2010. Differences in the Spatiotemporal Parameters of Transtibial and Transfemoral Amputee Gait. J. Prosthet. Orthot. 22 (1), 26–30.

Hunt, M.A., Simic, M., Hinman, R.S., et al., 2011. Feasibility of a gait retraining strategy for reducing knee joint loading: increased trunk lean guided by real-time biofeedback. J. Biomech. 44 (5), 943–947.

Hurley, M., Dickson, K., Hallett, R., et al., 2018. Exercise interventions and patient beliefs for people with hip, knee or hip and knee osteoarthritis: a mixed methods review. Cochrane Database Syst. Rev. 4 (4), Cd010842.

Hurwitz, D.E., Ryals, A.B., Case, J.P., et al., 2002. The knee adduction moment during gait in subjects with knee osteoarthritis is more closely correlated with static alignment than radiographic disease severity, toe out angle and pain. J. Orthop. Res. 20, 101–107.

Hurwitz, D.E., Sumner, D.R., Andriacchi, T.P., et al., 1998. Dynamic knee loads during gait predict proximal tibial bone distribution. J. Biomech. 31 (5), 423–430.

Jones, R.K., Nester, C.J., Richards, J.D., et al., 2013. A comparison of the biomechanical effects of valgus knee braces and lateral wedged insoles in patients with knee osteoarthritis. Gait Posture 37 (3), 368–372.

Kim, M.K., Yoon, J.R., Yang, S.H., et al., 2018. Unicompartmental knee arthroplasty fails to completely restore normal gait patterns during level walking. Knee Surg. Sports Traumatol. Arthrosc. 26 (11), 3280–3289.

Kuster, M.S., 2002. Exercise recommendations after total joint replacement: a review of the current literature and proposal of scientifically based guidelines. Sports Med. 32 (7), 433–445.

Lau, E.C., Cooper, C., Lam, D., et al., 2000. Factors associated with osteoarthritis of the hip and knee in Hong Kong Chinese: obesity, joint injury, and occupational activities. American Journal of Epidemiology 152 (9), 855–862.

Lindsey, B., Bruce, S., Eddo, O., et al., 2021. Relationship between kinematic gait parameters during three gait modifications designed to reduce peak knee abduction moment. Knee 28, 229–239.

Luo, Z., Zhou, K., Peng, L., et al., 2020. Similar results with kinematic and mechanical alignment applied in total knee arthroplasty. Knee Surg. Sports Traumatol. Arthrosc. 28 (6), 1720–1735.

Mandeville, D., Osternig, L., Chou, L.S., 2007. The effect of total knee replacement on dynamic support of the body during walking and stair ascent. Clin. Biomech. (Bristol, Avon) 22, 787–794.

Maradit Kremers, H., Larson, D.R., Crowson, C.S., et al., 2015. Prevalence of total hip and knee replacement in the United States. J. Bone Joint Surg. Am. 97 (17), 1386–1397.

Mazzoli, D., Giannotti, E., Longhi, M., et al., 2017. Age explains limited hip extension recovery at one year from total hip arthroplasty. Clin. Biomech. (Bristol), 48, 35–41.

McClelland, J.A., Webster, K.E., Feller, J.A., 2007. Gait analysis of patients following total knee replacement: a systematic review. Knee 14 (4), 253–263.

McFadyen, B. J., Winter, D. A., 1988. An integrated biomechanical analysis of normal stair ascent and descent. J. Biomech. 21, 733–744.

Miki, H., Sugano, N., Hagio, K., et al., 2004. Recovery of walking speed and symmetrical movement of the pelvis and lower extremity joints after unilateral THA. J. Biomech. 37, 443–455.

Milner, C., 2009. Is gait normal after total knee arthroplasty? Systematic review of the literature. J. Orthop. Sci. 14, 114–120.

Moyer, R., Ikert, K., Long, K., et al., 2017. The value of preoperative exercise and education for patients undergoing total hip and knee arthroplasty: a systematic review and meta-analysis. JBJS Rev. 5 (12), e2.

Moyer, R., Lanting, B., Marsh, J., et al., 2018. Postoperative gait mechanics after total hip arthroplasty: a systematic review and meta-analysis. JBJS Rev. 6 (11) e1

Nankaku, M., Tsuboyama, T., Kakinoki, R., et al., 2007. Gait analysis of patients in early stages after total hip arthroplasty: effect of lateral trunk displacement on walking efficiency. J. Orthop. Sci. 12, 550–554.

Nantel, J., Termoz, N., Vendittoli, P.A., et al., 2009. Gait patterns after total hip arthroplasty and surface replacement arthroplasty. Arch. Phys. Med. Rehabil. 90, 463–469.

Nha, K.W., Shon, O.J., Kong, B.S., et al., 2018. Gait comparison of unicompartmental knee arthroplasty and total knee arthroplasty during level walking. PLoS One 13 (8), e0203310.

Palmer, J.S., Monk, A.P., Hopewell, S., et al., 2019. Surgical interventions for symptomatic mild to moderate knee osteoarthritis. Cochrane Database Syst. Rev. 7 (7), Cd012128.

Perron, M., Malouin, F., Moffet, H., et al., 2000. Three-dimensional gait analysis in women with a total hip arthroplasty. Clin. Biomech. (Bristol, Avon) 15, 504–515.

Pollo, F.E., 1998. Bracing and heel wedging for unicompartmental osteoarthritis of the knee. Am. J. Knee Surg. 11 (1), 47–50.

Powers, C.M., Rao, S., Perry, J., 1998. Knee kinetics in trans-tibial amputee gait. Gait Posture 8, 1–7.

Pua, Y.H., Ong, P.H., Chong, H.C., et al., 2013. Knee extension range of motion and self-report physical function in total knee arthroplasty: mediating effects of knee extensor strength. BMC Musculoskelet. Disord. 14, 33.

Queen, R.M., Campbell, J.C., Schmitt, D., 2019. Gait analysis reveals that total hip arthroplasty increases power production in the hip during level walking and stair climbing. Clin. Orthop. Relat. Res. 477 (8), 1839–1847.

Redhead, R. G., Davis, B. C., Robinson, K. P., et al., 1978. Post-amputation pneumatic walking aid. Br. J. Surg. 65 (9), 611–612.

Richards, J., Payne, K., Myatt, D., et al., 2016. Do orthotic walkers affect knee and hip function during gait? Prosthet. Orthot. Int. 40 (1), 137–141.

Robson, E.K., Hodder, R.K., Kamper, S.J., et al., 2020. Effectiveness of weight-loss interventions for reducing pain and disability in people with common musculoskeletal disorders: a systematic review with meta-analysis. J. Orthop. Sports Phys. Ther. 50 (6), 319–333.

Sanderson, D.J., Martin, P.E., 1997. Lower extremity kinematic and kinetic adaptations in unilateral below- knee amputees during walking. Gait Posture 6, 126–136.

Sappey-Marinier, E., Pauvert, A., Batailler, C., et al., 2020. Kinematic versus mechanical alignment for primary total knee arthroplasty with minimum 2 years follow-up: a systematic review. Sicot. J. 6, 18.

Scarvell, J.M., Galvin, C.R., Perriman, D.M., Lynch, et al., 2018. Kinematics of knees with osteoarthritis show reduced lateral femoral roll-back and maintain an adducted position. A systematic review of research using medical imaging. J. Biomech. 75, 108–122.

Schafer, Z., Vanicek, N., 2021. A block randomised controlled trial investigating changes in postural control following a personalised 12-week exercise programme for individuals with lower limb amputation. Gait Posture. 84, 198–204.

Schafer, Z. A., Perry, J. L., Vanicek, N., 2018. A personalised exercise programme for individuals with lower limb amputation reduces falls and improves gait biomechanics: A block randomised controlled trial. Gait Posture. 63, 282–289.

Schipplein, O.D., Andriacchi, T.P., 1991. Interaction between active and passive knee stabilizers during level walking. J. Orthop. Res. 9, 113–119.

Schuitema, D.C., Creve, K., Postema, R., et al., 2019. Effectiveness of mechanical treatment for plantar fasciitis: a systematic review. J. Sport Rehabil. 29 (5), 657–674.

Scott, H., Condie, M. E., Treweek, S. P., et al., 2000. An evaluation of the Amputee Mobility Aid (AMA) early walking aid. Prosthet. Orthot. Int. 24 (1), 39–46.

Segal, A.D., Orendurff, M.S., Klute, G.K., 2006. Kinematic and kinetic comparisons of transfemoral amputee gait using C-LegW and Mauch SNSW prosthetic knees. J. Rehabil. Res. Dev. 43, 857–870.

Shaw, K.E., Charlton, J.M., Perry, C.K.L., et al., 2018. The effects of shoe-worn insoles on gait biomechanics in people with knee osteoarthritis: a systematic review and meta-analysis. Br. J. Sports Med. 52 (4), 238–253.

Shirota, C., Simon, A. M., Kuiken, T. A. et al., 2015. Transfemoral amputee recovery strategies following trips to their sound and prosthesis sides throughout swing phase. J. NeuroEngineering. Rehabil. 12(1), 79.

Shull, P.B., Lurie, K.L., Cutkosky, M.R., et al., 2011. Training multi-parameter gaits to reduce the knee adduction moment with data-driven models and haptic feedback. J. Biomech. 44 (8), 1605–1609.

Simic, M., Hinman, R.S., Wrigley, T.V., et al., 2011. Gait modification strategies for altering medial knee joint load: a systematic review. Arthritis Care Res. (Hoboken) 63 (3), 405–426.

Sloan, M., Premkumar, A., Sheth, N.P., 2018. Projected volume of primary total joint arthroplasty in the U.S., 2014 to 2030. J. Bone Joint Surg. Am. 100 (17), 1455–1460.

Soliman, S.B., Spicer, P.J., van Holsbeeck, M.T., 2019. Sonographic and radiographic findings of posterior tibial tendon dysfunction: a practical step forward. Skeletal Radiol. 48 (1), 11–27.

Sonoo, M., Iijima, H., Kanemura, N., 2019. Altered sagittal plane kinematics and kinetics during sit-to-stand in individuals with knee osteoarthritis: a systematic review and meta-analysis. J. Biomech. 96, 109331.

Sosdian, L., Dobson, F., Wrigley, T.V., et al., 2014. Longitudinal changes in knee kinematics and moments following knee arthroplasty: a systematic review. Knee, 21 (6), 994–1008.

Sun, X., Wang, J., Su, Z., 2020. A meta-analysis of total knee arthroplasty following high tibial osteotomy versus primary total knee arthroplasty. Arch. Orthop. Trauma Surg. 140 (4), 527–535.

Takahashi, K. Z., Kepple, T. M., Stanhope, S. J. et al., 2012. A unified deformable (UD) segment model for quantifying total power of anatomical and prosthetic below-knee structures during stance in gait. J. Biomech. 45(15), 2662-2667.

Telfer, S., Lange, M.J., Sudduth, A.S.M., 2017. Factors influencing knee adduction moment measurement: a systematic review and meta-regression analysis. Gait Posture 58, 333–339.

Totah, D., Menon, M., Jones-Hershinow, C., et al., 2019. The impact of ankle-foot orthosis stiffness on gait: a systematic literature review. Gait Posture 69, 101–111.

Tsai, T.-Y., Dimitriou, D., Li, J.-S., et al., 2015. Asymmetric hip kinematics during gait in patients with unilateral total hip arthroplasty: in vivo 3-dimensional motion analysis. J. Biomech. 48 (4), 555–559.

Umehara, T., Tanaka, R., 2018. Effective exercise intervention period for improving body function or activity in patients with knee osteoarthritis undergoing total knee arthroplasty: a systematic review and meta-analysis. Braz. J. Phys. Ther. 22 (4), 265–275.

van Tunen, J.A.C., Dell'Isola, A., Juhl, C., et al., 2018. Association of malalignment, muscular dysfunction, proprioception, laxity and abnormal joint loading with tibiofemoral knee osteoarthritis – a systematic review and meta-analysis. BMC Musculoskelet. Disord. 19 (1), 273.

Vanicek, N., Coleman, E., Watson, J., et al., 2021. STEPFORWARD study: a randomised controlled feasibility trial of a self-aligning prosthetic ankle-foot for older patients with vascular-related amputations. BMJ Open. 11(3), 13.

Vanicek, N., Strike, S., McNaughton, L., et al., 2009. Gait patterns in transtibial amputee fallers vs. non-fallers: Biomechanical differences during level walking. Gait Posture. 29(3), 415-420.

Vanicek, N., Strike, S. C., Polman, R. et al., 2015. Kinematic differences exist between transtibial amputee fallers and non-fallers during downwards step transitioning. Prosthet. Orthot. Int. 39(4), 322-332.

Vickers, D. R., Palk, C., McIntosh, A. S., et al., 2008. Elderly unilateral transtibial amputee gait on an inclined walkway: A biomechanical analysis. Gait Posture. 27 (3), 518-529.

Vrieling, A. H., van Keeken, H. G., Schoppen, et al., 2008. Uphill and downhill walking in unilateral lower limb amputees. Gait Posture. 28(2), 235-242.

Walter, J.P., D'Lima, D.D., Colwell, C.W., 2010. Decreased knee adduction moment does not guarantee decreased medial contact force during gait. J. Orthop. Res. 28 (10), 1348–1354.

Waters, R. L., Mulroy, S., 1999. The energy expenditure of normal and pathologic gait. Gait Posture. 9(3), 207-231.

Wong, D. W. C., Lam, W. K., Yeung, L. F., et al., 2015. Does long-distance walking improve or deteriorate walking stability of transtibial amputees? Clinical Biomechanics. 30(8), 867–873.

Xu, Q., Chen, B., Wang, Y., et al., 2017. The effectiveness of manual therapy for relieving pain, stiffness, and dysfunction in knee osteoarthritis: a systematic review and meta-analysis. Pain Physician, 20 (4), 229–243.

Yoo, J.-I., Cha, Y.-H., Kim, K.-J., et al., 2019. Gait analysis after total hip arthroplasty using direct anterior approach versus anterolateral approach: a systematic review and meta-analysis. BMC Musculoskelet. Disord. 20 (1), 63–63

Yoshida, Y., Mizner, R.L., Ramsey, D.K., et al., 2008. Examining outcomes from total knee arthroplasty and the relationship between quadriceps strength and knee function over time. Clin. Biomech. (Bristol, Avon) 23 (1), 320–328.

Zafar, A.Q., Zamani, R., Akrami, M., 2020. The effectiveness of foot orthoses in the treatment of medial knee osteoarthritis: a systematic review. Gait Posture 76, 238–251.

8

Gait Analysis of Running and the Management of Common Injuries

Kim Hébert-Losier and Komsak Sinsurin

Running is a popular form of physical activity and is associated with health-enhancing benefits, including a 27% reduction in the risk of all causes of mortality (Pedisic et al., 2019). Despite these benefits, the risk of sustaining a running-related injury is relatively high, with reported injury incidence rates ranging from 26.0% to 92.4% (Van Gheluwe and Madsen, 1997) and from 7.7 to 17.8 injuries per 1000 hours of running (Videbæk et al., 2015). Typically, 40% to 50% of runners experience an injury each year (Kakouris et al., 2021), with 75% these of injuries occurring at or below the knee and primarily due to overuse. Clinicians and researchers alike are still searching for the main risk factors associated with running-related injuries (van der Worp et al., 2015; Dillon et al., 2021), with the cause of running-related injuries being undoubtedly multifactorial (Esculier et al., 2020). However, risk factors have been linked to training errors and loads such as doing 'too much, too soon' (Soligard et al., 2016), and there is some evidence that suggests sudden changes in training loads increase the risk of running-related injuries (Damsted et al., 2019). The majority of clinicians and researchers agree that running biomechanics is part of the puzzle and an important aspect to consider, assess and train

or retrain in the context of prevention, management and rehabilitation of injuries, as well as performance (Harrast, 2019). This chapter provides a brief overview of running biomechanics, clinical assessment of running mechanics, as well as potential risk factors and key management strategies of common running-related injuries.

RUNNING BIOMECHANICS

Key Differences to Walking

Running is a form of bipedal gait, and adults typically transition from walking to running at a speed of approximately 2 m/s which is triggered by a number of factors, notably those related to mechanical efficiency and load (Kung et al., 2018). Several of the concepts and terminology used in walking gait covered in the previous chapters apply to running, including the usual delineation of a gait cycle (or running stride) from footstrike to footstrike of the same foot. The aim of this section is not to address all facets of running biomechanics in detail, but rather to highlight a few key distinguishing features of running compared to walking.

Walking has a double support phase where both limbs are in contact with the ground. An inverted pendulum is often used to model walking gait (Cavagna et al., 1977). In contrast, running has a float or flight phase where no limbs are in contact with the ground, and is modelled using a spring-mass model (McMahon et al., 1987) (Fig. 8.1). In both walking and running models, the centre of mass

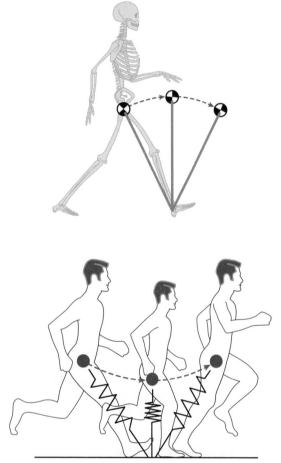

Fig. 8.1 Schematic representation of the 'inverted pendulum' model used in walking *(above)* (Source: Matthis Jonathan Samir and Fajen Brett R. 2013, Humans exploit the biomechanics of bipedal gait during visually guided walking over complex terrainProc. R. Soc. B.28020130700. https://doi.org/10.1098/rspb.2013.0700) and 'spring-mass' model used in running *(below)* (Source: The Gait Cycle in Running, Part II: Viscous-Spring-Dampeners, HealthyStep 2022. From: https://www.healthystep.co.uk/advice/the-gait-cycle-in-running-2/) . A point mass (centre of mass) connects to the ground at the foot via the limb and follows a ballistic trajectory through the gait cycle. In the spring-mass model, the leg 'spring' compresses during the first half of stance and rebounds during the second half, storing and releasing energy.

motion follows an arch trajectory from footstrike to toe off. These models are of course oversimplifications of the complexities of human locomotion. Nonetheless, these models provide a conceptual mechanical framework and apt pictorial representation of these cyclical locomotive tasks. The centre of mass during walking is lowest close to footstrike and highest near mid-stance, when the limb is relatively extended; in running the centre of mass is highest during flight and lowest at mid-stance, when the limb is flexed.

The stance and swing phases of the walking cycle represent about 60% and 40%, respectively, which can be further subdivided into seven periods (see Chapter 2, Normal Gait). On the other hand, the stance and swing phases of the running cycle represent about 35% and 65% respectively, which can be subdivided into five key periods: stance phase absorption, stance phase propulsion, early float (or swing phase generation), swing (or swing phase reversal) and late float (or swing phase reversal), as shown in Fig. 8.2.

To increase running speed, both stride frequency (also known as cadence) and stride length can increase. Whereas endurance running mainly relies on increases in stride length to increase speed (Bramble and Lieberman, 2004), increases in sprinting speed are primarily through increasing cadence, although it is worth noting that certain elite sprinters rely more on increases in stride length whilst others increase cadence to achieve top-end running speeds (Salo et al., 2011). At sprinting speeds, the proportion of time spent in stance can decrease to 20%. Concurrently with increases in speed from walking to running, peak vertical ground reaction forces increase from approximately 1.2 to 2.5, and reach up to 4.0 times body weight in elite sprinters (Čoh et al., 2018). Joint ranges of motion (ROMs) of the lower extremity, predominantly in the sagittal plane, increase as speed increases; additionally, the pelvis becomes more anteriorly tilted and the trunk becomes more flexed. The major muscle groups involved during walking, including the gluteus maximus, iliopsoas, hamstrings, quadriceps, triceps surae and tibialis anterior, all become more active in running, and joint moments and powers at the hip, knee, ankle and foot increase. Predictably, the mechanical and energetic demands of running are overall greater than walking.

Running Gait Analysis

The two main goals of addressing running biomechanics are injury management (prevention, rehabilitation, retraining) and performance enhancement. This chapter predominantly addresses the former aspect. The methods of running gait analysis parallel those presented in Chapter 4, Methods of Gait Analysis, but typically involve higher sampling frequencies. A minimum of 120 Hz or higher is recommended when conducting objective biomechanical

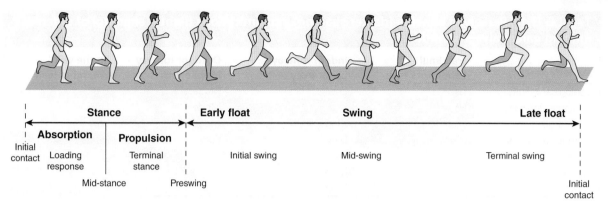

Fig. 8.2 Running gait cycle and subdivisions with key events.

assessment of running kinematics using two- or three-dimensional motion analysis methods (Souza, 2016). Visual running gait analysis is still common in clinical practice; however, even experts cannot accurately identify runners with an economical running gait using observations alone (Cochrum et al., 2020). This challenge might be due to the absence of an 'ideal' running style. Indeed, several running patterns can result in similar running economy outcomes.

The use of rating scales can assist in assessing runners' global running patterns along a continuum using visual observations (Lussiana et al., 2017), but when possible and for monitoring purposes, the use of objective measures to quantify running gait is recommended. Most commonly, biomechanical metrics of interest are grouped as *spatiotemporal* (e.g., speed, step/stride length, step/stride frequency or cadence, contact times, flight times, duty factor, etc.), *kinematic* (e.g., joint angles, angular velocities, angular accelerations, etc.) and *kinetic* (e.g., peak ground reaction forces, vertical loading rates, impulses, etc.). The duty factor reflects the proportion of the stride period during which time each foot is in contact with the ground. This measure is suggested to represent a more global biomechanical behaviour than the footstrike pattern, as it considers the duration of force production in relation to stride duration. External forces are lower in recreational runners who run with a higher duty factor (Bonnaerens et al., 2021), which could have implications for injury prevention. A higher duty factor reflects a runner who spends a proportionally longer time in contact with the ground when running and can be calculated as follows:

$$Duty\ factor = \frac{contact\ time}{contact\ time\ +\ swing\ time}$$

Most clinicians conduct running assessments on a treadmill. In this situation, treadmill speed is used to calculate some of the spatiotemporal parameters. For example, right step length (m) can be measured by multiplying the treadmill speed (m/s) by the time (s) taken from left footstrike to right footstrike. Conducting a running assessment on a treadmill has several advantages (Table 8.1), notably that it allows analysis of numerous cycles, permits standardisation of running conditions and requires limited space. In contrast, it necessitates financial investment, requires familiarisation of runners and is less ecologically valid. Reviews on the differences between overground and treadmill running highlight that spatiotemporal, kinematic, kinetic, muscle activity and muscle-tendon measures are largely comparable between the two modes of running (Van Hooren et al., 2019), with the exception of vertical displacement, knee flexion ROM and foot-ground angles at footstrike which are greater when running overground. Noteworthy, though, is that the mechanical properties of commercial-grade treadmills can markedly differ from one another as well as from outdoor running surfaces (Colino et al., 2020). Treadmills typically demonstrate higher shock absorption, greater vertical deformation and lower energy restitution than outdoor running surfaces. Since treadmill construction itself can significantly affect biomechanics, metabolic cost and perception of effort (Miller et al., 2019), clinicians undertaking treadmill analysis should attempt to select a treadmill that mimics the overground running conditions of their target population. A stiffer treadmill is recommended for running assessment given that most runners run on concrete or asphalt where vertical deformation and shock absorption are minimal, and energy restitution is high. In research, using an instrumented treadmill is ideal as this provides a stiff running platform in addition to ground reaction force data.

TABLE 8.1   Perceived benefits (darker shading) and limitations (lighter shading) of different running gait analysis methods

	Treadmill – Laboratory tech	Indoor runway – Laboratory tech	Outdoor runway – Mobile tech	'In the wild' – Wearable tech
Ecological validity	Low	Low	Moderate	High
Equipment validity	High	High	Moderate	Low
Standardisation	High	Moderate	Moderate	Low
Number of cycles	High	Low	Low	High
Accessibility	Low	Low	High	High
Familiarisation needs	High	Moderate	Moderate	Low
Hawthorne effect	High	High	High	Low

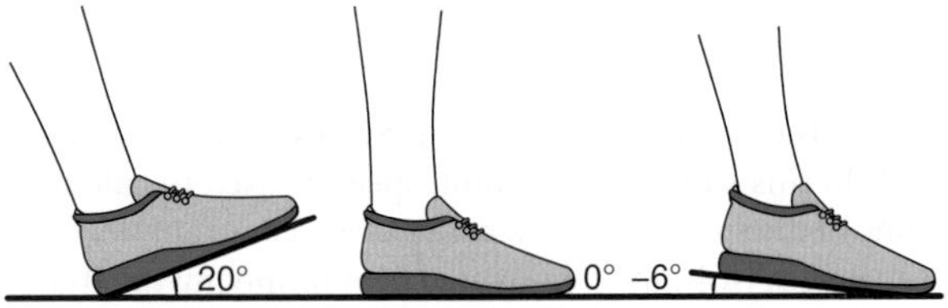

Fig. 8.3 Foot-ground angles for rearfoot *(left)*, midfoot *(centre)* and forefoot *(right)* footstrike patterns from two-dimensional analyses *(solid lines)*. Printed courtesy of: Hoenig T, Rolvien T, Hollander K. Footstrike patterns in runners: concepts, classifications, techniques, and implications for running-related injuries. Dtsch Z Sportmed. 2020, 71: 55-61. doi:10.5960/dzsm.2020.424. Figure 1: Rearfoot strike (RFS).

The foot normally contacts the ground with the heel or rear part of the foot during walking. In running, the footstrike pattern is typically classified in one of three discrete categories based on which part of the foot makes initial contact with the ground. Footstrike patterns are categorised as *rearfoot* when the first contact is with the heel or rear third of the sole; *midfoot* when the first contact is with the midfoot or entire sole; or *forefoot* when the first contact is with the forefoot or front half of the sole (Fig. 8.3). A foot-ground angle from two-dimensional videos is often also calculated as the line that joins the sole of the shoe from the point of first contact and the horizontal plane of the running surface, where positive angles represent more pronounced rearfoot striking and negative angles represent more pronounced forefoot striking (Fig. 8.3). The foot-ground angle when using three-dimensional motion analysis can be calculated as the angle between the anteroposterior laboratory axis and a vector formed between a heel marker and another placed on the second metatarsal head. Using this method, the foot-ground angle in stance is subtracted from that during running, so a 0-degree value reflects a flat foot. This foot-ground angle can be used to

categorise footstrike patterns; with rearfoot being greater than 8 degrees, midfoot from 8 to –1.6 degrees, and forefoot when less than –1.6 degrees (Altman and Davis, 2012).

There is controversy regarding which footstrike pattern is more or less injurious and more or less economical, and whether it even matters. Given their distinct structural and mechanical loading patterns, it is likely that certain types of injuries are more common in rearfoot strikers, such as patellofemoral pain syndrome and medial tibial stress syndrome, whereas others are more frequent in forefoot strikers, such as Achilles tendinopathies and metatarsal stress fractures. To date, however, there is limited evidence to support a causal relationship of footstrike pattern with injury risk in running (Anderson et al., 2020).

Kinematic Measures

In clinical settings, sagittal and frontal planes are most commonly examined (see Table 8.2). It is important to emphasise that humans are dynamic systems and move in a 'global' manner, so changes in one area are likely to lead to changes elsewhere. For instance, increasing cadence at a given running speed is typically linked with shorter stride lengths, lower vertical oscillations, an initial ground contact with the foot closer to the centre of mass, a smaller foot-ground angle and a more vertical tibia.

Kinetic Measures

The ground reaction forces during running are usually examined in research using instrumented treadmills or forceplates embedded into the ground. The vertical component of the ground reaction force is the most studied and typically presents one of two distinct shapes based on footstrike pattern (Fig. 8.4). Rearfoot strikers typically present an impact peak resulting from a sharp increase in the ground reaction force after the initial ground contact. In forefoot strikers, this impact peak is not always present. The peak vertical ground reaction force occurs at mid-stance in both

TABLE 8.2 Common running gait analysis parameters examined in clinical settings and plane of reference

Event	Sagittal	Frontal
Initial contact	Footstrike pattern	
	Foot-ground angle	
	Foot-to-centre of mass distance	
	Tibial inclination	
	Knee flexion angle	
Midstance	Knee flexion angle	Foot placement (or step width)
	Ankle dorsiflexion angle	Foot-to-centre of mass alignment
	Antero-posterior pelvic tilt	Pronation/supination[a]
	Trunk flexion	Knee separation
		Dynamic knee valgus[b]
		Pelvis lateral inclination
		Trunk lateral flexion
Toe-off	Knee flexion	
	Hip extension	
Gait cycle	Vertical displacement of the centre of mass	

[a]Pronation: rearfoot inwardly rotates about the subtalar joint. Supination: rearfoot outwardly rotates about the subtalar joint. In running gait, pronation is commonly considered a combined movement of eversion, dorsiflexion and forefoot abduction, whereas supination combines inversion, plantarflexion and forefoot adduction.
[b]Combination of hip adduction, hip internal rotation and knee abduction.

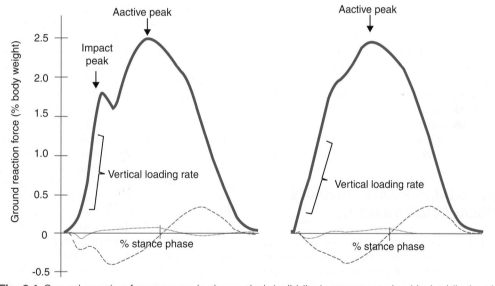

Fig. 8.4 Ground reaction force curves in the vertical *(solid line)*, anteroposterior *(dashed line)* and mediolateral *(dotted line)* directions (positive values represent vertical, anterior and lateral), respectively.

instances, is commonly referred to as the active peak and generally reaches 2.5 to 3.0 times body weight at endurance running speeds. In habitual rearfoot strikers, the active peak is generally slightly higher than nonrearfoot strikers. The vertical loading rate reflects how quickly the vertical ground reaction force is applied (body weights per second). Peak and average vertical loading rates are approximately two times lower in forefoot than rearfoot strikers. The precise vertical loading rate values depend on assessment and computational methods, but range from 30 to 90 body weights per second; however, vertical loading rates can be up to 460 body weights per second when running barefoot with a rearfoot strike pattern (Lieberman et al., 2010). The anteroposterior ground reaction forces reflect propulsion and braking forces, and are much smaller in magnitude than the vertical force. Peak anteroposterior force values during running range from 0.25 to 0.5 times body weight. Relatively little is known regarding the mediolateral forces and their impact on running gait, with peak values ranging from 0.10 to 0.20 times body weight and demonstrating numerous zero crossings.

There is again conflicting evidence regarding the role of kinetic parameters in running-related injury incidence, which might be due to the few prospective studies available. Currently, vertical loading rates and braking forces are the two variables that demonstrate potential links with certain running-related injuries, in particular in female recreational runners (Davis et al., 2016; Napier et al., 2018).

Note on Wearable Sensors

There is growing interest and promise in the use of wearable sensors to quantify and analyse running gait, predominantly in the use of inertial measurement units (IMUs), but also in pressure-sensing insoles and flexible textiles. There are currently a number of considerations in using such wearable sensors, including their sampling frequency, anatomical calibration method, fixation method, sensor capacity, durability, and validity and reliability of the derived metrics (Hughes et al., 2021). On the latter topic, the accuracy of metrics from wearable devices compared to laboratory-based methods is acceptable for spatiotemporal parameters (Horsley et al., 2021), but these are heterogeneous across studies and still suboptimal for numerous measures (Blazey et al., 2021), warranting further research before they are widely implemented within clinical practice.

COMMON RUNNING-RELATED INJURIES AND CLINICAL CONSIDERATIONS

As highlighted in this chapter's introduction, the risk of sustaining a running-related injury is considerable. Understanding the aetiology of injury is essential to implement successful injury prevention programmes. From a basic biomechanical standpoint, injuries happen when the mechanical load placed on a structure exceeds its load tolerance (McIntosh, 2005).

There are numerous sport-related injury aetiologies (McIntosh, 2005) and prevention (Finch, 2006) models. While it is beyond the scope of this chapter to address each one of these models, it is worth emphasising that all of them acknowledge the multifactorial nature of sport-related injuries, with more recent frameworks highlighting their complex and dynamic nature, and involvement of biological, physical, psychological and sociocultural factors (Wiese-Bjornstal, 2010). A framework specific to the aetiology of running-related injuries was proposed in 2017 (Bertelsen et al., 2017) which focused on their causal mechanisms. This framework considered the structure-specific load capacity at the start of a running session and the reduction in this capacity throughout the session as a product of the magnitude, distribution and number of load cycles (Fig. 8.5).

There have been numerous reviews on running-related injuries, which overall indicate that injuries to the lower extremities are the most common. Two of the most recent reviews identified the knee (28% to 31%), ankle-foot (26% to 28%), lower leg (16% to 20%) and hip-thigh (14%) regions accounting for the highest proportion of injuries in adult runners (Francis et al., 2019; Kakouris et al., 2021). The specific pathologies accounting for the highest proportion of overall injuries were patellofemoral pain syndrome (17%), Achilles tendinopathy (7% to 10%), medial tibial stress syndrome (8% to 9%), plantar fasciitis (7% to 8%) and iliotibial band syndrome (6% to 8%) (Francis et al., 2019; Kakouris et al., 2021), with stress fractures accounting for 4% to 6% of running-related injuries.

A key component in the management of running-related injuries is a comprehensive subjective assessment and history. One of the more consistently reported risk factors associated with running-related injuries is a previous injury (van der Worp et al., 2015). Another important clinical factor is training load and history, which should consider more than weekly distance (Paquette et al., 2020). Both too little and too much running have been associated with running-related injuries, with either insufficient or excessive loads impeding the biological adaptations needed for injury-free running. Some important external (mechanical) load metrics include volume, intensity, surface and terrain; internal (physiological) load metrics include perception of effort and heart rate (Paquette et al., 2020). It is well known that footwear and change in footwear can substantially affect running biomechanics and load distribution, which needs to be considered as a tool in the management of injuries. More often than not, something has changed and led to the development of a running-related injury where the load exceeded the capacity of the tissue. However, addressing purely the physical components of running-related injuries might be insufficient in certain cases, requiring a more holistic or interdisciplinary approach and involvement of other healthcare professionals.

There are numerous cross-sectional studies indicating the presence of certain movement patterns once an injury is present; but few prospective studies exist linking given movement patterns with the incidence of running-related injuries. For instance, runners with common

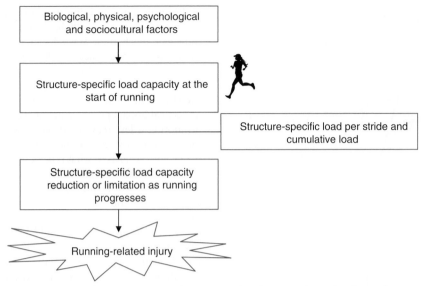

Fig. 8.5 Simplification of the conceptual framework for the causal mechanism of structure-specific running-related injuries proposed by (Bertelsen et al., 2017), complemented by the biopsychosocial injury risk profile (Wiese-Bjornstal, 2010).

running-related injuries have been shown to run with greater peak contralateral pelvic drop and forward trunk lean at midstance, and more extended knee and ankle dorsiflexion at initial contact compared to uninjured runners (Bramah et al., 2018). While insightful, these movements can often represent a consequence rather than a cause of injury. In fact, hierarchical cluster analysis on three-dimensional kinematic data performed on injured and healthy runners identified distinct subgroups of runners with similar running patterns; but these distinct running patterns were not related to injury location or injury status (Jauhiainen et al., 2020). These findings support the notion that there might be no 'ideal' or 'protective' running pattern. That is not to say that biomechanics does not play a role in the management of running-related injuries. Indeed, running gait retraining has been successfully used in the prevention (Chan et al., 2018) and treatment (Davis et al., 2020) of running-related injuries. The following sections address some of the most common running-related injuries and clinical considerations.

PATELLOFEMORAL PAIN

Clinical Presentations

Patellofemoral pain (PFP) is the most common running injury, representing around 17% of injuries in runners (Francis et al., 2019; Kakouris et al., 2021). Runners with

PFP typically present with pain around or behind the patella that is worsened in weight-bearing and dynamic knee flexion activities, such as stair climbing, squatting, running and jump-landing (Crossley et al., 2016). No 'gold standard' PFP diagnosis exists, although this clinical diagnosis should be considered in the presence of retro- or peri-patellar pain and in pain reproduction during activities loading the patellofemoral joint in a flexed posture or dynamic movements when tibiofemoral pathologies have been excluded (Willy et al., 2019). In runners with PFP, a number of kinematic, kinetic, muscle activity and muscle strength presentations have been reported. Runners with PFP typically present with one or more of the following:

- knee pain during running;
- weakness of lower limb muscles, notably knee extensors, hip abductors, hip external rotators and hip extensors (Duffey et al., 2000);
- increased peak hip adduction and internal rotation during the stance phase of running (Wirtz et al., 2012);
- increased contralateral pelvic drop during the stance phase of running (Bramah et al., 2018);
- increased rearfoot eversion in heel strikers (Duffey et al., 2000; Kulmala et al., 2013);
- greater peak lateral forces at the patellofemoral joint (Chen and Powers, 2014); or
- dynamic knee valgus during the stance phase of running (Petersen et al., 2014) (Fig. 8.6).

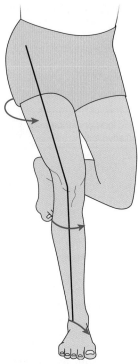

Fig. 8.6 Dynamic knee valgus posture.

Running gait retraining should be considered as a viable intervention, especially in the presence of altered running gait mechanics. Several gait retraining approaches exist and have been successfully used in the rehabilitation of runners with PFP. These approaches include the use of visual, tactile and auditory feedback aimed at increasing cadence, running more 'softly', reducing tibial acceleration or vertical impact peaks, reducing dynamic knee valgus or promoting a less rearfoot strike pattern to reduce patellofemoral joint stress. To date, there is no conclusive evidence with regards to what type of feedback and approach is best suited for an individual and condition; thus, clinicians need to work with their patients to identify the most cost-effective and implementable approach on a case-by-case basis.

Physical examinations should be performed for PFP cases to aid in individualised prescription (Table 8.3). Based on the clinical examination, clinical presentation and individual responses, numerous adjunct interventions can be integrated in the management of runners with PFP. These interventions can include hip and knee strengthening exercises, taping, foot orthoses and mobility/flexibility exercises. Running in minimal footwear has also been shown to reduce patellofemoral joint stress and may be beneficial in the treatment of runners with PFP.

Key Management Strategies

Patient education in terms of load management and activity modification plays a central role in managing PFP and is a key feature in best-practice guidelines for the conservative management of PFP (Collins et al., 2018; Willy et al., 2019). Runners have been shown to successfully self-manage rehabilitation of PFP by reducing their running distance and speed, increasing their running frequency and managing their training within acceptable clinical thresholds, such as by keeping pain levels less than 2 out of 10 with no worsening of symptoms (Esculier et al., 2017). Hence, it is important that clinicians educate patients regarding self-management strategies, the benefits of active rehabilitation and anticipated recovery and return-to-running times.

A holistic approach to the treatment of PFP is encouraged and should consider biological, physical, psychological and sociocultural factors (Fig. 8.5). Graded exercise and return to activity are one facet, but psychological stressors and lifestyle factors can also contribute to injury or slow rehabilitation. It is important for clinicians to help patients with PFP understand these potential contributing factors and assist them in accessing appropriate and suitable intervention options.

TABLE 8.3	PFP intervention strategies based on clinical assessment	
PFP presentation	**Intervention**
1. Overuse/Overload without other impairments	• Taping • Activity modification
2. PFP with movement coordination deficits	• Gait and movement retraining
3. PFP with muscle strength deficits	• Hip/gluteal muscle strengthening • Quadriceps muscle strengthening

4. PFP with mobility impairments	• Hypermobility
	  • Foot orthosis
	  • Taping
	• Hypomobility
	  • Patellar retinaculum/ soft issue mobilisation
	  • Stretching

Above patellofemoral pain (PFP) presentations and intervention guidelines based on Willy et al. (2019).

ACHILLES TENDINOPATHY

Clinical Presentations

Achilles tendinopathy reflects 7% to 10% of running-related injuries (Francis et al., 2019; Kakouris et al., 2021). Achilles tendinopathy is characterised by localised pain and swelling of the Achilles tendon, as well as loss of function. Symptoms can be reproduced during running, single-leg hopping or functional activities. Achilles tendinopathy is considered an overuse injury resulting from excessive mechanical loading of the tendon with impaired healing. Runners presenting with Achilles tendinopathy typically present with a recent increase in training volume, intensity or frequency, or a rapid change to more minimal footwear. Other clinical findings can include local tissue thickening (Maffulli et al., 2003), dorsiflexion ROM limitation and plantar flexor muscle weakness (Martin et al., 2018), stiffness and pain in the morning or after a prolonged rest, pain at the start of an activity that decreases as activity progresses, and reduced running performance (Janssen et al., 2018). There are few running kinematic differences in runners with compared to without Achilles tendinopathy (Mousavi et al., 2019), except for increased rearfoot eversion at ground contact. Changes in neuromuscular control have been reported, such as earlier soleus offset relative to lateral gastrocnemius during running (Wyndow et al., 2013). Other risk factors associated with Achilles tendinopathy of relevance to runners include previous lower limb tendinopathy or fracture, use of ofloxacin antibiotics, training in cold weather, use of compressive socks and use of a training schedule (Lagas et al., 2020).

Key Management Strategies

Early detection and intervention can help to prevent worsening or persistence of Achilles tendinopathies. Active treatments are more effective than the wait-and-see approach for Achilles tendinopathy (van der Vlist et al., 2021). Various domains can affect tendon health (Fig. 8.7), which should be considered in the planning and provision of interventions (Silbernagel et al., 2020; Vicenzino, B., et al., 2020). A holistic approach to treatment can contribute to restoring function and preventing recurrence.

There is emerging evidence that subgroups of Achilles tendinopathies exist which may require tailored approaches to rehabilitation (Hanlon et al., 2021). These subgroups can be categorised by activity, psychosocial and body structure considerations. The activity-dominant subgroup is the largest and contains patients with higher physical activity levels, functional abilities and quality-of-life scores than the other subgroups; moderate symptoms; and generally younger age. Rehabilitation methods for this subgroup should consider load management, progressive rehabilitation and gradual return-to-running scenarios to optimise recovery. The majority of runners who sustain an Achilles tendinopathy would fall under an activity-dominant subgroup; however, it remains important to consider all subgroups as potential causes of Achilles tendinopathy.

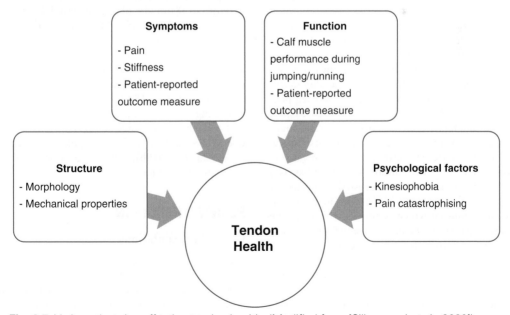

Fig. 8.7 Various domains effecting tendon health. (Modified from [Silbernagel et al., 2020]).

There is strong evidence for the effectiveness of exercise therapy for the treatment of Achilles tendinopathy, either alone or in conjunction with adjunct therapies. The Victorian Institute of Sport Assessment-Achilles questionnaire (VISA-A) along with a battery of tests, including the calf raise test for endurance, are recommended to assess and monitor individuals with Achilles tendinopathy. The number of calf raises an individual is expected to complete ranges from 20 to 50 repetitions based on age, physical activity levels, gender and body mass index (Hébert-Losier et al., 2017). The rehabilitation phase is important in the treatment of Achilles tendinopathy. It requires time and an individually progressed loading programme to allow the tendon to adapt and prevent injury recurrence (Magnusson and Kjaer, 2019). Early in the rehabilitation of runners, high-speed and uphill running should be avoided due to the load on the Achilles tendon; furthermore, the use of minimal shoes and forefoot striking in the acute phases of an Achilles tendinopathy might exasperate symptoms and should be considered later in the rehabilitation process or in chronic stages to promote adaptation and remodelling. Gait retraining aimed at increasing cadence should also be considered given that increasing step frequency lowers peak Achilles tendon stress and strain (Lyght et al., 2016).

MEDIAL TIBIAL STRESS SYNDROME

Clinical Presentations

Medial tibial stress syndrome (MTSS) is a common (8% to 9%) running-related injury (Francis et al., 2019; Kakouris et al., 2021) and typically presents as localised pain at the two-thirds distal portion of the posteromedial aspect of the tibia, but can also be located at the anterolateral aspect. MTSS is commonly referred to as *shin splints* and is categorised as an exercise-induced lower leg pain (Raissi et al., 2009). MTSS is often considered as part of a continuum, spanning irritation of the periosteum to stress fractures. MTSS is treated based on its clinical presentation due to lack of strong evidence regarding its aetiology (Winters, 2018), although bone stress as a result of tibial bending has been suggested as a cause of MTSS. Typically, runners with MTSS present with pain during or after running which improves with rest. The reproduction of pain upon palpation over a 5-cm or more area along the posteromedial tibia is used for clinical diagnosis (Winters, 2020). Prior use of orthotics, fewer years of running experience, previous history of MTSS, increased navicular drop, increased body mass index, increased plantarflexion and hip external rotation ROMs and female gender are identified risk factors for MTSS

in runners (Newman et al., 2013). These risk factors can inform the management strategies. Runners who develop MTSS have been reported to show greater rearfoot eversion, contralateral pelvic drop and pressure on the medial aspect of the foot during running (Becker et al., 2018). Case studies have also reported the incidence of MTSS when transitioning to shoes with more cushioning and a broader base of support (Hannigan and Pollard, 2021), warranting footwear considerations.

Key Management Strategies

Various modalities have been used to treat MTSS, including cryotherapy, shockwave therapy, massage, orthotics, pneumatic leg bracing, gait retraining and avoidance of high loading activities. However, there is yet to be strong evidence regarding the effectiveness of these interventions (Winters et al., 2013). For runners, education regarding load management and graded return to running is central to managing MTSS. Progressing running distance less than 30% from week to week has been suggested as appropriate to avoid running-related injuries (Damsted et al., 2019). In the presence of MTSS, a slower progression is advised, and should be symptom based.

A randomised control trial in runners with MTSS was conducted in 2012. All runners followed a graded return-to-running programme that allowed no more than 4 or more on a 10-point visual analogue scale. The addition of calf muscle stretching and strengthening exercises, or wearing sports compression stockings during running, did not speed up the return-to-run time, with the average time to return to 18 minutes of running at a difficult speed being approximately 3.5 months (Moen et al., 2012).

Gait retraining can also be considered in MTSS patients. A 6-week gait retraining programme aimed at adopting a forefoot strike pattern has been successfully used to treat exercise-induced lower leg pain in runners (Helmhout et al., 2015). Providing two to six running gait retraining sessions promoting landing more on the forefoot and a higher cadence has also been linked with positive MTSS results in military populations (Zimmermann et al., 2019a, 2019b), with a successful return taking approximately 5 months.

PLANTAR HEEL PAIN

Clinical Presentations

Plantar heel pain represents 7% to 8% of running-related injuries (Francis et al., 2019; Kakouris et al., 2021). Other commonly used terms to reference plantar heel pain include *plantar fasciitis*, *plantar fasciopathy* and *plantar fasciosis* (McNeill and Silvester, 2017). Plantar heel pain is a common condition in active populations and normally has a gradual onset (Hill et al., 2008). Typically, patients with plantar heel pain report a high intensity of pain in the first few steps of walking after sleeping or long resting (Buchbinder, 2004), and a worsening of symptoms when standing or walking for a long time or towards the end of the day (Petraglia et al., 2017). Common clinical presentations include one or more of the following:

- localised pain at the anteromedial aspect of the heel, especially at the origin of the plantar fascia (Buchbinder, 2004);
- increased ankle plantar flexion ROM (Hamstra-Wright et al., 2021);
- weak foot muscles (Osborne et al., 2019);
- less femoral internal rotation (Harutaichun et al., 2019);
- poor movement quality in the lateral step-down test (Harutaichun et al., 2019); or
- increased body mass index and body mass (Hamstra-Wright et al., 2021).

Key Management Strategies

There are three strategies reflecting the core approach to treating plantar heel pain in the first 4 to 6 weeks of care: individualised education, plantar fascia stretching and low dye taping (Morrissey et al., 2021). Education should be individualised and address load management, pain education, health-related conditions and footwear considerations. Psychosocial variables, such as depression, anxiety and job satisfaction, may increase levels of pain and loss of function in patients with plantar heel pain (Drake et al., 2018); hence, this aspect should be integrated within patient education, and referrals should be sought when needed. In the case of no or limited improvement, shockwave therapy and orthoses can be added as adjunct therapies.

Body weight is an important factor to address in the management and prevention of plantar heel pain. This consideration might be of relevance to runners who have taken a rest or who are getting back to training. A gradual increase in running load, intensity and volume can assist in tissue adaptation and improve load capacity (Hamstra-Wright et al., 2021). Combining calf muscle strengthening and shoe inserts showed superior outcomes in terms of pain and foot function at 3 months compared to combining plantar-specific stretching and shoe inserts (Rathleff et al., 2015). Given that individuals with plantar heel pain present with reduced foot muscle strength and volume, intrinsic foot muscle strengthening exercises can also be recommended (Osborne et al., 2019).

Running uphill or at high speeds can increase the strain on the plantar fascia and should be avoided during early rehabilitation. There are few studies on runners with plantar heel pain; hence, in terms of gait retraining and footwear, similar principles to those presented in the Achilles tendinopathy section are proposed until evidence specific to plantar heel pain is available.

ILIOTIBIAL BAND SYNDROME

Clinical Presentations

Iliotibial band syndrome (ITBS) represents 6% to 8% of running-related injuries (Francis et al., 2019; Kakouris et al., 2021) and is the second most common overuse injury in runners (Taunton et al., 2002). Tissue compression or impingement of the iliotibial band on the lateral femoral epicondyle is thought to be responsible for ITBS and associated lateral knee pain. Lateral knee pain is typically worse at 20 degrees to 30 degrees of knee flexion (Hamill et al., 2008). Usually, runners with ITBS report lateral knee pain onset a few kilometres into running. Training errors are common in the subjective history of patients, such as a sudden increase in running volume and downhill running. Such training errors can lead to a disruption in tissue homeostasis (Dye, 2005; Gabbett, 2016) and tissue overload (Fig. 8.8).

There are limited prospective studies on ITBS (Aderem and Louw, 2015), and no clear biomechanical causes of ITBS have been identified in runners (Louw and Deary, 2014). Runners with ITBS can clinically present with decreased hip abductor muscle strength and the following running gait kinematics (Aderem and Louw, 2015; Foch et al., 2015), particularly when fatigued:

- Increased hip adduction during the stance phase
- A narrowed step width
- Increased peak knee internal rotation
- Increased peak ipsilateral trunk flexion (lateral trunk bending)

Running with excessive hip adduction and knee internal rotation in stance may increase the tensile and torsional strains in the iliotibial band. This running pattern can

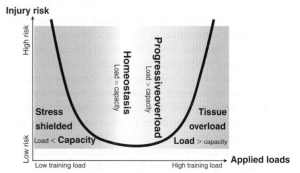

Fig. 8.8 Tissue homeostasis model (Dye, 2005; Gabbett, 2016).

maintain compression of the iliotibial band onto the lateral femoral epicondyle (Fairclough et al., 2006) and induce high strain rates on the iliotibial band (Hamill et al., 2008). Gait retraining methods that reduce these movement patterns may be beneficial in the treatment of ITBS, such as increasing cadence.

Key Management Strategies

ITBS symptoms in athletes can be effectively reduced using conservative management strategies (Bolia et al., 2020), despite the quality of available evidence being relatively low. Generally, pain management is a primary focus in the acute phases. Exercise or training while managing load should nonetheless be encouraged during this phase. After the pain-dominant phase, clinicians should progress running programmes and exercises to increase load tolerance. Lateral knee pain or irritation the following day should not exceed 2 on a 10-point visual analogue scale during the pain-dominant phase.

Running gait retraining is one strategy that can be used to address hip and knee coordination and running patterns (van der Worp et al., 2012) and can reduce knee loads while running. The gait retraining approaches highlighted in the earlier discussion of patellofemoral pain can be considered for ITBS. Incorporating running retraining using verbal and visual feedback into an 8-week conditioning programme was shown to be more effective than no feedback when attempting to influence some of the proposed risk factors to running-related injury, including average and instantaneous vertical loading rates, peak hip adduction, peak knee internal rotation and peak rearfoot invertor moments (Letafatkar et al., 2020). In this particular study, the feedback provided included running more softly, avoiding a rearfoot strike landing, and running with the knees apart and kneecaps pointing forwards. At the 1-year follow-up, the running gait retraining with feedback group had a lower injury incidence of 66.7% ITBS, 57% PFP, and 66.7% plantar fasciitis (Letafatkar et al., 2020).

Strengthening should also be considered in individuals with ITBS. Progressive hip exercises performed over 8 weeks have demonstrated superior outcomes in terms of pain, function and strength than stretching and conventional exercises (McKay et al., 2020). Complementing interventions with mobilisation and education regarding running surfaces (e.g., avoiding concrete surfaces and downhill running, and incorporating various running surfaces) can also contribute to positive treatment outcomes (van der Worp et al., 2012). Clinicians should prescribe intervention programmes individually, and consider including strengthening, especially the hip abductors; joint mobilisation; orthoses and the management of soft tissues (van der Worp et al., 2012; McKay et al., 2020).

KEY POINTS

- About one in every two runners experiences a running-related injury each year, with 75% of injuries occurring at or below the knee.
- Running-related injuries are multifactorial in nature. The most consistently reported risk factors include a previous injury and recent changes in running training.
- Numerous cross-sectional studies indicate the presence of certain movement patterns once an injury is present, but few prospective studies link specific movement patterns to injury incidence. Changes in movement patterns are often a consequence rather than a cause of injury.
- The key management strategies in treating the most common running-related injuries include patient education on load management, activity modification and footwear; gait retraining; and graded exercise and return-to-running programmes.
- Addressing purely the physical components of running-related injuries might be insufficient in certain cases, requiring a more holistic or interdisciplinary approach and referrals to other healthcare professionals when needed.

REFERENCES

Aderem, J., Louw, Q.A., 2015. Biomechanical risk factors associated with iliotibial band syndrome in runners: a systematic review. BMC Musculoskelet. Disord. 16, 356.

Altman, A.R., Davis, I.S., 2012. A kinematic method for foot-strike pattern detection in barefoot and shod runners. Gait & Posture 35 (2), 298–300.

Anderson, L.M., et al., 2020. What are the benefits and risks associated with changing foot strike pattern during running? A systematic review and meta-analysis of injury, running economy, and biomechanics. Sports Medicine 50 (5), 885–917.

Becker, J., Nakajima, M., Wu, W.F.W., 2018. Factors contributing to medial tibial stress syndrome in runners: a prospective study. Med. Sci. Sports Exerc. 50 (10), 2092–2100.

Bertelsen, M.L., et al., 2017. A framework for the etiology of running-related injuries. Scand. J. Med. Sci. Sports 27 (11), 1170–1180.

Blazey, P., Michie, T.V., Napier, C., 2021. A narrative review of running wearable measurement system accuracy and reliability: can we make running shoe prescription objective? Footwear Science 13 (2), 117–131.

Bolia, I.K., et al., 2020. Operative versus nonoperative management of distal iliotibial band syndrome—where do we stand? A systematic review. Arthrosc. Sports Med. Rehabil. 2 (4), e399–e415.

Bonnaerens, S., et al., 2021. Relationship between duty factor and external forces in slow recreational runners. BMJ Open Sport Exerc. Med. 7 (1), e000996.

Bramah, C., et al., 2018. Is there a pathological gait associated with common soft tissue running injuries? Am. J. Sports Med. 46 (12), 3023–3031.

Bramble, D.M., Lieberman, D.E., 2004. Endurance running and the evolution of Homo. Nature 432 (7015), 345–352.

Buchbinder, R., 2004. Clinical practice. Plantar fasciitis. N. Engl. J. Med. 350 (21), 2159–2166.

Cavagna, G.A., Heglund, N.C., Taylor, C.R., 1977. Mechanical work in terrestrial locomotion: two basic mechanisms for minimizing energy expenditure. Am. J. Physiol. 233 (5), 243–261.

Chan, Z.Y.S., et al., 2018. Gait retraining for the reduction of injury occurrence in novice distance eunners: 1-year follow-up of a randomized controlled trial. Am. J. Sports Med. 46 (2), 388–395.

Chen, Y.-J., Powers, C.M., 2014. Comparison of three-dimensional patellofemoral joint reaction forces in persons with and without patellofemoral pain. J. Appl. Biomech 30 (4), 493–500.

Cochrum, R.G., et al., 2020. Visual classification of running economy by distance running coaches. Eur. J. Sport Sci. 2020/09/16 edn, 1–24

Čoh, M., et al., 2018. Kinematics of Usain Bolt's maximal sprint velocity. Kinesiology 50 (2), 100–101.

Colino, E., et al., 2020. Mechanical properties of treadmill surfaces and their effects on endurance running. Int. J. Sports Physiol. Perform. 15 (5), 685–689.

Collins, N.J., et al., 2018. 2018 consensus statement on exercise therapy and physical interventions (orthoses, taping and manual therapy) to treat patellofemoral pain: recommendations from the 5th International Patellofemoral Pain Research Retreat, Gold Coast, Australia, 2017. Br. J. Sports Med. 52 (18), 1170–1178.

Crossley, K.M., et al., 2016. 2016 patellofemoral pain consensus statement from the 4th International Patellofemoral Pain Research Retreat, Manchester. Part 1: Terminology, definitions, clinical examination, natural history, patellofemoral osteoarthritis and patient-reported outcome measures. Br. J. Sports Med. 50 (14), 839–843.

Damsted, C., et al., 2019. The association between changes in weekly running distance and running-related injury: preparing for a half marathon. J. Orthop. Sports Phys. Ther. 49 (4), 230–238.

Davis, I.S., et al., 2020. Gait retraining as an intervention for patellofemoral pain. Curr. Rev. Musculoskelet. Med. 13 (1), 103–114.

Davis, I.S., Bowser, B.J., Mullineaux, D.R., 2016. Greater vertical impact loading in female runners with medically diagnosed injuries: a prospective investigation. Br. J. Sports Med. 50 (14), 887–892.

Dillon, S., et al., 2021. Do injury-resistant runners have distinct differences in clinical measures compared to recently injured runners? Med. Sci. Sport Exerc. [Preprint]. 2021/04/27 edn

Drake, C., Mallows, A., Littlewood, C., 2018. Psychosocial variables and presence, severity and prognosis of plantar heel pain: a systematic review of cross-sectional and prognostic associations. Musculoskeletal Care 16 (3), 329–338.

Duffey, M.J., et al., 2000. Etiologic factors associated with anterior knee pain in distance runners. Medicine & Science in Sports & Exercise 32 (11), 1825–1832.

Dye, S.F., 2005. The pathophysiology of patellofemoral pain: a tissue homeostasis perspective. Clin. Orthop. Relat. Res. (436), 100–110.

Esculier, J.F., et al., 2017. Is combining gait retraining or an exercise programme with education better than education alone in treating runners with patellofemoral pain? A randomised clinical trial. Br. J. Sports Med. [Preprint]. 2017/05/10 edn

Esculier, J.-F., et al., 2020. A contemporary approach to patellofemoral pain in runners. J. Athl. Train 55 (12), 1206–1214.

Fairclough, J., et al., 2006. The functional anatomy of the iliotibial band during flexion and extension of the knee: implications for understanding iliotibial band syndrome. Journal of Anatomy 208 (3), 309–316.

Finch, C., 2006. A new framework for research leading to sports injury prevention. J. Sci. Med. Sport 9 (1–2), 3–9.

Foch, E., et al., 2015. Associations between iliotibial band injury status and running biomechanics in women. Gait & Posture 41 (2), 706–710.

Francis, P., et al., 2019. The proportion of lower limb running injuries by gender, anatomical location and specific pathology: a systematic review. J. Sports Sci. Med. 18 (1), 21–31.

Gabbett, T.J., 2016. The training—injury prevention paradox: should athletes be training smarter and harder? Br. J. Sports Med. 50 (5), 273–280.

Hamill, J., et al., 2008. A prospective study of iliotibial band strain in runners. Clin. Biomech. (Bristol, Avon) 23 (8), 1018–1025.

Hamstra-Wright, K.L., et al., 2021. Risk factors for plantar fasciitis in physically active individuals: a systematic review and meta-analysis. Sports Health 13 (3), 296–303.

Hanlon, S.L., Pohlig, R.T., Silbernagel, K.G., 2021. Beyond the diagnosis: using patient characteristics and domains of tendon health to identify latent subgroups of Achilles tendinopathy. J. Orthop. Sports Phys. Ther. (0), 1–28.

Hannigan, J.J., Pollard, C.D., 2021. Biomechanical analysis of two runners who developed leg injuries during a six-week transition to maximal running shoes: a case series. J. Sports Sci. 2021/06/03 edn, 1–7

Harrast, M.A., 2019. Clinical Care of the Runner E-Book: Assessment, Biomechanical Principles, and Injury Management. Elsevier Health Sciences., Available at: https://books.google.co.nz/books?id=dnXADwAAQBAJ

Harutaichun, P., Boonyong, S., Pensri, P., 2019. Predictors of plantar fasciitis in Thai novice conscripts after 10-week military training: s prospective study. Phys. Ther. Sport 35, 29–35.

Hébert-Losier, K., et al., 2017. Updated reliability and normative values for the standing heel-rise test in healthy adults. Physiotherapy 103 (4), 446–452.

Helmhout, P.H., et al., 2015. The effectiveness of a 6-week intervention program aimed at modifying running style in patients with chronic exertional compartment syndrome: results from a series of case studies. Orthop. J. Sports Med. 3 (3) 2325967115575691

Hill, C.L., et al., 2008. Prevalence and correlates of foot pain in a population-based study: the North West Adelaide health study. J. Foot Ankle Res 1 (1), 2.

Horsley, B.J., et al., 2021. Does site matter? Impact of inertial measurement unit placement on the validity and reliability of stride variables during running: a systematic review and meta-analysis. Sports Med. [Preprint]. 2021/03/25 edn

Hughes, G.T.G., et al., 2021. Novel technology in sports biomechanics: some words of caution. Sports Biomech, 1–9.

Janssen, I., et al., 2018. Investigating Achilles and patellar tendinopathy prevalence in elite athletics. Res. Sports Med. (Print) 26 (1), 1–12.

Jauhiainen, S., et al., 2020. A hierarchical cluster analysis to determine whether injured runners exhibit similar kinematic gait patterns. Scand. J. Med. Sci. Sports n/a(n/a)

Kakouris, N., Yener, N., Fong, D.T.P., 2021. A systematic review of running-related musculoskeletal injuries in runners. J. Sport Health Sci [Preprint]

Kulmala, J.-P., et al., 2013. Forefoot strikers exhibit lower running-induced knee loading than rearfoot strikers. Med. Sci. Sports Exer 45 (12), 2306–2313.

Kung, S.M., et al., 2018. What factors determine the preferred gait transition speed in humans? A review of the triggering mechanisms. Hum. Mov. Sci. 57, 1–12. 2017/11/10 edn

Lagas, I.F., et al., 2020. Incidence of Achilles tendinopathy and associated risk factors in recreational runners: s large prospective cohort study. J. Sci. Med. Sport. 23 (5), 448–452.

Letafatkar, A., et al., 2020. Long-term efficacy of conditioning training program combined with feedback on kinetics and kinematics in male runners. Scand. J. Med. Sci. Sports 30 (3), 429–441.

Lieberman, D.E., et al., 2010. Foot strike patterns and collision forces in habitually barefoot versus shod runners. Nature 463 (7280), 531–535.

Louw, M., Deary, C., 2014. The biomechanical variables involved in the aetiology of iliotibial band syndrome in distance runners – a systematic review of the literature. Phys. Ther. Sport 15 (1), 64–75.

Lussiana, T., et al., 2017. Do subjective assessments of running patterns reflect objective parameters? Eur. J. Sport Sci., 1–11.

Lyght, M., et al., 2016. Effects of foot strike and step frequency on Achilles tendon stress during running. J. Appl. Biomech 32 (4), 365–372.

Maffulli, N., et al., 2003. Clinical diagnosis of Achilles tendinopathy with tendinosis. Clin. J. Sport Med. 13 (1), 11–15.

Magnusson, S.P., Kjaer, M., 2019. The impact of loading, unloading, ageing and injury on the human tendon. J. Phys 597 (5), 1283–1298.

Martin, R.L., et al., 2018. Achilles p, stiffness, and muscle power deficits: midportion Achilles tendinopathy revision 2018. J. Orthop. Sports Phys. Ther. 48 (5), A1–A38..

McIntosh, A.S., 2005. Risk compensation, motivation, injuries, and biomechanics in competitive sport. Br. J. Sports Med. 39 (1), 2–3.

McKay, J., et al., 2020. Iliotibial band syndrome rehabilitation in female runners: a pilot randomized study. J. Orthop. Surg. Res. 15 (1), 188.

McMahon, T.A., Valiant, G., Frederick, E.C., 1987. Groucho running. J. Appl. Physiol. 62 (6), 2326–2337.

McNeill, W., Silvester, M., 2017. Plantar heel pain. J. Bodyw. Mov. Ther. 21 (1), 205–211.

Miller, J.R., et al., 2019. A systematic review and meta-analysis of crossover studies comparing physiological, perceptual and performance measures between treadmill and overground running. Sports Med. [Preprint]. 2019/03/09 edn

Moen, M.H., et al., 2012. The treatment of medial tibial stress syndrome in athletes; a randomized clinical trial. Sports Medicine, Arthroscopy, Rehabilitation, Therapy & Technology: SMARTT 4, 12.

Morrissey, D., et al., 2021. Management of plantar heel pain: a best practice guide informed by a systematic review, expert clinical reasoning and patient values. Br. J. Sports Med. [Preprint]

Mousavi, S.H., et al., 2019. Kinematic risk factors for lower limb tendinopathy in distance runners: a systematic review and meta-analysis. Gait Posture 69, 13–24.

Napier, C., et al., 2018. Kinetic risk factors of running-related injuries in female recreational runners. Scand. J. Med. Sci. Sports 28 (10), 2164–2172.

Newman, P., et al., 2013. Risk factors associated with medial tibial stress syndrome in runners: a systematic review and meta-analysis. Open Access. J. Sports Med. 4, 229–241.

Osborne, J.W.A., et al., 2019. Muscle function and muscle size differences in people with and without plantar heel pain: a systematic review. J. Orthop. Sports Phys. Ther. 49 (12), 925–933.

Paquette, M.R., et al., 2020. Moving beyond weekly "distance": optimizing quantification of training load in runners. J. Orthop. Sports Phys. Ther. 50 (10), 564–569.

Pedisic, Z., et al., 2019. Is running associated with a lower risk of all-cause, cardiovascular and cancer mortality, and is the more the better? A systematic review and meta-analysis. Br. J. Sports Med. bjsports-2018-100493

Petersen, W., et al., 2014. Patellofemoral pain syndrome. Knee Surg. Sports Traumatol. Arthrosc. 22 (10), 2264–2274.

Petraglia, F., Ramazzina, I., Costantino, C., 2017. Plantar fasciitis in athletes: diagnostic and treatment strategies. A systematic review. Muscles Ligaments Tendons J. 7 (1), 107–118.

Raissi, G.R.D., et al., 2009. The relationship between lower extremity alignment and medial tibial stress syndrome among non-professional athletes. Sports Medicine, Arthroscopy, Rehabilitation, Therapy & Technology: SMARTT 1 (1), 11.

Rathleff, M.S., et al., 2015. High-load strength training improves outcome in patients with plantar fasciitis: a randomized controlled trial with 12-month follow-up. Scand. J. Med. Sci. Sports 25 (3), e292–e300.

Salo, A.I., et al., 2011. Elite sprinting: are athletes individually step-frequency or step-length reliant? Med. Sci. Sports Exerc. 43 (6), 1055–1062.

Silbernagel, K.G., Hanlon, S., Sprague, A., 2020. Current clinical concepts: conservative management of Achilles tendinopathy. J. Athl. Train 55 (5), 438–447.

Soligard, T., et al., 2016. How much is too much? (Part 1) International Olympic Committee consensus statement on load in sport and risk of injury. Br. J. Sports Med. 50 (17), 1030–1041.

Souza, R.B., 2016. An evidence-based videotaped running biomechanics analysis. Phys. Med. Rehabil. Clin. N. Am. 27 (1), 217–236.

Taunton, J.E., et al., 2002. A retrospective case-control analysis of 2002 running injuries. Br. J. Sports Med 36 (2), 95–101.

Van Gheluwe, B., Madsen, C., 1997. Frontal rearfoot kinematics in running prior to volitional exhaustion. J. Appl. Biomech. 13 (1), 66.

Van Hooren, B., et al., 2019. Is motorized treadmill running biomechanically comparable to overground running? A systematic review and meta-analysis of cross-over studies. Sports Medicine [Preprint]

Vicenzino, B., et al., 2020. ICON 2019-International Scientific Tendinopathy Symposium Consensus: There are nine core health-related domains for tendinopathy (CORE DOMAINS): Delphi study of healthcare professionals and patients. Br. J. Sports Med. 54 (8), 444–451.

Videbæk, S., et al., 2015. Incidence of running-related injuries per 1000 h of running in different types of runners: a systematic review and meta-analysis. Sports Medicine 45 (7), 1017–1026.

van der Vlist, A.C., et al., 2021. Which treatment is most effective for patients with Achilles tendinopathy? A living systematic review with network meta-analysis of 29 randomised controlled trials. Br. J. Sports Med. 55 (5), 249–256.

Wiese-Bjornstal, D.M., 2010. Psychology and socioculture affect injury risk, response, and recovery in high-intensity athletes: a consensus statement. Scand. J. Med. Sci. Sports 20 (Suppl 2), 103–111.

Willy, R.W., et al., 2019. Patellofemoral pain. J. Orthop. Sports Phys. Ther. 49 (9) CPG1–CPG95.

Winters, M., et al., 2013. Treatment of medial tibial stress syndrome: a systematic review. Sports Med. (Auckland, N.Z.) 43 (12), 1315–1333.

Winters, M., 2018. Medial tibial stress syndrome: diagnosis, treatment and outcome assessment (PhD Academy Award). Br. J. Sports Med 52 (18), 1213–1214.

Winters, M., 2020. The diagnosis and management of medial tibial stress syndrome: an evidence update. Unfallchirurg 123 (Suppl 1), 15–19.

Wirtz, A.D., et al., 2012. Patellofemoral joint stress during running in females with and without patellofemoral pain. Knee 19 (5), 703–708.

van der Worp, M.P., et al., 2012. Iliotibial band syndrome in runners. Sports Med. 42 (11), 969–992.

van der Worp, M.P., et al., 2015. Injuries in runners: a systematic review on risk factors and sex differences. PloS One 10 (2) e0114937–e0114937

Wyndow, N., et al., 2013. Triceps surae activation is altered in male runners with Achilles tendinopathy. J. Electromyog. Kinesiol. 23 (1), 166–172.

Zimmermann, W.O., et al., 2019a. Conservative treatment of anterior chronic exertional compartment syndrome in the military, with a mid-term follow-up. BMJ Open Sport Exerc. Med 5 (1), e000532.

Zimmermann, W.O., et al., 2019b. Gait retraining reduces vertical ground reaction forces in running shoes and military boots. Transl. Sports Med. 2 (2), 90–97.

INDEX